*Debates and Dilemmas
in Promoting Health*

This book forms part of the Open University course *Promoting Health: Skills, Perspectives and Practice* (K301) and a new qualification, the Certificate in Health Promotion. It has been produced with support from the Health Education Authority and Health Promotion Wales, although the content of the course is the sole responsibility of The Open University.

If you are interested in studying the course and gaining the new Certificate please write to the Information Officer, School of Health and Social Welfare, Walton Hall, Milton Keynes MK7 6AA, UK.

Other texts required for the course and also published by Macmillan in association with The Open University are:

- the first core text, *Promoting Health: Knowledge and Practice*, edited by Jeanne Katz and Alyson Peberdy

- the second core text, *The Challenge of Promoting Health: Exploration and Action*, edited by Linda Jones and Moyra Sidell

- the set book, *Health Promotion: Professional Perspectives*, edited by Angela Scriven and Judy Orme.

Debates and Dilemmas in Promoting Health

A Reader

Edited by

Moyra Sidell

Linda Jones

Jeanne Katz

and

Alyson Peberdy

MACMILLAN

The Open University

First published 1997 by
MACMILLAN PRESS LTD
Houndmills, Basingstoke, Hampshire RG21 6XS
and London
Companies and representatives
throughout the world

ISBN 0–333–69416–3 hardcover
ISBN 0–333–69417–1 paperback

A catalogue record for this book is available
from the British Library.

This book is printed on paper suitable for recycling and
made from fully managed and sustained forest sources.

10   9   8   7   6   5   4   3
06   05   04   03   02   01   00   99

Printed and bound in Great Britain by
Creative Print and Design (Wales), Ebbw Vale

Contents

Section Two: Questioning the evidence base of health promotion

Section Three: Promoting health in a wider context

Section 4: Looking beyond 2000: dilemmas in health promotion

List of figures and tables

Figures

Tables

Acknowledgements

The editors and publishers wish to thank the following for permission to use copyright material: Baywood Publishing Co., Inc. for material from Wendy Farrant, 'Addressing the contradictions: health action in the United Kingdom', *International Journal of Health Services*, 21:3 (1991) pp. 423–39; BMJ Publishing Group for material from Paola Dey, Stuart Collins, Sheila Will and Ciaran B. J. Woodman, 'Randomised controlled trial assessing effectiveness of health education leaflets in reducing incidence of sunburn', *British Medical Journal*, 311, 21 October 1995, pp. 1062–3, and Jean-Claude Desenclos, Philippe Bouvert, Elizabeth Benz-Lemoine, Francine Grimont, Hélène Desqueyroux, Isabelle Rebière and Patrick A. Grimont, 'Large outbreak of *Salmonella enterica* serotype *paratyphi B* infection caused by goats' milk cheese, France, 1993: a case finding epidemiological study', *British Medical Journal*, 312, 13 January 1996, pp. 91–4; Michael L. Burr for his article, 'Explaining the French paradox', *Journal of the Royal Society of Health*, August 1995, pp. 217–19; Churchill Livingstone for material from C. Godfrey, 'Is prevention better than cure?' from *Purchasing and Providing Effective Health Care*, ed. M. Drummond and A. Maynard (1993) pp. 183–97; Elsevier Science Ltd for material from Regina H. Kenen, 'The at-risk health status and technology: a diagnostic invitation and the "gift" of knowing', *Social Science and Medicine*, 42:11 (1996) pp. 1545–53, and Charlie Davison, Stephen Frankel and George Davey Smith, 'The limits of lifestyle: reassessing "fatalism" in the popular culture of illness prevention', *Social Science and Medicine*, 34:6 (1992) pp. 675–85; Health Education Authority for material from Keith Tones, 'Health education as empowerment' from *Health Promotion Today* (1995) pp. 38–51; Health Education Journal for Alan Beattie, 'Evaluation in community development for health: an opportunity for dialogue', *Health Education Journal*, 54 (1995) pp. 465–72, Andrew Tannahill, 'Health eduction and health promotion: planning for the 1990s', *Health Education Journal*, 49 (1990) pp. 194–8, and Linda J. Jones and Adrian L. Davis, 'Health and environmental constraints: listening to children's voices', *Health Education Journal*, 55 (1996) 4; Stephen Jan for his article, 'How community preferences can more effectively shape equity policy', *Critical Public Health*, 6:3 (1995) pp. 12–18; King's Fund Policy Institute for material from Michaela Benzeval, Ken Judge and Margaret Whitehead, 'Summary' from *Tackling Inequalities in Health*, ed. Michaela Benzeval *et al.* (1995) pp. xvii–xxv, copyright © King's Fund 1995; Macmillan Press Ltd for material from Martin Bradford and Sandra Winn, 'Practice nursing and health promotion', pp. 119–31, and Alison Dines, 'A case study of ethical issues in health promotion – mammography screening: the nurse's position', pp. 43–50, from *Research in Health Promotion and Nursing*, ed. J. Wilson-Barnett and J. Macleod Clark (1994) pp. 119–31, and Angela Everitt and Pauline Hardiker, 'Towards a critical approach to evaluation' from *Evaluation for Good Practice* (1996) pp. 83–104; Oxford University Press for material from Trudi Collins, 'Models of health: pervasive, persuasive and politically charged', *Health Promotion International*, 10:1 (1995) pp. 317–24, John Catford, 'The mass media is dead: long live multimedia', *Health Promotion International*, 10:4 (1995) pp. 247–50, R. C. Lefebvre, 'The social marketing imbroglio in health promotion', *Health Promotion International*, 7:1 (1992) pp. 61–4, Ronald Labonté, 'Econology: integrating health and sustainable development', *Health Promotion International*, 6:2 (1991) pp. 147–56, Billie Corti, C. D'Arcy, J. Holman and Robert J. Donovan, Shirley K. Frizzell and Addy M. Carroll, 'Using sponsorship to create health environments for sport, racing and arts venues in Western Australia', *Health Promotion International*, 10:3 (1995) pp. 185–97, Russell Caplan, 'The importance of social theory for health promotion: from description to reflexivity', *Health Promotion International*, 8:2 (1993) pp. 147–57, Roger Burrows, Robin Bunton, Steven Muncer and Kate Gillen, 'The efficacy of health promotion, health economics and late modernism', *Health Education Research*, 10:2 (1995) pp. 241–9, and figure from T. Hancock, 'Health, human development and the community ecosystem: three ecological models', *Health Promotion International*, 8 (1993) pp. 41–7; Royal College of General Practitioners for Norman Beale and Susan Nethercott, 'Job-loss and family morbidity: a study of a factory closure', *Journal of the Royal College of General Practitioners*, 35, November 1985, pp. 510–14; Routledge for material from John Sketchley, 'Counselling people affected by HIV and AIDS', from *Handbook of Counselling in Britain*, ed. W. Dryden, C. Charles-Edward and R. Woolfe (1989) Tavistock, pp. 347–58, 362, and Jenny Douglas, 'Developing health promotion strategies with Black and minority ethnic communities which address social inequalities' from *Working for Equality in Health*, ed. P. Bywaters and E. McLeod (1996) pp. 179–96; Sheed & Ward Ltd for material from Paulo Freire, *Pedagogy of the Oppressed*, tran. Myra Bergman Ramos (1972) pp. 150–5, 159, 180–3; Peter Townsend for material from his article, 'Think globally, act locally', *European Labour Forum*, June 1994, pp. 2–8; John Wiley & Sons Ltd for material from Dan Beauchamp, 'Life-style, public health and paternalism', from *Ethical Dilemmas in Health Promotion*, ed. S. Doxiadis (1987) pp. 69–83.

Every effort has been made to trace all the copyright-holders, but if any have been inadvertently overlooked the publishers will be pleased to make the necessary arrangement at the first opportunity.

Introduction

The turn of a century is a good time to take stock, to re-appraise and to move on. This is particularly apposite for health promotion as the year 2000 approaches. At Alma-Ata the World Health Organization set us all the task of achieving 'health for all' by the year 2000. For some this was an impossible dream, naively optimistic and unrealistic. For others it was a vision thwarted by lack of political will, global economic recession, third world debt and the greed of the 'haves' over the 'have nots.' Perhaps the time scale was just too short. But we also need to question whether health for all will ever be an achievable goal, whether we yet have a shared understanding of priorities or even a clear vision of 'what health is'. Part of the difficulty for health promotion has been that there are no straightforward answers to such questions.

Through the Ottawa Charter (WHO, 1986) and the Sundsvall Conference (1992) the health promotion movement has arguably set out more of a strategic checklist than a formal strategy for health promotion (Levin and Ziglio, 1996). In identifying five key priority areas – building healthy public policy, creating supportive environments, strengthening community action, developing personal skills and reorienting health services – it has offered scope for innovation and imagination but also for confusion and doubt. The discourse of health promotion has fuelled many debates and dilemmas; it has its advocates as well as its adversaries, there are believers and sceptics. Health promotion has sometimes been projected, rather like health itself, as an example of an unmitigated good. After all which groups would not wish to have their health protected and promoted? Who would not want to live longer and live better? In this view, the rise of health promotion is unproblematic, a response to changing knowledge about epidemiology and risk. Whether engaged in modifying people's behaviour or protecting the public through regulatory change, health promotion emerges as a justifiable and necessary enterprise.

In contrast to this, health promotion has been seen by critics as beset with problems. It has been criticised by those on the political right for its 'nanny state' attachment to policy interventions. Others have questioned its role in creating an apparatus of 'surveillance' which constructs and monitors the 'worried well' in its attempts to limit risk-taking. For some critics, health promotion approaches feed what is seen as an unhealthy contemporary consumerist obsession with health.

Much criticism has come from within health promotion itself, particularly about the narrow focus and superficiality of much health promotion work. One concern has been about its over-emphasis on

1

modifying individual behaviour and its construction of 'lifestyle' as a set of personal choices unrelated to the socio-cultural and economic influences on people's lives. Increasingly the knowledge base on which people are being asked to change their behaviour is questioned as the advice becomes more complex and often conflicting. The overwhelming evidence of the influence of social and economic disadvantage on health and disease has led many health promoters to recognise that the choice to change behaviour is not an easy one for many people and the phrase 'making healthy choices the easy choices' sums up the aim of health promotion. One identified way to do this is through influencing public policy at all levels to create supportive environments for health, an approach which resonates very much with the Ottawa Charter and Sundsvall agreement.

It is often said that health is everybody's business. But responsibility for the health of individuals, communities and populations is the subject of much debate. Tied up with notions of responsibility are notions of control. How far can people have responsibility for their health if the means to health are outside of their control? Those who advocate empowerment as the most appropriate means to promote health see education and participation in the decisions which affect health as a means to that end. Sharing of knowledge and listening to people have long been the tradition within community development but in the last ten years this has become increasingly advocated by government and policy makers. Initiatives such as 'Listening to Local Voices' and community oriented primary health care have put these issues on the agenda but many are sceptical about the motives behind such initiatives (Farrant, 1994).

Another focus of debate has been on the poverty of theory in health promotion, or rather the failure to make explicit the extent to which the health promotion agenda inevitably involves an acceptance of more thorough-going social, economic and political change. A related criticism has been of the vague and all-embracing nature of positive definitions of health and of the difficulties encountered in using a 'social change' approach, once the notion of health as 'absence of disease' has been found lacking.

Health promoters are increasingly being asked to evaluate their activities in cost-effective terms. Yet the diverse nature of the activity and the uncertainty about its parameters make a simple cost-benefit analysis unrealistic. The dilemma for health promoters is to find indicators for their work which reflect the process as well as the outcome.

The 38 articles that make up this collection testify to the fact that debate is alive and well in health promotion. Some of the articles are classics, others represent new thinking at the cutting edge of theory. Section One addresses key issues about the foundations of health and health promotion and the means through which it is practised. In Section Two questions are raised about the knowledge base of health promotion interventions. Evidence about the outcomes of such interventions and how they can be evaluated is subjected to scrutiny. Section Three explores wider debates around the interplay between local action and public policy and Section Four looks to the future and raises ethical, sociological and political dilemmas as health promotion moves into the 21st century.

This Reader was compiled to accompany an Open University third level course 'Promoting health: skills, perspectives and practices' which has been produced in collaboration with the HEA and leads to a certificate in Health Promotion. While the Reader forms an essential element in the 'Promoting Health' course it also stands alone as a coherent and wide ranging source book for those who would like to engage in some of the debates and dilemmas inherent in promoting health. Although purposely arranged in four coherent sections the individual articles stand alone and the book could be consumed *à la carte*. The contributors come from a wide range of backgrounds and include academics, practitioners and policy makers. We would like to thank the authors for their co-operation in reviewing and agreeing the sometimes extensive edits, amendments and revisions. We are assured that the substance and style of the original papers has been retained. We hope that the articles in this book will engage the reader in the fundamental dilemmas about health and its promotion and stimulate yet more debate.

References

Farrant, W. (1994). 'Addressing the contradictions: health promotion and community health action in the United Kingdom', *Critical Public Health*, 15, (1), 5–19.

Levin, S. and Ziglio, E. (1996). 'Health promotion as an investment strategy: considerations on theory and practice', *Health Promotion International*, 11, (1), 33–39.

World Health Organization (WHO) (1986). *Ottawa Charter for Health Promotion*.

Key issues in health and health promotion

Promoting health will remain at best a diverse, complex and multi-faceted activity. At worst it can be irritatingly jargon-ridden, impossibly idealistic and seemingly confused. This first Section of the Reader is designed to help explain, if not expunge, the jargon, temper the idealism of health promotion with hard ethical and political questioning and shed some light on the confusion.

Underlying the confusion is a basic uncertainly about the parameters of health promotion work. What is health promotion, beyond the specialist health promotion service? What should they be doing, these health, welfare, education and environmental professionals, lay people, community groups and policy makers pressed into service in the name of 'intersectoral collaboration' and 'healthy alliances'?

One key response, introduced in this Section and expanded on in the rest of the book, is to argue that these generalist health promoters should be continuing to undertake their usual work – *but in a more health promoting way*. This requires process changes: improved communication skills, increased sensitivity to socio-cultural issues, heightened awareness of environmental constraints, greater clarity about ethical problems, a more robust assessment and evaluation cycle and a more systematic understanding of concepts of health and its promotion. Add to this a clearer understanding of the contribution that others, lay or professional, might make which would complement and extend their own efforts. What it does not mean is a 'product' approach; that is, the addition of yet more tasks and roles, more clinics, visits, inspections, interactions, collaborations, undertaken to demonstrate that health promotion is 'really happening'.

The articles that follow address some of these central issues. We start with two chapters which highlight the relationship between health concepts and health promotion strategies. Moyra Sidell (Chapter 1) explains how moving beyond a disease-focused model of health to a salutogenic approach begins to open up the potential for exploring older

5

people's health in terms of Antonovsky's health-ease-dis-ease continuum. She explores how meaningfulness, comprehensibility and manageability in people's daily lives can assist in maintaining their health. The challenge to health promoters is to find ways in which such a 'sense of coherence' can be created.

The contribution from Michael Benzeval, Ken Judge and Margaret Whitehead (Chapter 2) builds on this theme by exploring the policy dimensions of health. Arguing that health inequalities have increased since the 1980s, they suggest that these can be tackled by housing, employment and health policies which strengthen individuals and communities. Beyond this, they call for broader structural changes such as more effective income maintenance, more equitable income distribution and enhanced social support. One consequence of such changes, we would suggest, would be the enhancement of people's health and 'sense of coherence' as their lives became more manageable and meaningful.

In contrast to this broad agenda for health improvement, health promotion has often appeared to be preoccupied with narrow lifestyle-related change. Charlie Davison, Stephen Frankel and George Davey Smith in Chapter 3 are critical of the 'lifestyle' approach, arguing that it ignores the influence of heredity, social conditions and environment on health and is seriously out of step with popular culture and lay beliefs about illness. This criticism finds a response in the new agenda in health education advocated by Keith Tones in Chapter 4 in this Section. He argues that the fundamental focus of health education should now be empowerment of individuals and communities. A major aspect of health promoters' work must be to raise public consciousness of health issues, to enable people to gain autonomy and to provide them with information and support to work for change at a local and policy level. This is a far cry from behaviour modification and opens up more general issues about conflicting approaches to health promotion, which form the focus for the next pair of articles.

Russell Caplan and Trudi Collins in Chapters 5 and 6 focus on health promotion models and challenge the prevailing view that a 'pick and mix' approach to models is realistic. Both emphasise the (often inexplicitly) political and economic agendas that underlie contemporary models, arguing that models and theories inevitably express deep seated beliefs about the social world. Health promotion models should be connected to wider social theories, with the complexity of socio-cultural and economic relationships at an individual and community level more clearly identified. In illustration of this, Chapter 7 by Martin Bradford and Sandra Winn demonstrates the everyday dilemmas faced by practice nurses as they undertake health promotion tasks. While a significant number of the nurses identify a 'social change' model as their preferred approach, only a tiny minority actually use it in practice. For most a medical approach best characterises their practice.

This gap between theory and practice is a matter of concern if contemporary health promotion is to develop or enhance the skills of health promoters. Gordon Macdonald in Chapter 8 raises the question of how innovation in theory and practice can be disseminated. He explores a range of research evidence which asks how new ideas can be communicated and adopted more widely. The final group of chapters in Section One respond to the theory–practice challenge by addressing two key aspects of health promotion: communication and ethics. At an individual level John Sketchley and Alyson Peberdy in Chapters 9 and 10 raise important issues about sensitivity and empathy in communication. The ability to put oneself in the other's shoes is the essence of empathy. John Sketchley discusses how counselling for people affected by HIV and AIDS assumes a special significance in the absence of cure. Alyson Peberdy, in discussing communication across cultural boundaries, argues that it is not only about getting the language right. Communication is about understanding the cultural context, and building relationships based on trust.

At a very different level, Ralph Lefebvre's contribution in Chapter 11 questions whether mass communication of health promotion messages through 'social marketing' is realistic or ethical. Should health promoters be in the business of selling health just as other producers market their goods? Is it ethically justifiable to convince people to change their habits through persuasive media messages? This leads us into an initial consideration of ethical issues in health promotion, through a case study by Alison Dines in Chapter 12 of mammography screening. In exploring the different ways in which health workers might respond to women's requests for advice, Dines highlights some of the dilemmas present in health promotion work. What are the boundaries of advice and information-giving? Where should professional intervention end and lay autonomy begin? We will return to such questions in the later Sections of this book.

1 Older people's health: applying Antonovsky's salutogenic paradigm *

Moyra Sidell

Introduction

If we take morbidity data as the yardstick, older people's health on the whole is not very good. Evidence from the General Household Survey has for the last ten years shown that about 60 per cent of all people over the age of 65 suffer from some form of chronic illness or disability and this rises to 70 per cent for those over 75 (Sidell, 1995). Yet when asked in the same survey how they rate their health less than 25 per cent rate it as poor. One possible explanation is that they are using different accounts of health. When asked to define 'health' well over half talked in terms of psychological wellbeing or feeling good, another 12 per cent said that it was about having energy. Only about 12 per cent saw health as the absence of disease with about a quarter defining health as the ability to function.

Accounts of health

Morbidity statistics which describe 60 per cent of the older population as diseased operate within a biomedical account of health. This is still the most influential of the health accounts in Western societies. It sees health as the absence of diagnosed disease. This view of health is both sanctioned and supported by the health care system. Biomedical explanations relate to the physical body and health is explained in terms of biology. It is a mechanistic view which concentrates on the structure of the body, its anatomy, and the way it works, its physiology. This functional view of health sees the human being as a complex organism which can be best understood by breaking it into isolated parts, each with a 'normal' way of working. Disease can then be narrowed down to the malfunction of a particular part of the body. Medical treatment focuses on the diseased part and the tendency is to concentrate on discrete parts

---

* Commissioned for this volume. This chapter draws on material published by the author elsewhere (see Sidell, 1995).

or organs and pay less attention to the whole or the interaction of the parts.

This mechanistic and disease orientated view of health inevitably paints a bleak and negative view of the prospects for health in old age. Later life is portrayed as a time of declining strength and increased frailty as organs and tissues wear out or succumb to disease and degeneration. It views individuals narrowly in terms of their bodies which are in decline as the natural consequence of growing older. Hope for better health in old age will come from maintaining the body in better shape, eradicating the diseases to which the ageing body is prone and replacing defective organs. Increasingly medicine is accepting wider social and psychological influences on health and reflecting elements of other models of health. But most doctors and research scientists still believe that the way our bodies work can be understood within a biological framework and that a cause and therefore a treatment can be found for all disorders, even mental disorders.

But biomedicine with its emphasis on the functioning of individual bodies has little to say about emotional and psychological health. Some strands of biomedicine have tended to see mental illness as some form of malfunctioning of the brain. Yet the separation of mind and body in explanations of health is a fairly recent phenomenon. In earlier historical periods in western society and in some contemporary eastern cultures the mental and physical health are inseparably linked.

The humanistic psychology tradition developed the notion of a healthy personality with an ideal of health as a thinking, feeling and reflecting being, able to change and grow – a rounded, balanced personality (Stevens, 1990). Maslow and Carl Rogers have explored more positive aspects of psychological health with an ideal of health moving from fulfilling basic human needs to reaching a state of 'self-actualisation' or 'becoming what one is capable of becoming' (Maslow, 1954)). In this model self-esteem and the ability to express one's emotions are important elements of healthy growth in people.

A holistic account of health is more concerned with the whole person as a unique individual. The older person is not seen as a collection of bodily ills but as a thinking, feeling, creative being who has strengths and weaknesses of body, mind and spirit. It is possible to be healthy in mind and spirit even though the body may be frail. Holism is often linked with equilibrium or a state in which bodies, minds and spirits are in balance. These are concepts drawn from ancient eastern traditions and have become very popular in the west, particularly in the alternative health movement. But as with biomedicine the focus of attention is on the individual. Critics of a holistic account of health argue that this ignores the impact on the individual of the wider physical and social environment

There is now widespread support for a more overarching social model of health which extends the medical model and draws attention to the adverse effects on health in the physical and social environment, such as poor housing, poverty, pollution, unemployment and poor working conditions (Beattie *et al*, 1992). This represents a challenge to orthodox medical views and puts health concerns on wider agendas, emphasising the link between the economic, political and social environment and health.

The social model of health puts less emphasis on decline and decay of the organism and more on the interactions with the physical and social environment. So disease and decline are not inevitable in old age and not attributable to age *per se* but to the conditions in which people age and in which they have lived their lives. Disease is never just 'due to your age' but to hostile forces in the environment such as poverty and poor housing.

All the accounts of health explored so far see the normal state of affairs to be one of homoeostasis. Any disruption of this homoeostasis is considered abnormal and if homoeostasis is not restored then the organism is said to be in a state of pathology or disease. Aaron Antonovsky (1984) has called this 'the pathogenic paradigm' and he claims that all our models of health, even the biopsychosocial models, are dominated by this paradigm.

Moving to a salutogenic paradigm

Antonovsky (1984) points out some of the consequences of the domination of the pathogenic paradigm. The first is that 'we have come to think dichotomously about people, classifying them as either healthy or diseased' (p.115). Those categorised as 'healthy' are normal, those categorised as non-healthy or diseased are deviant. If 60 per cent of older people have some form of chronic illness or disability then the majority of older people are not healthy. There is no place in this dichotomy for those who have a chronic illness yet are able to function perfectly well or for those who have a handicap yet are well satisfied with life. Secondly, and this echoes the holistic account, we have come to think of specific diseases such as cancer or heart disease instead of being in a state of dis-ease. We have become obsessed with morphology instead of relating to generalised dis-ease and its prevention. This leads to Antonovsky's third concern which is that we look for specific causes for these specific diseases in order that the causes can be eradicated instead of accepting that 'pathogens are endemic in human existence' (p.115). He believes that we need to explore the capacity of human beings for coping with pathogens. Fourthly the pathogenic paradigm deludes us into thinking that if we can eliminate 'disease' we will have health. This 'mirage of health' (Dubos, 1961) has been the driving force behind the 'technological fix' and 'magic bullet' attitude to eradicating disease. This attitude leads to the fifth consequence which Antonovsky identified, which is that the pathogenic paradigm concentrates on 'the case' and identifies high risk groups instead of studying the 'symptoms of wellness'(p.116). Adopting this approach would entail studying the smokers who do not get lung cancer or the 'fat eaters' who do not have heart trouble.

Antonovsky believes that we should think 'salutogenically'. He claims that instead of assuming that the normal state of the human organism is one of homoeostasis, balance and equilibrium it makes more sense to acknowledge that the 'normal state of affairs for the human organism is one of entropy, of disorder, and of disruption of homoeostasis' (p.116). He suggests that none of us can be categorised as either healthy or diseased but that we all can be located somewhere along a continuum which he calls 'health-ease–dis-ease'. He explains:

> we are all somewhere between the imaginary poles of total wellness and total illness. Even the fully robust, energetic, symptom-free, richly functioning person has the mark of mortality: he or she wears glasses, has moments of depression, comes down with flu, and may well have as yet nondetectable malignant cells. Even the terminal patient's brain and emotions may be fully functional. (p.116)

This way of thinking would have profound effects on the way we view health in old age. It would discourage a percentage approach to assessing the health of older people. Instead of assuming that because 60 per cent have a chronic illness or disability they are therefore in poor health whilst the other 40 per cent are in good health, we would need to look behind those figures to ask how those 60 per cent are actually affected by their chronic illness or disability and to explore their wellness. We would have to ask questions such as why do some people cope whilst others do not, why some consider themselves to be healthy in spite of their chronic illness whilst others do not . We would also need to ask about the dis-ease of the 40 per cent without chronic illness or disability. Do they have non-classifiable aches and pains, discomforts and feelings of unwellness?

Antonovsky is anxious that this reorientation towards health does not minimise the achievements of medical science, nor would he wish to impede the progress of technological change. Rather his purpose is to redress an imbalance inherent in the way we view health, not to abandon the struggle against disease but to widen the armoury and explore other ways of achieving health. We need the availability of hip replacement surgery but we also need to understand why one person copes well with the operation and fully regains mobility while another does not. We need to identify all the factors which might help us move along the continuum and not just focus on the disease. We ask not so much how we can eradicate certain stressors but how we can learn to live with them, concentrating on the ability to adapt.

Another feature of the salutogenic paradigm which helps in our understanding of health in later life is that it turns on its head the notion that older people are a high risk group. As Antonovsky says, all of us *by virtue of being human are in a high risk group* (p.117). If we locate people dynamically along a continuum of health then we are less likely to stereotype 'the elderly' as diseased. By adopting a salutogenic paradigm we can reconceptualise questions about health in later life to concentrate on why and how people cope well with chronic illness and disability. The questions change from what stops people becoming sick to what helps them to become healthy in spite of disease.

In an attempt to define the mechanisms which help people to cope with adverse health conditions Antonovsky developed a construct which he calls a *Sense of Coherence* which he abbreviates to SOC. He describes it as follows:

> The sense of coherence is a global orientation that expresses the extent to which one has a pervasive, enduring though dynamic feeling of confidence that one's internal and external environments are predictable and that there is a high probability that things will work out as well as can reasonably be expected. (Antonovsky, 1979, p.123)

In a later refinement he identified three main components – comprehensibility, manageability and meaningfulness. Comprehensibility is the ability to see one's own world as understandable, to *have confidence that sense and order can be made of situations* (p.118). One views the future as reasonably predictable rather than chaotic, disordered or unpredictable. Meaningfulness is the *emotional counterpart of comprehensibility . . . life makes sense emotionally* (p.119). Life is worth living for those who see their lives as comprehensible and meaningful. Manageability reflects the extent to which people feel that they have adequate resources, mental, physical, emotional, social and material to meet whatever demands are put upon them. He believes that wherever a person is located on the health-ease–dis-ease continuum at any particular time those with a stronger SOC are more likely to move towards the health end of the continuum.

A person's SOC is built up from a range of experiences and sources through the life cycle and should be well developed by adulthood. Antonovsky sees the SOC developing from the degree to which our life experiences provide 'consistency', an 'underload/overload balance' and provide for participation in decision making. We experience consistency when a given behaviour results in the same consequences whenever we exhibit it and when people respond to us in consistent ways. This allows us to predict the outcome of behaviour and therefore our lives seem reasonably predictable. Underload/overload balance is achieved when the demands made upon us are appropriate to our capacities. Underused capacity due to lack of challenges can be as harmful as not having sufficient capacity to meet the challenges with which we are faced. The extent to which we participate in decision making is important to the emergence of a strong SOC and is the basis of the meaningfulness component. When every thing is decided for us and we have no say in the matter, when the rules are set by others without consultation, then the experience is alien to us. The issue is not so much having control over the events of our lives but in having some part in the decision making process.

Antonovsky's theory provides a useful framework for analysing the health status of older people both collectively and individually. The health-ease–dis-ease continuum allows us to locate older people along the continuum rather than categorising them in terms of either health or disease. It allows us to explore how people move along the continuum towards the health end in spite of chronic illness disability.

It is possible that Antonovsky's theory of SOC could be interpreted in a very individualistic way and thus be 'victim blaming': if only those older people with chronic illness had developed a strong SOC they would cope better with their lot. This was clearly not Antonovsky's intention, and in a paper presented at the WHO seminar on 'Theory in Health Promotion: Research and Practice' held in September 1992, he makes a case for seeing the SOC as a theoretical basis for health promotion. He asks

> Can it be contended that strengthening the SOC of people would be a major contributor to their move toward health? (1996, p.16).

He goes on to make it clear that this strengthening of the SOC is not aimed at individuals but at a given population and frames the question for health promotion programmes:

> What can be done in this 'community' – factory, geographic community, age or ethnic or gender group, chronic or even acute hospital population, those who suffer from a particular disability, etc. – to strengthen the sense of comprehensibility, manageability and meaningfulness of the persons who constitute it?

It is important to remember that older people are a very diverse group, each with a unique biography and different life experiences and access to social and economic resources. But old age is a time when the threat to a sense of coherence can be great. Manageability, comprehensibility and meaningfulness can be hard to maintain in the face of much loss and change. This is particularly true of those old people who spend their last years in institutions where it is likely to be even more difficult to maintain any sense of coherence.

Antonovsky's theory presents a way of both understanding health in old age and of helping older people to move towards the health end of the continuum whatever their circumstances. In order to do this they require ageing-friendly environments which must be both prosthetic and stimulating at the same time. Unfortunately many older people experience extremely ageing-unfriendly or ageist environments which are a threat to any sense of coherence.

References

Antonovsky, A. (1979). *Health, Stress and Coping: New perspectives on mental and physical well-being.* San Francisco: Jossey-Bass.

Antonovsky, A. (1984). The sense of coherence as a determinant of health. In Matarazzo, J. P. (ed.), *Behavioural Health.* New York: Wiley.

Antonovsky, A (1996). The salutogenic model as a theory to guide health promotion' *Health Promotion International 11 1* 11–18.

Beattie, A., Jones, L. and Sidell, M.(1992). *Health and Wellbeing.* K258, 2nd level distance learning course. Milton Keynes: Open University.

Dubos, R. (1961). *Mirage of Health.* New York: Andor Books.

Maslow, A. (1954). *Motivation and Personality.* New York: Harper & Row.

Sidell, M. (1995). *Health in Old Age: Myth, mystery and management.* Buckingham: Open University Press.

Stevens, R. (1990). Humanistic psychology. In I. Roth (ed.) *Introduction to Psychology.* Milton Keynes: Open University and Lawrence Erlbaum Associates.

2 Tackling inequalities in health: extracts from the summary[*]

Michaela Benzeval, Ken Judge and Margaret Whitehead

The international evidence on inequalities in health is compelling. People who live in disadvantaged circumstances have more illnesses, greater distress, more disability and shorter lives than those who are more affluent. Such injustice could be prevented, but this requires political will. The question is: can British policy makers rise to the challenge?

Extent and nature of inequalities in health

In Britain death rates at all ages are two to three times higher among disadvantaged social groups than their more affluent counterparts. Most of the main causes of death contribute to these differences, and as a result, people in the least privileged circumstances are likely to die about eight years earlier than those who are more affluent. People living in disadvantaged circumstances can also expect to experience more illness and disability.

There is nothing new or unique about the existence of inequalities in health. They were first documented in Britain in the 1860s and are evident in countries across the developed world. Evidence that such inequalities exist is based on numerous studies that measure health and socio-economic circumstances in a variety of ways. They include data on mortality, morbidity, self-reported health status and professionally measured fitness, from official statistics, cross-sectional and longitudinal surveys and numerous small-scale studies.

What is particularly worrying, however, is that economic inequality appears to be growing more quickly in Britain than at any time since the Second World War. Moreover, during the 1980s social divisions accelerated at a rate not matched for such a sustained period by any other rich industrialised country. Not surprisingly, the impact that this increase has had on health is now beginning to emerge. Death rates in some of the most disadvantaged areas in Britain not only worsened in relative terms between 1981 and 1991 when compared with the most affluent areas, but

---

[*] King's Fund (1995), pp. xvii–xxv.

16

among some age groups, such as young men, the rates actually rose. As death rates in Britain have been declining since the 1930s, this rise signals a new and disturbing development.

Explanations about the causes of inequalities in health are complex, but it is likely that a combination of factors is at work reflecting people's living and working conditions, their resources, social relationships and lifestyles. However, since much health-related behaviour itself is socially determined, it is people's circumstances that are the most important determinant of health.

What could be done?

A detailed review of interventions in various countries at different times, by Margaret Whitehead, suggests that policy initiatives that can influence inequalities in health exist at four different levels:

- Strengthening individuals;
- Strengthening communities;
- Improving access to essential facilities and services;
- Encouraging macroeconomic and cultural change.

Policies that attempt to strengthen individuals aim to change people's behaviour or coping skills through personal education and/or empowerment. General health education messages have had a limited impact on people from disadvantaged environments because the pressures of their lives constrain the scope for behavioural change. However, more sensitive interventions that combine education and support can have a positive effect on the health of people in disadvantaged circumstances if they are carefully tailored to their needs and combined with action at other policy levels.

Policies that aim to strengthen communities have either focused on strengthening their social networks or they have adopted a broader strategy that develops the physical, economic and social structures of an area. Such initiatives can, through involving the community itself in the determination of priorities, change the local environment, services and support systems in ways that promote equity in health.

Despite some successes, however, efforts to strengthen individuals and communities have had a minimal impact on reducing inequalities in health. Much greater influence is possible at the other policy levels. Some of the greatest gains in health in the past have resulted from improvements in living and working conditions – better housing, improved water supply and sanitation, safer conditions in the workplace, education, the alleviation of poverty and general provision of health and welfare services. Western countries must guard against changes that undo these successes. At the same time, further changes in these areas will continue to be needed to reflect the pace of social change.

Macroeconomic and cultural changes are also important determinants of health because they influence the overall standard of living in a country and its distribution; attitudes to women, minority groups and older people; and major environmental factors such as international pollution. Policies at this level have been shown to have differential effects on the various groups in society, creating major implications for tackling inequalities in health. For example, some of the early structural adjustment policies, to deal with countries in economic crisis, hit the most disadvantaged sections of the population hardest. Conversely, macroeconomic policies in various countries that have protected or improved the standards of living of poorer groups have had a beneficial impact on the population's health.

A worthwhile agenda for tackling inequalities in health must therefore include a strong focus on reducing poverty and a commitment to the careful monitoring of the impact of major public policies on health, particularly among the most vulnerable groups.

What should be done?

The more the determinants of health are recognised and understood the more inescapable is the conclusion that a person's health cannot be divorced from the social and economic environment in which they live. Factors that are increasingly recognised to be of critical importance . . . include:

- The physical environment, such as the adequacy of housing, working conditions and pollution;
- Social and economic influences such as income and wealth, levels of unemployment, and the quality of social relationships and social support;
- Barriers to adopting a healthier personal lifestyle;
- Access to appropriate and effective health and social services . . .

An example of each factor – housing, income maintenance, smoking prevention and access to health care – has been selected to illustrate new policy initiatives that should form part of a strategy to tackle inequalities in health . . .

Housing

The housing problems facing Britain today . . . include:

- The rapid rise in homelessness in the 1970s and 1980s among both families and single people;

- The large numbers of properties in bad condition suffering from problems such as damp, inadequate heating, infestations, poor design and lack of play space;
- The social isolation caused by high-rise blocks and the social segregation apparent in many deprived estates.

Such problems can have adverse effects on people's health. For example:

- People sleeping rough are three times as likely to have chronic chest conditions;
- Families in bed-and-breakfast accommodation have higher rates of infections, gastro-enteritis, child accidents, parental stress, poor child development and nutritionally unsatisfactory diets;
- Inadequate or unaffordable heating almost certainly contributes to hypothermia and excess winter mortality among older people;
- Damp housing has been shown to cause respiratory and other illnesses in children and stress among adults.

A range of policies needs to be developed that tackles these housing problems in ways that reduce inequalities in health. Investment in new social housing and improving the existing housing stock should be promoted as a matter of urgency. Similarly, community regeneration schemes should be introduced in areas of high deprivation to improve the environmental, economic and social structures of disadvantaged neighbourhoods. In addition, tax concessions should be given to private landlords to encourage the expansion of the private rented sector.

Such policies could be financed by transferring public housing out of the public sector to enable capital to be raised and removing mortgage interest tax relief . . .

Family poverty

The latest evidence for 1991–92 suggests that families with children are over-represented at the lower end of the income distribution, comprising 57 per cent of households with incomes below 40 per cent of the UK average, but only 45 per cent of the total. There are three main causes of family poverty: unemployment; lone parenthood; low wages...

A strong association between low income and poor health has been demonstrated across the developed world. In Britain, people in the lowest income quintile are four times as likely to report their health as not as good as those in the highest income quintile.

Poverty can affect health in a number of different ways:

- Income provides the prerequisites for health, such as shelter, food, warmth and the ability to participate in society in society;

- Living in poverty can cause stress and anxiety which can damage people's health;
- Low income limits people's choices and militates against desirable changes in behaviour.

The best way of reducing family poverty is to tackle its causes by ensuring that all people who wish to be economically active have access to well-paid jobs. Useful steps in this direction would include better training opportunities and improved childcare facilities . . . However, given that it is unlikely that all families will be able to escape from a reliance on benefits in the foreseeable future, the social security system also needs to be reformed.

. . . One way of . . . reducing family poverty would be to increase means-tested benefits such as income support and family credit. Other policies that would reduce some of the pressures on people with low incomes should include:

- Tackling problems of low uptake of benefits;
- Replacing the social fund loans scheme with a grants system;
- Ensuring that all households have access to vital utilities – such as heat, light and water – without the threat of disconnection.

In addition, the drift to greater economic inequality that has been exacerbated by recent tax changes benefiting the most affluent needs to be reversed. Measures could include:

- Abolishing the upper limit on employee national insurance contributions;
- Restricting the value of the main personal tax allowances to the lowest rate, i.e. 20 per cent for all taxpayers;
- Increasing the highest rate of income tax;
- Shifting the balance of taxation away from spending and toward income.

Not only might these measures reduce inequalities in health but they would also raise the resources necessary to finance a comprehensive strategy to promote social justice and equity in health.

Smoking

Smoking-related diseases are the greatest single cause of premature mortality and excess morbidity in the UK.

Although the number of people who smoke has fallen substantially over the last three decades, this reduction has mainly occurred among more affluent social groups so that smoking is now predominantly a habit of people in disadvantaged circumstances. . . . Three times as many people in unskilled occupations smoke compared to those from professional groups. Particularly high smoking rates are found among people who are unemployed and young adults with children, especially lone parents.

Smoking increases the risks of most major killers such as lung cancer and heart disease. For example, smokers are twenty times more likely to die of lung cancer than non-smokers. Such diseases are much more prevalent among disadvantaged social groups. However, it should not be assumed that the health divide has a single cause. Substantial socio-economic gradients in mortality and morbidity exist among non-smokers. It is also important to note that behaviours are determined by the social environment in which people live, and so encouraging behavioural change requires much more than exhortation.

Policies to reduce smoking may include health education and cessation advice, controlling tobacco advertising, restricting the availability of cigarettes, creating smoke-free environments and increasing taxation on tobacco-related products.

- Health education and cessation advice have had a limited impact on smoking rates among the more disadvantaged social groups. However, these interventions can be made more effective by being made more sensitive to the pressures of people's lives and being backed up by wider policies to create a supportive environment.
- New resources should be invested in developing and evaluating innovative interventions, in health education, cessation support clinics and advice by primary care workers, targeted at vulnerable groups. Nevertheless, other wider strategies need to be adopted to have any major impact on smoking prevalence among the most disadvantaged groups.
- One priority for action is a ban on the advertisement and promotion of cigarettes and tobacco-related products. It is estimated that this would reduce smoking by approximately 7.5 per cent. In particular, given that young people are thought to be more influenced by advertising and that advertising is more prevalent in tabloid papers and on posters in disadvantaged areas, a ban would have most effect on teenagers and those with low incomes.
- A further priority is to increase the real price of cigarettes. This would reduce both the number of people who smoke and the number of cigarettes smoked by those who continue. However, the cost would fall disproportionately on people with low incomes and should not be lightly contemplated in isolation from a broadly based anti-poverty strategy.

The NHS

It is important not to exaggerate the role of health services in tackling health inequalities. It is equally important, however, that they do not abdicate those responsibilities which properly fall on them. Health care systems do have a useful even if relatively minor role to play in promoting social justice and equity in health . . . The Department of Health and the NHS at large have three key obligations:

- To ensure that resources are distributed between areas in proportion to their relative needs;
- To respond appropriately to the health care needs of different social groups;
- To take the lead in encouraging a wider and more strategic approach to developing healthy public policies.

Existing resource allocation mechanisms in the NHS have done much to address some of the historical inequities in health care provision, but further reforms are needed. A unified weighted capitation system should be introduced to ensure that all resources are allocated to areas in relation to the need for them.

In addition, as purchasing decisions are devolved to more local areas, two safeguards are required:

- Substantial resources need to be top-sliced for local health authorities to enable them to take the broad population approach – to assessing needs, monitoring access to care and providing community-based services – that is required to deliver equitable services;
- A fairer system of allocating resources to GP fundholders needs to be established.

Evidence about equitable access to care in Britain is patchy. There is some highly aggregated evidence that implies the NHS does surprisingly well in ensuring that resources are distributed between social groups in proportion to their relative needs. On the other hand, this is countered by a number of small-scale studies that suggest that among a range of specific services and at local levels more disadvantaged social groups do appear to be under-served.

Perhaps most worrying, however, is how little is actually known about the social characteristics of patients and their response to treatment. The NHS needs to make much greater efforts to assess whether it is achieving equal access for equal need for all social groups. Local health authorities need to develop equity audits as a matter of urgency.

Where there is evidence that people with poor socio-economic circumstances are inadequately served in relation to their needs, a new approach that empowers communities and individuals needs to be adopted. Some studies suggest that barriers to access to health care can be reduced through the introduction of more sensitive and appropriate community-based services.

The NHS should also take the lead in developing policies at both the national and local level to promote equity in health.

- At the national level, mechanisms are needed to facilitate inter-departmental co-operation and multi-sectoral action to tackle health inequalities. Health impact assessments should also be introduced to monitor the effects of all public policies on health.
- Equity-orientated health targets should be set to maintain a strong national focus on reducing inequalities.
- At the local level, the promotion of initiatives that develop structural links between different agencies can enable the health service to take part in policy making on issues that affect population health, such as the local environment, housing, education and transport . . .

Conclusion

Observed social inequalities in health are amenable to purposeful policy interventions. The problem is well documented and the solutions become clearer every day. What is needed is a determined effort to mobilise the political will to create a fairer society that embraces all sections of the community.

3 The limits of lifestyle: re-assessing 'fatalism' in the popular culture of illness prevention *

Charlie Davison, Stephen Frankel and
George Davey Smith

Introduction: fatalism and control in contemporary health promotion

One of the most important changes in twentieth century medical culture in industrial societies has been the shift in emphasis from acute and infectious diseases to chronic and multi-factorial disorders as the major causes of morbidity and mortality. This transition has been paralleled by the development of a stronger emphasis on the prediction and prevention of disease in both policy and practice circles.[1] This tendency has led professional and lay discourse increasingly to adopt the notion of risk as a central, guiding concept in constructing responses to disease. The aspect of this cultural process which forms the background of the present discussion is the heightened profile of disease prophylaxis as an organising motive in the everyday activities of the healthy population.

The gradual shift towards prevention in the general medical culture has meant that the circumstances and attributes of those who suffer and die from chronic disease have taken on a particular importance in the construction of risk. The central role of scientific epidemiology in identifying associations between disease and the various individual conditions of sufferers has been matched by the attempt to prevent people developing these dangerous or risky attributes. Perhaps the most striking feature of this process has been the development of a strong, officially-sponsored ideological perspective which emphasises the personal responsibility of the individual citizen in the maintenance of their own health and the avoidance of chronic disease.[2]

Informing the public of the risks associated with certain behaviours, and exhorting the adoption of a 'good' diet, regular exercise and abstention from society's two main legally sanctioned non-medical drugs has become

* From *Social Science and Medicine, 34 (6)* (1992), pp.675–685. Oxford: Pergamon Press. © Pergamon Press Plc 1992.

an important part of both General Practice and the newer state sectors of Health Education and Health Promotion. The overall responsibility of the individual in these areas has crystallised into the somewhat amorphous idea of the importance of following a 'healthy lifestyle'.

The term 'lifestyle' has recently come to be used widely in many contexts, and a brief clarification of the use of the term here is in order. Aside from its direct association with health-related behaviour, the word (or words) have been used to denote general conditions of living, as a product brand name, and to describe a type of television programming. Here we concentrate on the idea of 'lifestyle' issues as the aspects of health-related behaviours and conditions which entail an element of personal action at the individual level. The main fields covered by the rubric are diet, leisure activities (especially those involving exercise), intake of drugs, and personal body maintenance (hygiene, sleep, etc.). Our aim in this usage is to limit the term to those behaviours and conditions which official and commercial health promotion has strongly associated with the possibility of individual choice and the triumph of self control over self indulgence.[3]

One of the major problems facing the professions and institutions involved at the behavioural end of contemporary preventive medicine is the apparent failure of many individuals to comply fully with healthy lifestyle advice. In the developing discourse of health education, this situation has been attributed to two major causes. In the first place, it was suggested that there was a lack of accurate knowledge among the general public concerning the potential harm associated with certain aspects of everyday behaviour.[4] An image was canvassed that saw people with heart disease as "victims of their own ignorance".[5] This perspective assumed that, if knowledge were increased (or ignorance dispelled), rational people would decide to change their daily habits. In recent years, this approach has been labelled as out-moded by those with an academic or quasi-academic interest in lifestyle modification. Data gathered during ethnographic fieldwork, however, showed that many of those involved in the concrete business of giving health advice to the general public still regard ignorance as an important barrier to the adoption of healthy behaviour.

A second, slightly more sophisticated, line of analysis suggests that a major cause of non-compliance is the existence of an attitude which sees health as being largely determined by forces outside the control of the individual, and thus denies the possible relevance of personal behavioural change. As previous research and critique in this field has pointed out, the 'locus of control' trend in psychology has operated within an ideological perspective which takes as axiomatic that belief in individual control is 'correct', while belief in other agencies requires some kind of rectification (usually education). This type of analysis has led to the production of the idea that health promotion is involved in a battle for the hearts and minds of the population, a struggle between a modern belief in lifestyle and an atavistic culture of "fatalism".[6]

Two recent definitions of fatalism from quite different ends of the academic literature on lifestyle and health illustrate the currency of the concept:

> some members of the public have a fatalistic attitude to health and therefore do not believe that they have much control over their health status.[7]

> [their] attitudes were fatalistic: health was, as a general principle, the consequence of behaviour, but this did not apply to them; health was extremely important, but they themselves had no control over it.[8]

The first definition is taken from a report of survey data analysed in the somewhat partial fashion all too common in health promotion research. Having already decided on the moral status of smokers (reprehensible), the researchers proceed to 'prove' that which they plainly believed already. Their 'finding' is that people who smoke tobacco are also 'fatalistic' – a term they use against the backdrop of a barely-concealed contempt for a group of their informants they see as ignorant and/or culturally defective. We cite this paper as an extreme, though not unusual, example of the uncritical acceptance of the 'locus of control/fatalism' complex which pervades much British research and practice in the field of illness prevention.

The second definition, while coming from a study informed by a more proper scientific detachment, also includes the key notion that lies at the heart of the fatalism label – the idea that the individual feels that he/she cannot necessarily exercise control over his/her health . . .

Lifestyle and coronary heart disease

Our examination of the construction of personal control in the realm of CHD (coronary heart disease) prevention is based on extensive survey and ethnographic research in three communities in South Wales: Plasnewydd (a socially mixed ward of the City of Cardiff), Porth (an industrial and service town in the Rhondda Borough) and Llangammarch Wells (a village and rural district in the Borough of Brecknock). In total, extended semi-structured interviews were carried out with a randomly selected set of 180 adults of both sexes and a full range of socio-economic circumstances. The interviews covered general ideas of what 'health' might be, explanations of the causes of good and poor health, issues of control, prevention, illness avoidance, fault and blame, and a number of more specific topics concerning the heart and CHD . . .

The conceptual place of lifestyle

Aspects of life which, in the perception of our informants, have an effect on individual health status but cannot be individually controlled in any obvious way can be grouped, for the purposes of analysis, into three inter-locking fields:

- Fields involving the self-evident personal differences between individuals (e.g. heredity, upbringing, inherent traits).
- Fields involving the social environment (e.g. relative wealth and access to resources, risks and dangers associated with occupation, loneliness).
- Fields involving the physical environment (e.g. climate, natural dangers, environmental contamination).

To these three, a fourth conceptual area must be added. The fourth field exists, however, not as a substantive or concrete area in its own right, rather as a process or mechanism governing the first three. This fourth field concerns the operation of luck, chance, randomness and personal destiny. As the aspect of popular culture which gave its name to 'fatalism' itself, this fourth area is of obvious importance. But over and above this, our analysis indicates that, as a theoretical area involved with the explanation of the distribution of misfortune in an overall system based essentially on probability, these beliefs play a crucial role in the construction of culturally appropriate behaviour. We shall return to this area after examining the implications of the basic model .

While we have, thus far, followed the roughly orthodox path of placing an analytical or categorical division between lifestyle and these three sets of 'non-control' forces, the conceptual landscape we have observed during field research contains no such hard and fast barrier. Each of the three categories of areas outside personal control has a more complex relation-ship with individual health status and individual participation in healthy lifestyles than the fatalism/lifestyle dichotomy implies. In each case there is, on the one hand, a direct influence on health status, and on the other, an indirect influence, mediated through an effect on the possibility or ease of voluntary participation in healthy lifestyles.

The model can best be illustrated with an example. In the popular explanatory culture of CHD, being a 'worrier by nature' (a character trait widely recognised by our informants in Wales as being inherited via both genetic and social routes) can have various direct effects on the health of the individual. These are caused by the clenching of internal organs and muscles ('always being tensed up'), the disruption of normal blood chemistry ('too much adrenalin') and the consequent disruption of regular heart beat. Over and above these mechanisms, there exists the possibility of indirect health damage brought about through an effect of the condition on lifestyle. In the case of the 'worrier by nature' this occurs through combating worry with tobacco and alcohol and allowing worry to dictate inappropriate eating habits.

Lifestyle, then, as is the case with other elements of this model, did not really exist as an independent category for our informants. Rather it was only articulated in terms of its intimate but varied relationship with the other elements. As an issue concerning voluntarism and the possibility of individual choice and freedom, the relationship between health and lifestyle is of evident political importance. This political issue has resided at the centre of contemporary British debates concerning the social distribution of mortality and morbidity since the publication of the Black Report.[9]

If, as our simple model suggests, the entire lifestyle and health relationship is embedded in the wider operation of forces recognised as being outside individual control, there are strong implications for the construction of personal attitudes. Data from our three Welsh samples suggest that the key process involved is the assessment of the relevance of personal lifestyle change in the context of the unique position of the individual *vis-à-vis* the three substantial 'non-control' fields. Because diet, exercise, and drug consumption cannot be seen as being independent of the social and economic structures within which behaviour (and culture) are sited, they must also be involved with the realities of relative inequality in a stratified society . . .

General principles and individual events

Whether examined from the perspective of medical science or popular knowledge, prevention and control imply knowledge about cause. Attempts to exercise control over the timing and nature of events presuppose the existence of an explanation or set of explanations which account for the occurrence and distribution of the events themselves.[10] It has long been a commonplace observation in the discipline of social anthropology that cultural systems of explanation or accountability need to address two distinct issues. In the first place the general kind of misfortune requires explanation: how and why does it happen? In the second place, the site and time of particular misfortune require explanation: how and why did it happen to this person at this time?[11]

The healthy lifestyles movement within preventive medicine represents an attempt to reduce the second area of explanatory culture to a subset of the first. Indeed, as Gifford points out, the central concept of prevention (that of medical 'risk') is actually produced by the uncritical transposition of epidemiological associations derived from whole populations to the field of an individual life.[12]

The particular refinement of the healthy lifestyles movement as applied to heart disease has been to go to great lengths to place one set of general epidemiological principles (those involving behaviour open to personal control) at the centre of explanatory culture. Because the various 'non-control' mechanisms described here have been largely ignored in the publicity of the prevention movement, they have acquired an unofficial and even 'dissident' image.

A concomitant of this process is that these non-control areas have become somewhat marginalised in the explanatory culture associated with heart trouble. This marginalisation is exhibited by the fact that they often enter public discussion as subsidiary agents in the onset of illness and death, only after the assessment of the more scientifically mainstream and 'fashionable' lifestyle areas. Non-control areas in general, and the luck/fate field in particular, were observed to take centre stage most strikingly when illness and death struck individuals who 'should not have been victims' if the principles of lifestyle were always reliable . . .

An integral part of the modern prevention movement has been the public lowering of the threshold of risks concerning personal lifestyle. Although this process is ostensibly involved in extending the bounds of explicability and control, it has the paradoxical effect of highlighting anomalies. This has happened because aspects of life hitherto considered normal and safe (chip eating. lounging about, etc.) have become labelled as pathogenic. Because so many other factors are involved in illness causation and distribution, a result of this ideological development is that the number of people who survive dangerous lifestyles and do not get ill grows. Simultaneously, the cases of individuals who do all the 'correct' healthy things and yet still succumb to heart trouble become very well known.[13]

Because the everyday practice of lay epidemiology detects both anomalous deaths and unwarranted survivals, the tension or conflict between general principles and individual events is constantly made plain to members of society and has to be dealt with. An extremely common explanation of an anomaly thus becomes 'it was just one of those things', the full but unspoken version of which is 'it was just one of those things which violates general principles'.

Implications for health education and health promotion

Our investigation of the popular culture of illness avoidance and the protection of good health in three South Wales communities concentrated on the idea of control. By the very nature of the current social and political movements taking place in the public health field in all of Britain, we were led to focus on the interaction between popular culture and an intense official interest in promoting voluntary behavioural change.

In overall terms, we found that, by concentrating so heavily on the fields of diet, drug use and exercise, official health education messages and health promotion initiatives in the localities studied were quite seriously out of step with popular culture in those areas. We contend that this position is not unique to South Wales and that the same point could be made of the United Kingdom in general and quite possibly of other parts of the world. Our tentative recommendations for changes in health promotion practice are thus couched in relatively general terms.

If a greater cultural sensitivity could be achieved in health promotion practice, it is our view that some important areas of conflict could be eased. There are three specific areas in which health promotion could feasibly move towards a more culturally appropriate position.

First. the content of health education messages could be re-assessed. The effect of personal behaviour on health is apparently well understood by the vast majority of the population. While this does not necessarily imply that all individuals actually behave in concert with this knowledge. neither does it automatically indicate that repeated applications of the same propaganda would be beneficial. Indeed, a reassessment of the scientific epidemiology concerning lifestyle and the various non-control areas discussed in this paper may be revealing. In our observation, popular belief and knowledge concerning the relationship of health to heredity, social conditions and the environment may be more in step with scientific epidemiology than the lifestyle-centred orientation of the health promotion world.

A second step towards a more culturally appropriate health promotion stance concerns the conceptual division between the controllable and the uncontrollable. At present, the official line is sharply drawn: lifestyle is controllable, everything else is not. Public concern with environmental matters, however, indicate that a willingness to attempt to control some aspects of these areas does exist within society at large. It is revealing, however, that local and national movements aimed at environmental improvements operate outside the health promotion sphere and little institutional interest on the part of health promotion in bridging this gulf is in evidence. An easing of the stark official division between spheres open or closed to human control and a greater institutional interest in collective as well as individual action could be productive .

Finally, it is clear from our investigations that the existence of a random distribution of illness and death formed a central part of popular understanding in South Wales. Furthermore it is constantly and effectively re-affirmed by the workings of lay epidemiology. We believe that this finding from one small area of Europe will strike chords in many other places.

If a more effective collaboration between health promotion and the general public is to be achieved, a method of dealing with this area needs to be developed. In the branch of bio-medical culture concerned with individual diagnosis and cure, practitioners are satisfied to accept a certain level of mystery and use the label 'idiopathy'. The branch which focusses on prevention, however, is much more threatened by lacunae in the understanding either of causation or of distribution. This may have led to a counter-productive discourse in which exaggerated claims for predictability, regularity and certainty are made.

The fact remains, however, that, within the general statistical tendencies that can be observed within populations, there lies a more chaotic distribution of illness and death. Some fat smokers really do live till advanced old age, and some svelte joggers really do 'fall down dead'.

Falling back on the albeit honest defence that lifestyle advice is based on probability rather than certainty is plainly an inadequate response when the complexities of popular culture are properly taken into consideration. In this field more than any other, the fact that lay epidemiology is so firmly embedded in popular health culture poses a serious problem for health promotion. If the coronary prevention movement desires a good working relationship with society at large, both the true position of lifestyle and the real-life events addressed by fatalism need to be re-evaluated.

Notes

1. The conceptual conformity of British government policy spanning administrations run by both major political parties is illustrated in: Secretary of State for Health. *The Health of the Nation: a consultative document for health in England*, London: HMSO (1991), and in: Department of Health and Social Security. *Prevention and Health: Everybody's Business*, London: HMSO (1976).
2. Crawford R. You are dangerous to your health: the ideology and politics of victim blaming, *International Journal of Health Services* 7(4), 663–680 (1977). Radical Statistics Health Group Health Education: Blaming the victim? In *Facing the Figures – What is Really Happening to the National Health Service?* London: Radical Statistics (1987).
3. Areas of life which have sometimes been described as 'involuntary lifestyle', which include behaviours and conditions routed in a collective field and therefore not directly open to change at the individual level. such as being exposed to industrial pollution, appear in our analysis as 'environmental' factors.
4. *Health Education News*, Heart disease risks ignored, London: HEC (September 1981).
5. A. Dillon Director of the Coronary Prevention Group, speaking on BBC Radio 4 (October 1986).
6. Pill, R. and Stott, N. C. H., Development of a measure of potential behaviour: a Salience of Lifestyle Index. *Social Science Medicine 24(2)*, 125–134 (1987). Farrant W. and Russell J., The Politics of Health Education, *Bedford Way Papers, 28*, University of London Institute of Education, 1986. Naidoo, J., Limits to individualism. In *The Politics of Health Education – Raising the Issues* (edited by Watt, A. and Rodmell, S.). Routledge & Kegan Paul, London, 1986.
7. Lewis, P. A., Charny, M., Lamber, D. and Coombes, J. A fatalistic attitude to health among smokers in Cardiff. *Health Education Research 4(3)*, 361–365, 1989.
8. Blaxter, M., Health and Lifestyles. Tavistock/Routledge, London, 1990.
9. Townsend, P. and Davidson, N. *Inequalities in Health: The Black Report*. Penguin, Harmondsworth, 1982. Davey Smith, G., Bartley, M. and Blane, D. The Black Report on socio-economic inequalities in health 10 years on, *British Medical Journal 301*, 373–377, 1990.

10.   In Social Anthropology this aspect of cultural life has generally been discussed in terms of 'accounting for misfortune'; in Social Psychology as 'attribution theory'.

11.   Evans Pritchard, E. *Witchcraft, Oracles and Magic among the Azande of Anglo-Egyptian Sudan*. Clarendon Press, Oxford, 1937.

12.   Gifford, S. M. The meaning of lumps: a case study of the ambiguities of risk. In *Anthropology and Epidemiology* (edited by Janes, C. R. *et al.*), pp. 213–246. Reidel, The Hague, 1986.

13.   Davison, C., Davey Smith, G. and Frankel, S. Lay epidemiology and the prevention paradox – the implications of coronary candidacy for health promotion. *Sociology of Health and Illness 13(1)*, 1991.

4 Health education as empowerment[*]

Keith Tones

The discussion of health promotion in this chapter will centre on the dynamic interaction of health education and health policy and will argue that ethically and practically the main goal of the educational endeavour should be empowerment. The empowerment strategy helps to resolve an important dilemma in health promotion: the need, on the one hand, to prevent disease and safeguard the public health while, on the other hand, respecting individual freedom of choice – including the freedom to adopt an 'unhealthy' lifestyle.

For reasons of economy, the major focus of this chapter will be on health education rather than the equally relevant domain of policy development and implementation. . . .

Health promotion: anatomy and ideology

The term 'ideology' is used here in its simplest form and merely describes the complex of values inherent in belief systems and underpinning personal and professional practice. The conceptualisation of health promotion in this chapter incorporates the ideological canons of WHO which are central to its Health for All by the Year 2000 (HFA 2000) initiative and embodied in many landmark developments such as primary health care (PHC) and the Ottawa Charter. The ethical and moral view of humanity enshrined in WHO's perspective may be summarised as follows:

- Health should be viewed holistically. It is a positive state and an essential commodity which people need in order to achieve a socially and economically productive life.
- Health will not be achieved nor illness prevented and controlled unless existing health inequalities between and within nations and social groups have been eradicated.
- A healthy nation is not only one which has an equitable distribution of resources but one which also has active empowered communities which are vigorously involved in creating the conditions necessary for a healthy people.
- Health is too important to be left to medical practitioners: there must

[*] From *Health Promotion Today*. London: HEA (1995), pp.38–71.

33

be a 'reorientation of health services'. It is important also to recognise that a wide range of public and private services and institutions influence health for good or ill. Moreover, medical services frequently do not meet the needs of the public; they often treat people as passive recipients of care and are thus fundamentally depowering. The main *modus operandi* of health promotion is one of enabling not coercing; the focus should be on co-operation rather than on compliance.

- People's health is not just an individual responsibility: our health is, to a large extent, governed by the physical, social, cultural and economic environments in which we live and work. To cajole people into taking responsibility for their health, while at the same time ignoring the social and environmental circumstances which conspire to make them ill, is a fundamentally defective strategy – and unethical. It is, in short, victim-blaming. For these reasons, the process of 'building healthy public policy' is at the very heart of health promotion (Tones and Tilford, 1994, pp. 4–5).

It is important to acknowledge that this list of principles is a mix of verifiable fact and value-judgement. It should also be noted that WHO's major health promotion principles are incorporated in the Ottawa Charter (WHO, 1986). A majority of nations, therefore – including the UK – have apparently committed themselves to these principles as signatories of the Charter.

There is still, in some quarters, a degree of uncertainty about the difference between health education and health promotion. For some people they are synonymous. Indeed, within the UK health service, the assumption seems to be that the purpose of health promotion is primarily to influence lifestyles by means of education. However, health promotion is much broader than this, and Figure 4.1 seeks to demonstrate the nature of the educational contribution.

Traditional preventive models of health education place great emphasis on individual lifestyle changes. This may constitute blaming the victims of the social and environmental factors which create unhealthy circumstances in the first place. Alternatively a more radical approach is envisaged which will seek to bring about social and political change in order to make the healthy choice a more viable option (and doubtless to replace a dominant right-wing ideology with a more congenial radical alternative).

The radical option is fully compatible with the Ottawa Charter which brought the matter of health policy centre-stage and argued that there would be a global improvement in health only when governments made serious attempts to deal with the environmental and social circumstances which militated against health and nurtured disease. As may be seen from Figure 4.1, health education operates in a kind of partnership with policy development. Its role is two-fold. First of all, it seeks to influence individual lifestyle – but not in the traditional way. Its main purpose is not

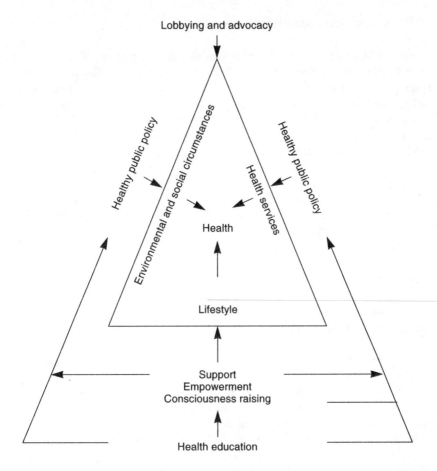

Figure 4.1   *The contribution of education to health promotion*

to coerce cajole or persuade, but rather to facilitate choice by providing people with empowering competences and support. This empowering function also extends to the utilisation of health services by helping patients interact assertively with practitioners.

The second and, perhaps, more challenging function for health education is about community rather than individual empowerment. Its rationale is simple: lobbying and advocacy alone will not materially influence policies which benefit powerful individuals and corporate interests. Accordingly vigorous public pressure and even the ballot box are prerequisites for substantial social changes. The underlying principles for this 'radical' approach have been established for some time and can be encapsulated in Freire's term 'critical consciousness raising' (CCR) (see Freire, 1974). However, CCR must be supported by the technology of empowerment if indignation is to be translated into community action.

Ethics and voluntarism

There are sufficient ethical issues in health education to justify the Society of Public Health Educators (SOPHE) of America establishing its own code of ethics (Faden and Faden, 1978). Of course since health education unlike medicine is undertaken by a wide range of practitioners – both skilled and unskilled – it is not possible to make generalisations about the nature and extent of ethical or unethical practice. However, SOPHE (1976) has unequivocally affirmed the importance of voluntarism:

> Health educators value privacy, dignity and the worth of the individual, and use skills consistent with these values. Health educators observe the principle of informed consent with respect to individuals and groups served. Health educators support change by choice, not by coercion.

Nevertheless, it is ingenuous in the extreme to assume that people normally have anything approaching complete freedom of choice – or indeed that such a state is desirable. Before considering the extent to which health education can actually facilitate choice in accordance with SOPHE principles, let us acknowledge the existence of important impediments to action. There are two significant barriers to individual freedom of choice. The first of these comprises those several environmental factors which healthy public policy is designed to remedy. The second kind of barrier is better described as psychological and operates in an often less obvious and more subtle way.

At the individual, psychological level, it is also apparent that complete freedom of choice is a relatively rare commodity and unequally distributed. Apart from lack of information, there may be many factors militating against people's capacity to choose freely. Those who are 'addicted' to some substance or other are not as free to choose to indulge in their habit as they were prior to their habituation – a fact amply illustrated by the very high proportion of smokers who claim that they would rather not be smoking. Again, there is consistent evidence that many people both know what is involved in healthy lifestyles and are motivated to improve their health status. What they lack is in part the skills and support needed to do so and in part the belief that they are actually capable of exercising any influence over often debilitating social circumstances. Accordingly, it is either extremely cynical or extraordinarily naïve to pronounce that health education should not interfere in other people's lives and leave them to choose their own pathway to health or to elect for a short but gratifying life! It is almost equally ingenuous to give the impression that only health educators are inclined to interfere with people's liberty.

These rather stirring statements of intent might reasonably bring accusations of empty rhetoric. However contrary to some opinion health education has a substantial corpus of theoretical wisdom with which to translate the rhetoric of empowerment into reality and an attempt will now be made to provide some insight into this process.

A theory and technology of empowerment

So far our references to health education have tended to be of an ideological nature: that is they have centred on its overriding purpose in terms of professional or moral values. We will now give some consideration to what best be termed the 'technological' aspects – the technical details involved in translating any given ideology into practice. In this respect, a definition of health education is not hard to formulate. It is conceptualised in this chapter as follows:

> Health education is any intentional activity which is designed to achieve health- or illness-related learning i.e. some relatively permanent change in an individual's capability or disposition. Effective health education may   therefore produce changes in knowledge and understanding or ways of thinking. It may influence or clarify values; it may bring about some shift in belief or attitude; it may facilitate the acquisition of skills; it may even effect changes in behaviour or lifestyle.

Although this definition is doubtless unsurprising to those who are professionally skilled there still exists in those who are not an often remarkably naïve conception of what is involved in influencing people's health-related behaviours. There are still those who appear to believe that unhealthy lifestyles are due to ignorance and are, consequently, thoroughly surprised when individuals persist in their irresponsible ways despite having been provided with large quantities of information! Other self-styled experts will acknowledge the limitations of this simplistic notion that knowledge leads to practice (K———P) and will insert an 'A ' into the 'formula' (K——A——P) arguing that attitudes must be changed before healthy practices are adopted. Frequently the result of such an analysis is a mass media message containing simplistic information in a form designed to change attitudes (perhaps by a measured dose of fear appeal). If they have the courage to evaluate the success of the initiative they are highly likely to record failure. Others will then confidently report yet another example of the ineffectiveness of health education.

Ironically, health education has a rich and sophisticated theoretical base on which to draw. The fact that this is often ignored by non-specialists is of some interest in its own right. It doubtless represents a lamentable tendency to assume that education is a quite simple and commonsense process – a point of great irritation to the teaching profession for very many years! Moreover, since health education has had a more or less close relationship with the medical profession over the years, it might also have something to do with the imbalance between the relative power and status of education and medicine!

Be that as it may, although there is a range of different social and behavioural science models and theories on which to draw, we do have a good understanding of what influences people's behaviours in health and illness – an observation which we will now seek to illustrate.

Making health-related decisions

Many of the factors influencing individual decision-making are incorporated in the above definition of health education – explicitly or implicitly. Let us, for instance, consider what might influence a hypothetical individual's decision to respond to an educational interaction which is concerned with prudent use of drugs. It is doubtless clear that some knowledge and understanding of the nature and effects of the given substance would be necessary: people would need to understand about units of alcohol and the recommended healthy limits to consumption. Although necessary, such knowledge would not be sufficient. In addition, the individual in question would have to believe this 'healthy message' and might also need a number of supportive skills. He or she would undoubtedly benefit from social interaction skills training in order to resist pressure from peers in a 'round-buying culture' to have unwanted drinks. First-aid skills would also be useful for occasions when friends may have over-dosed!

The importance of people's beliefs in the decision-making process cannot be over-estimated; indeed ensuring that individuals' health-related beliefs correspond to current realities might well be the main concern of the educational endeavour. For instance, the celebrated health belief model (Janz and Becker, 1984) offers useful guidance for those seeking to persuade clients to adopt safer sex practices. Before, for example, condom use becomes a more attractive proposition clients must be reasonably convinced that they are susceptible to HIV infection; they must believe the outcome of infection will be serious: they must accept that condoms are actually beneficial in acting as a barrier to the virus; they need to balance this (and any other) perceived benefits against the costs which they might believe condom use will incur.

Although useful the health belief model has its limitations. For instance we must certainly reckon with another category of belief in addition to those highlighted by the model. We must take into account people's beliefs about the nature and cause of diseases (sometimes described in terms of attributions of causality). The relevance of this theoretical construct is well illustrated by the many reviews of myths about cancers. If for instance, people believe that cancer is a single undifferentiated disease or that it lies dormant within each person as a seed only waiting for one of many 'triggers' to generate overt disease, then it is hardly surprising that pessimism about treatment and prevention prevail and delay in seeking medical help is not uncommon. Accordingly, health educators need to acknowledge these various 'theories of illness'; indeed Tuckett *et al.* (1985) argued that the exploration of patients' concepts and beliefs about their condition should be a sine qua non of effective medical consultations.

Any respectable theory must of course take account of people's motivational state. Decisions about sexual practices will, for instance, inevitably be influenced by individual value systems. As would be expected, moral values will be particularly relevant but paradoxically may prove a handicap unless they are sufficiently powerful that they enable individuals to 'resist temptation'. The worst possible scenario is where, say, a moral imperative prevents a young woman even contemplating anticipatory purchase of a condom but is not quite strong enough to prevent her yielding to the power of the sex drive!

Further consideration of the health belief model's central concept of perceived susceptibility requires more sophisticated analysis. It is self-evident that some people are actually motivated by a belief in susceptibility to certain kinds of risk: they may be 'sensation seekers'; they may enjoy the experience of maintaining control 'at the edge'(Lyng, 1990). At all events they will not co-operate with health education messages emphasising the risk of damage to their health. Indeed, one of the more revealing conceptualisations of the reasons why adolescents frequently engage in health-threatening behaviours is embodied in Jessor and Jessor's (1977) theory of problem behaviour. In short health-compromising activities (like delinquent or anti-social behaviour) is symptomatic. Accordingly, health promotion must again address root causes – a point to be revisited when we later note the disadvantages of 'vertical' programmes.

All we can hope to do here is to provide a vignette which supports our earlier assertion that we have a rich theoretical tapestry at our disposal if we care to use it to explain individuals' decision-making processes in health and illness. However, even a brief review must give some consideration to those psycho–social and environmental factors which contribute directly to the *empowerment* of decisions. This we will now attempt to provide.

The dynamics of empowerment

The concept of empowerment is central to the philosophy and practice of health promotion. In one sense it parallels the concept of health: it can be said to be both a desirable end in itself and a means to an end. And so, just as WHO has come to regard health as a means to achieving a socially and economically productive life, empowerment of individuals and communities acts instrumentally to facilitate 'healthy' decision-making. The concept of empowerment is both complex and 'slippery' and only some of its bare bones can be mentioned here. In short, empowerment has to do with the relationship between individuals and their environment; the relationship is reciprocal. This reciprocity factor is central to social learning theory and Bandura (1982 and 1986) has emphasised the importance of recognising the phenomenon of 'reciprocal determinism'. Clearly the environment may exercise a powerful controlling influence on people but people may also influence their environment. For instance, as a collective, a community might put pressure on authorities – local or national – in order to achieve change (see Figure 4.1). Communities might also take direct action to improve their environments. Again, individuals may exert pressure for change (perhaps after a process of critical consciousness raising) by lobbying or through the ballot box.

At the micro level empowerment is also a key health promotion goal. For instance as part of client contract behaviour modification, people might learn how to avoid environmental circumstances which trigger their consumption of tobacco or alcohol; they might acquire skills in resisting social pressure; they might learn how to control 'temptation' by applying self-regulatory skills and by rewarding themselves with some substitute gratifications. As we will note later such techniques need to be incorporated into many health promotion consultations – either face-to-face or within a group context. They also provide a clear example of how the rhetoric of empowerment can be operationalised and translated into specific educational objectives.

As should be evident from the preceding discussion these empowering tactics draw on a corpus of sophisticated research and psychological constructs. A comprehensive account is not possible here but key self-empowerment concepts include beliefs about control (e.g. perceived locus of control and self-efficacy beliefs), values such as self-esteem and a variety of specific social and personal skills which might be encapsulated in the terms 'health and life skills'. Some of these may be seen in Figure 4.2.

Figure 4.2 may be interpreted in the light of early observations about the limitations of the 'K——A——P' formula. First, the provision of knowledge must be supplemented by a process of values clarification in order to facilitate decision-making. Secondly, and in order to fulfil the criterion of empowerment, mere knowledge must be accompanied by the state of heightened and critical awareness which is the goal of critical consciousness raising.

This 'superior brand' of knowledge is, nonetheless, not sufficient to influence intention and attitude in a satisfactory health-promoting fashion. Individuals must also believe they are capable of achieving what they

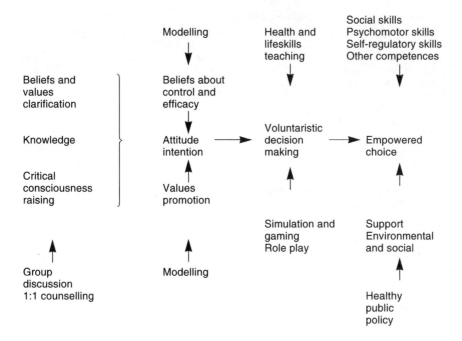

Figure 4.2   *An empowerment model of health education*

would like to achieve: in short they will need to acquire self-efficacy beliefs. We should also note that the educational process is not value-free in the sense that any decision is acceptable so long as it is empowered! Figure 4.2 emphasises the need for active 'values promotion': for example, decisions should be 'responsible'. Although responsibility frequently seems to mean behaving in accordance with the often rather narrow moral principles espoused by the communicator, its definition here is quite broad. The moral imperative is essentially voluntaristic and utilitarian: the guideline is that people's decisions are ethical provided that they do not harm others and do not impinge on others' freedom to act.

Figure 4.2 also incorporates the central requirement of a supportive environment. Apart from demonstrating the need to provide supportive health and lifeskills – as mentioned above – it asserts the principle that healthy public policy is necessary to ensure that the healthy choice is the easy choice.

References

Bandura, A. (1982). Self efficacy mechanism in human agency, *American Psychologist, 37(2)*, 122–47.

Bandura, A. (1986). *Social Foundations of Thought and Action: A social cognitive theory.* Englewood Cliffs, N. J.: Prentice-Hall.

Faden, R. R. and Faden, A. I. (1978) The ethics of health education as public health policy,

Health Education Monographs, 6 (2), 180–97

Freire, P. (1974). *Education and the Practice of Freedom*. London. Writers and Readers Publishing Cooperative (originally published in Portuguese. 1967).

Janz, N. K. and Becker, M. H. (1984). The health belief model: a decade later, *Health Education Quarterly, 11*, 1–47.

Jessor, R. and Jessor, S. L. (1977). *Problem Behavior and Psychosocial Development: a longitudinal study of youth*. New York: Academic Press.

Lyng, S. (1990). Edgework: a social psychological analysis of voluntary risk taking, *American Journal of Sociology, 95(4)*: 851–36.

SOPHE (Society for Public Health Education) (1976), *Code of Ethics, 15 October, 1976*. San Francisco, California.

Tones, B. K. and Tilford, S. (1994). *Health education: effectiveness, efficiency and equity*. London: Chapman & Hall.

Tuckett, D. *et al.* (1985). *Meetings between experts*. London: Tavistock.

WHO (1986). *Ottawa Charter for Health Promotion*. Copenhagen. WHO Regional Office for Europe.

For a fuller review, see Tones, B. K. (1992), Health promotion, empowerment and the concept of control. In *Health Education: Politics and Practice*. Victoria: Deakin University Press; and Tones and Tilford (1994)

5 The importance of social theory for health promotion: from description to reflexivity*

Russell Caplan

Situating the problem

In trying to understand what health education/promotion is, and what those involved in it do, we have constructed various models. These models aim to capture in words some of the sense of what happens in practice. As such, they tend to describe in imaginative terms peculiar to the person doing the describing. The limitations of this form of understanding health education/promotion rest on the fact that people frequently use different terms/adjectives to describe similar health education/promotion situations or processes. Consequently, the more important similarities among health education/promotion models appear as differences, and fundamental differences are rarely considered. The net result of all this confusion is a failure to spell out more precisely what it is one means by health education/promotion, and more importantly what one is doing when one claims to be practising health education/promotion.

This confusion can be best understood as an inability to move beyond describing what one is doing to the more fundamental theoretical level, which explains more fully the nature and choice of particular models. In health promotion, as in many other fields of social intervention, descriptive models all too often take on the appearance of a theory. This blocks the possibility of deeper forms of understanding and evaluation. Access to knowledge about health education/promotion approaches, I believe, rests on a structure of abstract theoretical constructs and categories which serve to make up a theoretical map on which a wide range of health education/promotion approaches can be rationally located and explained as a series of paradigms or exemplars (Gallie, 1956; Kuhn, 1970; Chalmers, 1985). However, these exemplars or paradigms can only be uncovered through a rigorous analysis of those abstract theoretical and philosophical assumptions/categories which lie hidden in the terms health

* From *Health Promotion International*. *8(2)* (1993), pp. 147–157. Oxford: Oxford University Press. © Oxford University Press 1993.

education/promotion is presented in. This is what I shall call *reflexive analysis*, in the sense that these abstract categories or assumptions are read back from the initial descriptive terms in which health education/promotion is presented (Holland, 1977). These abstract theoretical and philosophical assumptions constitute a basic structure which determines all our descriptions, concepts and theories about health education/promotion. This is the area of *social theory* proper.

The theoretical and philosophical assumptions

Theoretical and philosophical assumptions contained in the various health education/promotion models consist of two fundamental questions or dimensions.

The first question or dimension concerns the evidence or data on which we plan our interventions. Within health education/promotion the question revolves around the nature of scientific knowledge with competing theories of causality regarding individual and community health status laying claim to the mantle of scientific rationality. Does the medical view of health and illness as the presence or absence of an *objective* pathological entity provide the basis for a rational grasp of the causal links necessary to plan an effective programme of health promotion/education? Or, do we need to draw on less tangible categories of *subjective* human experience such as the cultural and personal meanings and definitions which would appear to connect with people's individual and collective health status?

Clearly, the question of causality within this latter position is much more complex and less linear and mechanical than its medical counterpart which has tried to bridge the gap by focusing on individual behaviour as an objective causal entity. But behaviour does not equate with this latter view of experience since it remains within the objectivist fold of medical explanations as a mechanical cause of health damaging effects, whereas the opposing position from the point of view of meaningful human experience would suggest individual human behaviour as a consequence or effect of a complex socio-economic, cultural and ecological system the rationality of which must be understood in different terms from that of the natural sciences. Thus, it can be argued that effective health education/promotion in reducing the incidence of coronary heart disease in the population needs to focus on categories of social and cultural experience which give meaning to the eating, drinking and smoking habits of people. Preventable heart disease cannot be effectively addressed as a consequence of unhealthy behaviour. Rather unhealthy behaviour must be made intelligible in the light of people's experience of living in a social system defined by many layers of meaning ranging from family experience to the impact of social class.

The knowledge base around which we plan our programmes for action is thus a crucial dimension in determining what we do in the name of health promotion/education, how we do it and most importantly how we compete for scarce resources. The problem of knowledge on which we base our programmes for action remains the fundamental philosophical question of immense practical import in the struggle over competing systems of rationality.

This struggle over competing systems of rationality in the design and adoption of health promotion policies and strategies can be represented on a horizontal plain as opposing views or polarities about the nature of scientific knowledge, and how we acquire knowledge about human affairs (see Figure 5.1).

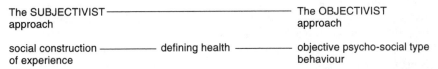

The SUBJECTIVIST ———————————————— The OBJECTIVIST
approach   approach

social construction ————— defining health ————— objective psycho-social type
of experience   behaviour

Figure 5.1   *Philosophical positions: the subjective–objective dimension about the nature of scientific knowledge*

The second dimension or question implicit in the various models of health education/promotion can be represented on a vertical plane which has to do with assumptions concerning the nature of society. These assumptions range from theories of Radical Change at the top to theories of Social Regulation at the bottom (see Figure 5.2).

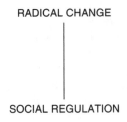

RADICAL CHANGE

SOCIAL REGULATION

Figure 5.2   *Assumptions' spectrum*

Radical change
Views related to theories of *radical change* argue that our society is essentially unstable with a basic tendency towards change. It is governed by basic conflicts such as that between capital and labour, and the domination of ideas, rules and objectives of some groups over others. For example, the domination of men over women expressed in a patriarchal ordering of society, and, a Eurocentric value system which is both culturally and racially insensitive to ethnic and cultural differences, expressed in the many forms of discrimination and racism in our society. The consequences of this is the exploitation, deprivation and alienation of certain groups within our society.

Theories of *radical change* are therefore concerned with finding explanations which demonstrate the need for fundamental change in the way our society is organised, that is, by social conflicts, tension and domination. Radical change then, is concerned with emancipation from structures which constrain and limit human potential. It consequently focuses on questions which look at human deprivation in both social and psychological terms. Its major concern is with what is *possible*, more than with what *is* . . .

Social regulation

Ideas associated with theories of *social regulation* argue that we live in a predominantly stable society which is integrated and holds together well. This it is argued is reflected in a general consensus on rules and objectives. Social institutions such as the family, education, health and welfare all exist for the satisfaction of both individual and social needs.

Ideas about *social regulation* are therefore concerned with providing explanations of society in terms which emphasise its underlying unity and integration. This view seeks to understand why society holds together instead of falling apart. It is consequently concerned with the need for regulation in human affairs . . .

The two dimensions of Subjectivist and Objectivist approaches to knowledge and Radical Change or Social Regulation assumptions about the functioning of society, which all models of health education/promotion entail, can be combined as shown in Figure 5.3. Each quadrant represents a major approach or paradigm to the understanding of health and the practice of health education/promotion. It also provides the necessary concepts with which to assess more deeply and fundamentally what the differences are between the various health education/promotion models, and what they have in common with one another.

While Figure 5.3, and the more comprehensive map shown in Figure 5.4 is not a simple 'mechanical device' for piecemeal identification,

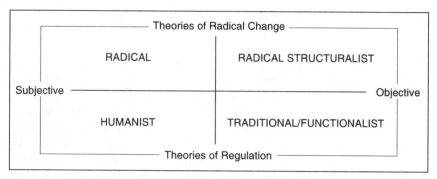

Figure 5.3   *Major paradigms*

Source: Burrel and Morgan (1985).

RADICAL HEALTH EDUCATION

Core view
Society is oppressive and alienating, It is characterised by hierarchical and authoritarian institutions of the state, business corporations, the professions, science, work and the family, which cognitively dominate people, (political and ideological domination). The very language we have to speak creates and sustains our participation in this form of oppression.

Sources of problems
Institutions we inhabit, which socialise and train us, and in which we work. The order which these institutions define devalues, discredits or invalidates alternatives. It affects huan consciousness, relationships and potential, producing alienation and frustration of full personal and communal fulfilment.

Health education aims
Self-discovery through mutual aid and non-hierarchical cooperative projects which challenge the necessity of institutional processes. Radical self-help and deprofessionalism of health care which changes social control systems instead of so-called deviants. Reveal and challenge the 'political' in health.

RADICAL STRUCTURALIST HEALTH EDUCATION

Core view
Fundamental conflicts and contradictions arising from the economic system which give unequal wealth, power and opportunity to different classes. This determines broadly, the form of social institution and the state, of which the health and welfare services are but one example. Society is characterised by class conflict and struggle to redress the economic basis of class inequality.

Sources of problems
The demands of production and the reproduction of the conditions for capital accumulation (of which profits are part). Production – occupational diseases and injuries; unemployable and unemployed; occupational stress. Consumption – lifestyle patterns and consumer habits determined by what is produced, e.g. advertising which induces consumer preferences. Distribution – artificially maintained scarcity for basic needs, e.g. inadequate housing, heating, food and clothing.

Health education aims
Provide a theoretical analysis of the relationship between health, illness and the economic class structure. Link health education to those initiatives which challenge capitalism.

Subjective

Objective

Core view
Social life is meaningful and proceeds on the basis of the subjective interpretations of participants. Social structures, institutions, roles and concepts of normality are socially created, sustained and changed by people through their interactions with one another. Implicit orientation to integrated, harmonious and enduring social units since it does not focus on political or economic consequences, or causes.

Sources of problems
Meanings and definitions that people give to their actions or identities are disrupted by events, or reinterpreted or so labelled by others that disorganised or deviant roles, identities and health careers are created. Loss and disruption of taken-for-granted reality produces disorientation and distress.

Health education aims
Improve understanding of self and others; improve communication by exploring the meanings of problems and events to all relevant parties, reconstruct identities by reframing accounts, representing unheard or unexpressed versions, challenging key labellers, correcting stereotypes.

Core view
An enduring and integrated system based on a harmony of interests and common value system. Models and methods of natural science applied to the understanding of human affairs (medical science and epidemiology). The social whole is sustained by social institutions which function in the interests of individual and society, and which is adaptable to change.

Sources of problems
Pathological, maladaptive or incorrect (irresponsible) behaviour, habits or lifestyle; or, pathological or faulty functioning of orgainsational and environmental processes.

Health education aims
Behaviour and attitude modification; or, administrative, legislative and environmental change (social engineering). Social change is not precluded so long as it is based on acceptance of the rules and legitimate institutions of liberal democracy.

HUMANIST HEALTH EDUCATION

FUNCTIONALIST HEALTH EDUCATION

Figure 5.4   *Theoretical approaches in health education*

Source: Caplan (1990), adapted from Whittington and Holland (1985)

categorising and cataloguing of the various aspects of a model, it does nevertheless help us to assess whether there is anything of substance about a particular model, and its general direction. Again, while the approaches are not mutually exclusive with regard to certain assumptions, there are nevertheless certain limits beyond which to hold one position or approach must necessarily preclude the adoption of some other approaches . . .

By understanding the nature and purpose of health education/ promotion models in this way, it becomes possible to examine the degree of overlap and fundamental differences far more adequately and meaningfully.

The two abstract theoretical and philosophical dimensions (*Subjectivist–Objectivist* and *Radical Change–Social Regulation*) translate at a more concrete level into three pre-eminently practical questions which are implicit beacons, a type of cognitive compass guiding policy makers and practitioners alike in their quest to understand just what the determinants of health are, and what exactly constitutes a health promotion intervention.

Thus in each of the four approaches or paradigms which appear in Figure 5.4 the following questions provide the necessary evaluative mechanism by which various ideas, policies and plans can be properly analysed and mapped: (i) What is the core view of society? (ii) What are the principal sources of health problems? (iii) What are the health education/promotion aims? (Whittington and Holland, 1985).

Presented in this way, it becomes possible to construct a comprehensive map as set out in Figure 5.4 which summarises the position of each of four approaches or paradigms. This systematised approach to theory in health promotion/education provides strong refutation of the conventional wisdom current within health promotion/education circles which argues that we are extremely unlikely to reach a point when a definitive map of health education will be possible (French and Adams, 1986).

Reflexivity in action–using social theory

The 'Ottawa Charter for Health Promotion' 1986, building on the 'Targets for Health for All 2000' (WHO, 1985), is the clearest statement of principles of a new public health movement which permeates much of the thinking and practice in the field. This statement of principles brings together a broad spectrum of descriptive terminology and categories which appear to be novel, radical and above all capable of providing the sort of understanding about health necessary for building effective action to promote it.

The view, however, as expressed in the Ottawa Charter, that you can build a new public health movement out of the rhetoric of disparate and contradictory ideological positions, constitutes an unwitting instrument for the imposition of an uncritical consensus incapable of mounting the necessary political and ideological challenges to the status quo so crucial for a health engendering society. In the final analysis the Ottawa Charter in the interests of consensus means all things to all people and precisely because of that is unlikely to provide the means for a clear strategy of action in raising the public health . . .

Much of what appears in the Ottawa Charter is an amalgamation of various models of health education/promotion which demand a proper analysis of their theoretical and philosophical underpinning . . . At least four models or methods which predate the Charter can be readily identified: the educational model, self-empowerment, the political economy model and the community development model (Tones, 1981, 1984, 1985; Beattie, 1984; Keeley-Robinson, 1984). While it is true that the terms in which they are presented are not always identical with that of the language used in the Charter, they nevertheless reflect with greater analytical precision the key notions embraced by the Charter. These notions relate to the development of personal skills as a means of self-empowerment through education and advocacy; the building of healthy public policy through political and economic means; and the empowerment of communities through community development (Ottawa Charter, 1987).

More often than not both the *educational* and *self-empowerment* notions or models, are presented as a radical antidote to the mechanical *objectivism* of the medical view based on simple disease prevention or individual behaviour change (Keeley-Robinson, 1984; Tones, 1985). However, if the preventive view of promoting health is 'by encouraging individuals to move away from unhealthy life styles and to adopt healthy behaviours' (Keeley-Robinson, 1984) then the educational and self-empowerment methods, while appearing to be more sensitive to the ideas of not imposing the professional's view of the right kind of health-related behaviour on individuals, nevertheless do not quite escape this line of reasoning.

Firstly, in the case of the educational model, who provides individuals with information, and secondly, who decides what informed decisions about health related behaviours are? This *objectivist* tendency within the self-empowerment framing of the model, while hidden by terms such as 'self-esteem' and 'informed healthy choices' (Keeley-Robinson, 1984; Ottawa Charter, 1987) is nevertheless all too present in the notion conveyed that there are *objectively identifiable skills*. Thus, it is argued that 'the purpose of health promotion is to enable people to achieve the personal skills and understanding of the environment that will allow them to exercise more control over their own health and make healthful choices' (Ottawa Conference Report, 1987).

What is clearly evident here on closer inspection is 'the existence of a priori concepts of the professional that are directive and strongly implicated in the succeeding action'. There is a preconceived model of 'how things should be which is implicit in the attitude of professionals' (Grace, 1991) and which is indicative of an *objective* purpose outside the individual . . .

In addition the preventive model, like the other two models, focuses on 'encouraging individuals to move away from 'unhealthy life-styles' (Keeley-Robinson, 1984). In fact, I would strongly suggest that these three models are really aspects of a more complex *medical model* with *education* concerned with the ethics and obligations of the health educator, which is respect for and protection of individuals' health interests; prevention providing the scientific basis or *objective knowledge* about what has to be changed, health-related behaviour of individuals; and *self-empowerment* being the actual activity taught, conducted, or prescribed . . .

The *core view of society* which these approaches seem to hold is one of social integration and harmony where individuals need to change if their health status is going to be improved. The *principal source of health problems* lies somewhere between pathological, maladaptive or incorrect behaviour and disrupted life events forcing a dysfunctional set of roles and meanings to the behaviour of individuals. The *aim* conveyed here is a sense of individuals needing to be regulated or regulating themselves to a pre-defined goal of healthy behaviour. There is very little in these approaches which impresses upon the reader the sense of *collective action* borne of the essential class tensions and conflicts which is the real stuff of *radical change*. The overall position of these approaches lies somewhere between the Traditional or Functionalist and Humanist as set out in Figure 5.4 . . .

The Ottawa Charter also argues the case for combining 'diverse but complementary approaches including legislation, fiscal measures, taxation and organizational change' (Ottawa Charter, 1987). 'Public health legislation, better housing, an improved food supply and greater purchasing power are acknowledged as the most significant contributions to improvements in health status' (Keeley-Robinson, 1984). The view conveyed by this approach is that a package of legislative and administrative reforms is what is needed to improve people's health. Health education/promotion as *social engineering* is the strategy proposed to bring about the desired social changes.

The difference between this model and the educational and self-empowerment approaches is that the emphasis here is on administrative and legislative machinery to bring about the changes which will impact on the health related behaviour of individuals. The *objectivism* of individual behaviour has been substituted for the *objectivism* of public policy which is once again outside the locus of individual control.

And, even though 'powerful interests which profit from the products not conducive to health' (Keeley-Robinson,1984) are identified as part of the problem, they are nevertheless considered within an overall framework of a stable and enduring social consensus. They simply need to be reformed through the same legislative, administrative and fiscal measures which have been used in the past and even presently to secure these very same profits . . .

This fits quite easily into a *Functionalist* or *Traditional* approach. Political and economic indicators in this approach are a recapitulation of the traditional logic of incrementalism which simply adds 'new' indicators to an already bulging edifice of 'accumulated findings, like pebbles which if stacked up in sufficient quantity are bound to reach the sky eventually' (Ingleby, 1981). What is required is 'a "critical theory" that reconstitutes what needs to be indicated' (Stevenson and Burke, 1991) namely, radical *political economy*.

Perhaps the best attempt at constructing a truly radical practice in health education/promotion lay in the invocation of community action through *community development*. 'Community development draws on existing human and material resources in the community to enhance self-help and social support, and to develop flexible systems for strengthening public participation and direction of health matters. At the heart of this process is the empowerment of communities, their ownership and control of their own endeavours and destinies' (Ottawa Charter, 1987). 'The first step for the health educator/promoter' therefore 'would be to elicit the felt needs of the community. The formation of community groups would then be facilitated as a means of responding to identified needs' (Keeley-Robinson, 1984).

The *Radical* approach themes of domination in both its cognitive and institutional sense is implicit here (see Figure 5.4). In other words the community identifies what it considers to be its health problems (cognitive appropriation) and forms its own community groups (organisational ownership and control). However, while identifying health problems 'as one aspect of poverty and multi-deprivation' (Keeley-Robinson. 1984) it does not go further than this.

The *community development* model presented here, is more readily identified with the *Humanist* approach, belonging with the other three models to a theory of *social regulation*. It is in the final analysis about competing more effectively within the defined social consensus. It is a piecemeal attempt at solving social and political issues of poverty and multi-deprivation through local community activity.

This is well demonstrated by the use of the term *community*. Community implies unity, togetherness, as opposed to social divisions which the *radical change* approaches are concerned with. Consequently, if a model is concerned with *radical change* then it cannot reflect the overall interests of everyone, as if they all had the same interest implied by the term *community*. This is because power, wealth and opportunity are unequally spread among the population, in the view of *radical change* adherents. If health is a consequence of this, then it is only the interests of a certain class or group of people that the *radical* or *radical structuralist* approaches are concerned with. . . .

Conclusion

It would appear that all the models have a very similar view of society even though they seem to differ with regard to what they consider to be the *principal sources of health problems* and the *health education/promotion aims*. However, by showing how similar they are in their view of society we can come to an understanding of their differences at the level of sources of health problems and health education/promotion aims, as differences in degree and emphasis rather than fundamental differences of approach.

The analysis of the models is necessarily schematic. It does not represent a definitive analysis, but provides a common method and language through which to conduct a more thorough and informed debate. This points to, and draws on, a theoretical framework more definitive and enduring than has hitherto been realised within health education/promotion. This is not simply a matter of semantical refinement. For what is at stake is the very practice of health education/promotion and the positions it adopts based on a particular view of the world we live in. . . .

Unless we understand more fully the theoretical and philosophical assumptions which underlie our methodological preferences, the link between health education/promotion and political processes remains unclear.

References

Beattie. A. (1984). Health education and the science teacher: invitation to a debate, *Education and Health*, (January) 9–15.

Burrell. G. and Morgan, G. (1985). *Social Paradigms and Organisational Analysis*. Aldershot: Gower, 18.

Chalmers, A. F. (1985). *What is this thing called Science?* Milton Keynes: Open University Press.

French, J and Adams L. (1986). From analysis to synthesis: Theories of health education, *Health Education Journal*, 45, 71–74.

Gallie, W. B. (1956). Essentially contested concepts, *Reports of meeting of the Aristotelian Society* (21 Bedford Square, London, 12 March).

Grace, V. M. (1991). The marketing of empowerment and the construction of the health consumer: a critique of health promotion, *International Journal of Health Services*, 21, 329–343.

Ingleby, D. (ed.) (1981). *Critical Psychiatry: The politics of mental health*. Harmondsworth: Penguin.

Holland, R. (1977). *Self and Social Context*. London: Macmillan, 267.

Keeley-Robinson, M. (1984). Adult education issues for health promotion, *Occasional Paper*, 1. Hull University, 12–14.

Kuhn, T. S. (1970). *The Structure of Scientific Revolutions.* Chicago: University of Chicago Press.

Ottowa Charter for Health Promotion (1987). *Health Promotion,* 1, iii–v.

Ottowa Conference Report (1987). First International Conference on Health Promotion, *Health Promotion,* 1, 443–462.

Stevenson, H. M. and Burke, M. (1991). Bureaucratic logic in new social movement clothing: the limits of health promotion research, *Health Promotion International,* 6, 281–289.

Tones, B. K. (1981). Health Education: prevention or subversion? *Journal of the Royal Society of Health,* 3, 114–117.

Tones, B. K. (1984). Health education: present prospects and future potential, *TACADE Monitor,* 66, 6–9.

Tones, B. K. (1985). Health promotion – a new panacea? *Journal of the Institute of Health Education,* 3, 17–422.

WHO (1985). *Targets For Health For All 2000,* Copenhagen: World Health Organization.

Whittington, C. and Holland R. (1985). A framework for theory in social work, *Issues in Social Work Education,* Summer, 1–54.

6 Models of health: pervasive, persuasive and politically charged*

Trudi Collins

Introduction

The use of models clearly has the potential to be problematic. Each user has their own (or their agency's) political agenda and will interpret the model in their own, and possibly in their class, interest. Model developers can do little to protect against this except to include detailed explanations/interpretations of the model. Even then, the model developer's intentions can be ignored, misunderstood or misinterpreted. It is useful, therefore, to consider some established models of the determinants of health and to explore both the ways it appears their developer intended their use and some other possible interpretations. The implications of the political ideology underpinning these models and its explicitness will also be addressed. The intent of this exercise is to consider ways in which models can be 'safeguarded' from misuse (if, indeed, that is possible) and, in addition, to assist in the development of an alternative way to conceptualise the determinants of health.

An established model of health

Hancock (1993) has been involved in the development of three ecological models of health, human development and the community. The third and most comprehensive of these, the model of health and the community ecosystem (Hancock, 1993), attempts to show the interactions between community, environment and the economy as they relate to health (see Figure 6.1). It emphasises concepts such as conviviality in communities (social support, public participation, equity), generation of adequate wealth by the economy in a manner that is both socially and environmentally sustainable, and a liveable and viable built and natural

* From *Health Promotion International*, 10, (4) (1995), pp. 317–324. Oxford: Oxford University Press. © Oxford University Press 1995.

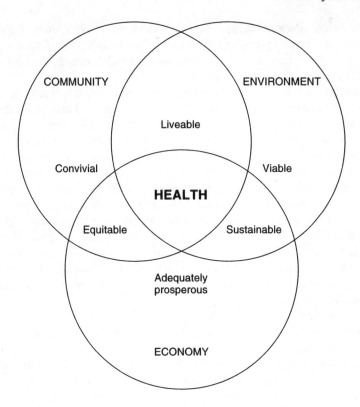

Figure 6.1   *Interactions between community, environment, economy and health*

Source: Hancock (1993)

environment (Hancock, 1993). This model has a clear emphasis on economics being required to meet standards of environmental sustainability and thus implicitly rejects the concept of economic growth at any cost, which has been gaining popularity in the wake of the ongoing recession experienced in the industrialised world. However, the model is less clear about the political implications of constraints on economic activity. For example, the notion of an *adequately* prosperous economy which is equitably distributed, as described by Hancock, is anathema to competitive, profit-motivated capitalist production. As noted in Tesh (1990), there are implicit political assumptions in the *status quo* (individualism, *laissez-faire* government, control by technocrats rather than lay people) and in challenges to the *status quo*. None of these issues or considerations of the impact and potential resolution of the political conflict suggested by this concept of environmental sustainability, are made explicit in Hancock's (1993) description of his model of health and the community ecosystem. Thus, while Hancock's model is an innovative and attractive attempt to link macro factors such as economic growth, environment and community conviviality to health, its silence on the public-policy implications of adopting such a model, may restrict its utility as a tool for change.

A similar but less pronounced de-politicising of the equity concept occurs in Hancock's (1993) description of his model. Thus while there is mention made of the need to distribute wealth more fairly, the political implications of this statement are not made explicit and neither are the appropriate policy items that would follow from such an understanding. While to some extent these implications may be self-evident, they become a question of interpretation rather than intent, as each user applies their own political understanding and agenda in deciding what appropriate programmes or policy would look like. Again, by not making explicit a political ideology for the model to be interpreted within, Hancock essentially locates his model within the *status quo* and falls short of making the political connections between a society organised on an understanding of the determinants of health as he has shown them and the one we currently inhabit.

This is not to say that Hancock does not possess that understanding, merely that he has not made it explicit. Indeed his models represent an excellent attempt to introduce the concept of sustainability of economic and environmental practices to the health debate. Yet they fall short of their potential as a result of Hancock's failure to 'root' them in an explicit political ideology or explanatory account for why we do not have a 'healthy' society. As a result of this, it is not clear if structural socio-economic change is even on Hancock's agenda, or whether his models are calling for a conceptual re-ordering rather than a political re-structuring. This leaves their interpretation to the undeclared biases of the user . . .

It is from the context of the analysis of [this] established model of health (and others not described in this paper) that an alternative approach to conceptualising health has been developed.

An alternative way to conceptualise health

A model within a model

This model of health is composed of two 'levels' of activity at which health interventions could occur: the individual and the community (see Figure 6.2). This division was created primarily with the intention of 'forcing' model users to be aware of both the target and type of health determinants on which they are focusing their intervention *and* the other determinants (and level) that they are not addressing. i.e. to make explicit the limitations of their chosen intervention. This structure is intended to discourage programme developers from focusing on the least contested

INDIVIDUAL MODEL

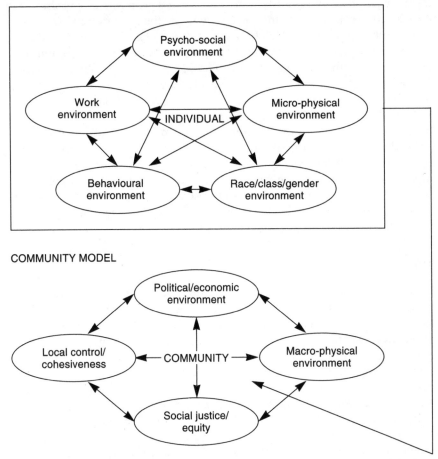

COMMUNITY MODEL

Figure 6.2   *A nested model of health (note that the individual is located within the Community model)*

determinants of health (e.g. social support) to the exclusion of other less tractable but equally important areas (e.g. political and economic factors related to equity).

The intent of the 'model within a model' construction shown in Figure 6.2 is, then, to ensure that users are *explicitly* aware of the focus of their programme and the political implications of what that focus both includes and excludes. This is in direct contrast to the established models of health discussed above, which allow the user to focus on any determinant of heath and which do not address the individual–community interaction. Conceptually, the 'individual' portion of the model is located *within* the 'community' at the centre of the community model. The 'model within a model' concept asserts the importance of the structural factors such as the economic and political environment without suggesting a deterministic hierarchical structure. In addition, this 'nested' concept emphasises the effects of social justice and equity within the community on both community and individual health. A consideration of the individual determinants of health is expected to lead to an evaluation of the community determinants of health and then a re-consideration of the individual level. [O]ne level of the model cannot be considered without also contemplating the other, for they are logically linked and inter-dependent.

The model's nested format also addresses the issue of reconciling a 'personal' model of health with a political model of health. The 'individual' part of the model relates well to the lived experiences of test cases used in model development, while the 'community' part of the model provides an avenue by which the over-riding macro or societal determinants of health can be emphasised. The intent of the model's construction is, therefore, to make it both personally and politically relevant, without being internally contradictory.

What is community?

In using the category 'community', however, one must be careful to be explicit as to its meaning. In the model described above, community is simply used to represent an aggregation of individuals with some shared experience. Therefore it could refer to a geographic community (towns, neighbourhoods), cultural community (ethnic groups, women's groups) or societal community (for example, Canadians). This concept has been deliberately left broad in order to encompass all levels of group behaviour and thus to make the model's application as wide as possible.

It is also noted that the nested construction is culturally specific to Western 'developed' societies, in that it accentuates a division between the individual and the community. In other societies less suffused with individualism, this division, would probably not be appropriate. This approach to conceptualising health arises from the context of an industrialised, advanced economy country and may not be appropriate for application in a developing country setting.

Model components

Individual model

The individual model is comprised of five broad categories or 'environments' of health determinants. These include the psycho-social environment (e.g. social support), the micro-physical environment (e.g. quality of indoor air, individual housing, etc.), the race/class/gender environment (e.g. the social construction of an individual's race, class or gender, education level, socio-economic level, effect of culture, etc.), behavioural environment (e.g. alcohol use, smoking behaviour, fitness, sexual practices, etc.) and the work environment (including workplace physical and chemical hazards, level of control over work scheduling and workplace demands). Each of these environments is thought to have influence on each other and also to both influence and be influenced by the individual in question. The health of the individual located at the centre of the model, will, then, be affected by some combination of these factors plus that person's biological makeup.

Thus, fitness behaviour is known to be affected by the class (Calnan and Williams, 1991) and gender (Saltonstall, 1993) environment as well as the safety of one's location (micro-physical environment). The micro-physical environment is, in turn, expected to be affected by one's socio-economic status (class environment), both of which have an effect on one's psychosocial environment. The simple schematic representation in Figure 6.2 can be seen, therefore, to mask a complex and changing set of interactions between factors. It is further expected that the 'environments' will differ in importance for different individuals and for the same individual over time. Therefore the model is expected to be temporally dynamic and to be able to accommodate the experience of a wide variety of people.

Community model

The individual model is then 'nested' within the community at the centre of the community determinants of health model. This community model consists of four broad categories of influential factors. These include the political and economic climate within which the 'community' is located (e.g. this may be as broad as global political trends and as specific as local by-laws, local unemployment levels or power-sharing within a support group), the macro-physical environment (e.g. outdoor air quality, transportation options, availability of good quality subsidised housing, global climate change, contamination of food sources, sustainable local environment, etc.), the degree to which there is a social justice and equity in the community (e.g. fair income distribution, a robust social security net, publicly insured health care, etc.) and the extent of community control and cohesiveness (e.g. the existence of vibrant community groups addressing community-identified needs, community involvement in local planning, an ethic of mutual-aid rather than competition).

Again, the linkages between each of these key categories of social determinants of health are designed to suggest the inter-relatedness of the categories. It is further conceptualised that there will be reciprocal interactions between the determinants of a healthy community and the community at the centre of the model. In addition, the determinants of a healthy community are expected to have an impact on the determinants of individual health and, thus, indirectly on individuals themselves. Again, this is perceived as a reciprocal relationship, with individual change leading to community change as well. Hence the model has been designed to allow a role for human agency (Arnoux and Grace, 1991; City of Toronto, 1991) while still maintaining an explicit political stance regarding macro-economic, political and equity issues. Again, the established model of health reviewed earlier does not provide a way to conceptualise this interaction between 'levels' of health.

A discussion of the implications of the model for both health promotion practice and policy development is provided here, but first it is necessary to locate the model in a theoretical context. This essentially outlines the model developer's 'agenda', an issue not always made explicit in published models.

Brief theoretical underpinnings

Using Caplan's (1993) framework of health education as a guide (see Chapter 5 in this volume), the overall model can be located towards the radical change end of the spectrum. What is important about this theoretical location is its recognition of the surfacing of the political, both in the model's inclusion of the political/economic climate as a determinant of community health and, hence, individual health, and also in the model structure which makes explicit to the user the areas both selected and avoided in designing health-promotion programmes or public policy, thus reducing the user's ability to omit a consideration of the political and economic determinants of health.

This inclusion of political/economic factors provides a direct link between the dominant political ideology and community and individual health. This is strengthened by the inclusion of the social justice/equity compartment, which is designed to encourage the user to consider the mitigative effects of the welfare state and social democracy on health in capitalist societies (Navarro, 1992). The inclusion of the community control/cohesiveness compartment is also designed to focus attention on issues of local rather than corporate control. Together, it is hoped that these elements will orient the user to challenge the political and economic *status quo*.

Implications for health promotion practice

From the perspective of health-promotion practice, the model has a number of implications, some of which follow directly from its theoretical base discussed above. Thus health-promotion programmes challenging the political and economic *status quo* at either level of the model would be expected to be developed by model users. For example, planned socio-political change as described in McKinlay (1993), programmes designed to increase equity in the society by providing economic activity for marginalised groups usually excluded from mainstream employment, and environmental health-promotion projects advocating for changes to environmental legislation or company operating procedures, would all constitute appropriate health-promotion programmes based on this model.

It is hoped that programme developers with a strict behaviour focus (e.g. smoking cessation) would be prompted by the model structure to consider other aspects of the issue. For example, a programme developer might consider the psycho-social (class-specific) benefits of smoking as well as the political and economic aspects of tobacco production and cigarette advertising and thereby propose a multi-faceted approach to the issue rather than the more common focus on individual behaviour. As with the other models reviewed, however, the focus of any programming developed with the aid of the model remains at the discretion of the user.

Implications for healthy public policy

The four influential categories of health determinants at the community level (political/economic, macro-physical environment, social justice/equity, local control/cohesiveness) are expected to provide the main focus for policy makers using the 'model within a model' concept. Thus like Hancock's (1993) model of health and the community ecosystem, equity, adequate economic prosperity and environmental sustainability might be key policy goals. Local control that truly involved power-sharing and local skills development would also be an appropriate policy development using the model.

In keeping with the political orientation of the model, it is intended that state regulation would be given precedence over free-market policies although this would likely occur within the constraints of balancing the contradictory roles of the state (Fitzpatrick, 1987). Healthy public policy developed using the 'model within a model' concept is expected to extend to market regulation, environmental protection and equity measures.

Use of models: problems or panacea?

. . . The strength of the 'model within a model' conceptualisation of health arises not from its components, which can be found in many ecological health models of health, but in the way these determinants of health are organised into interactive, nested 'levels' of activity. The nested model attempts to provide a fluid representation of both individually and societally relevant determinants of health and tries to keep the user aware of the multiple 'levels' of health determinants and their implications for health-promotion practice and policy development.

It is worthwhile, however, to consider the more general utility of attempting to develop models of health. Indeed, models are, by their nature, reductionist generalisations that obscure detail and invite interpretation. They can be viewed as a product of positivist thinking that seeks a single or defined 'truth' to the problem' of the determinants of health. They provide a simple representation of a situation that is both temporally and spatially varying (i.e. from person to person and with time).

Further, since health and its determinants are vexedly complex issues, in the face of increasing (or increasingly touted) financial insecurity of the state and rising health costs, a 'simple' understanding of health that allows resources to be moved from the expensive medical care system to other model-validated (and presumably less expensive, although undoubtedly less tried) determinants, is by its nature attractive. All models including the 'model within a model', can be seen in this broader political and economic context of the crisis of the welfare state and they need to be interpreted with care as a result of this context . . . How better to justify change than by using theory as exemplified by a satisfyingly simple model? Models of health therefore have the potential to become dangerous political tools.

This analysis notwithstanding, models have many uses, some of them relatively benign. These include education, planning and concep-tualisation of health. Beyond these formalised uses, unarticulated 'models of health' underpin our understanding of health as health workers, policy makers and health-care receivers, and inform our approach to health-related matters in an unconscious but powerful manner. Indeed, one can attempt to develop, safeguard and use models in a manner that remains true to their developers' intent, and explicitly surfaces the ideology intrinsic to every model.

Recommendations

A number of possible approaches to 'safeguarding' models of health have been provided below. These are intended as a starting point for 'critical' health-model building and include:

- The need to make explicit both the political underpinnings and the policy or health-promotion practice implications of the model;
- The need for accompanying text detailing the theoretical basis of the model, its anticipated use, and contraindicated uses;
- A consideration of the potential for models to be applied in such a manner as to emphasise some determinants of health over others;
- The provision of examples of the contrary or ambiguous application of the model with respect to its goals. For example, does a model with an emphasis on community-based care provide some consideration of both the positive aspects of this approach (humanised health care, pre-servation of client's independence, etc.) and the potential negative consequences (potential for privatisation and 'feminisation' of care leading to an unhealthy burden on women as caregivers)?;

- A clear representation of the goals (beyond mere representation of the determinants of health) of the model;
- And, in the absence of such a clear representation on the part of the model developers, a critical analysis by the model user of the policy implications suggested by the model structure.

It is not enough, therefore, to merely provide a schematic representation of one's current understanding of the social determinants of health without qualifiers about what informs those beliefs and a clear indication of the agenda the model intends to advance.

References

Arnoux, L. and Grace, V. (1991). From physical to critical epidemiology. New Zealand Public Health Association presentation, mimeo.

Calnan, M. and Williams, S. (1991). Style of life and the salience of health: an exploratory study of health related practices in households from differing socio-economic circumstances. *Sociology of Health and Illness, 13*, 506-529.

Caplan, R. (1993). The importance of social theory for health promotion: from description to reflexivity,*Health Promotion International, 8*, 147-157.

City of Toronto (1991). *Advocacy for Basic Health Prerequisites*. Toronto: Department of Public Health.

Fitzpatrick, R. (1987). Political science and health policy. In Scambler, G. (ed.), *Sociological Theory and Medical Sociology*. New York: Methuen.

Hancock, T. (1993) Health, human development and the community ecosystem: three ecological models, *Health Promotion International, 8*, 41-47.

McKinlay, J. P. (1993). The promotion of health through planned sociopolitical change, *Social Science and Medicine, 36*, 109-117.

Mustard, J. F. and Frank, J. (1991). *The Determinants of Health*, CIAR Publication, 5. Toronto: Canadian Institute of Advanced Research.

Navarro, V. (1992). Has socialism failed? An analysis of health indicators under socialism. *International Journal of Health, 2*, 583-601. Premier's Council on Health Strategy (1991). *Nurturing Health: A framework on the determinants of Health*. Toronto: The Ontario Premier's Council.

Saltonstall, R. (1993). Healthy bodies, social bodies: men's and women's concepts and practices of health in everyday life, *Social Science and Medicine, 36*, 7-14.

Tesh, S. (1990). *Hidden Arguments*. New Brunswick, N.J.: Rutgers University Press, 154-177.

7 Practice nursing and health promotion: a case study*

Martin Bradford and Sandra Winn

Introduction

The volume of work undertaken in general practice has increased considerably as a result of the 1990 GP contract (Fry, 1991; Hannay *et al.*, 1992) . . . Much of this health promotion work is carried out by practice staff other than GPs, in particular practice nurses (Fry, 1991; Stilwell, 1991).

The way in which health promotion activities are delivered in general practice is likely to be affected by the attitudes and values of the providers, of whom practice nurses are a key group. The attitudes and values of health promotion providers will in turn be influenced by a multitude of factors including peer groups, psychological and sociological theories encountered during professional training, as well as personal and political philosophies (Muntz, 1988). Thus the attitudes and values of practice nurses, who have a central role in the provision of health promotion, may affect the nature of the health promotion in general practice.

Health promotion strategies employed by health professionals differ according to varying definitions of health (Bechoffer, 1989). Ewles and Simnet (1988) have outlined five models on which health can be promoted ranging from a conservative medical approach to social change, a more radical method. Other models include: the client directed approach, in which action is centred on the clients' stated needs; the behaviour change model which encourages a healthy individual lifestyle; and the educational model which aims to increase the understanding of health issues. Although these models are not separate entities and it is recognised that overlap occurs, they provide a useful tool with which to investigate the preferences of health professionals in the way that they promote health.

Our research examines the nature of the work carried out by practice nurses in one health district and, using the models outlined above, investigated practice nurses' views about health promotion.

* From J. Wilson-Barnett and J. Macleod Clark (eds) (1994) *Research in Health Promotion and Nursing*, Chapter 14, pp. 119–131. London: Macmillan.

Research methods

A questionnaire was sent to all practice nurses in the Brighton Health District asking for three types of information. First, basic data about the characteristics of practice nurses was elicited (age, sex, qualifications, training, number of years in practice nursing). Second, the nature of the health promotion work undertaken by practice nurses was investigated. Following on from this, practice nurses' views about health promotion were explored by asking respondents to rank in order of personal preference five models of promoting health (medical, client-directed, educational, behaviour change and social change), and to select the model which best described their working practice. Respondents were then given four short statements about the nature of health promotion with which they were asked to agree or disagree using Likert response scales . . .

Results

Sample characteristics

The response rate was 63 per cent (65 responses from a population of 103). A total of 80 per cent of practices which employ a practice nurse was represented in the sample.

The characteristics of the Brighton sample are broadly similar to those of the practice nurses in a 1987 survey undertaken by Greenfield *et al.* in the West Midlands. However, a much larger proportion of the present sample was aged under 30 (16 per cent, compared with 7 per cent in the 1987 survey), and a larger proportion in the present survey had a health visiting qualification (14 per cent, compared with 3 per cent in the 1987 survey). The balance between RGN (92 per cent) and SEN (10 per cent) qualified practice nurses is similar to those recorded in other surveys (Selby, 1992).

The majority of respondents had entered practice nursing relatively recently. This is in accordance with national data trends (DHS, 1990; Stilwell, 1991) and corresponds with the increased GP workload ensuing from the 1990 contract. Practice nursing in this district is a predominantly part-time profession with 67 per cent of respondents indicating that they were employed on this basis. Eighty-nine per cent of respondents worked in a group practice and of those practices with five or more GPs, 75 per cent employed three or more practice nurses.

Current responsibilities of practice nurses

High levels of activity were reported for clinical tasks such as collecting samples, suture removal and immunisations (Table 7.1). Although the

Table 7.1   *Current responsibilities of respondents*

	Percentage of respondents (n = 65)
Immunisations	91
Health promotion clinincs	88
Sutures	85
Collecting samples	83
Cervical cytology screening	77
Administration	74
Health checks on elderly people	71
New registration checks	69
Counselling/advice	51
Minor surgery	51
Family planning	39
Health checks on non-attenders	32
Ante-natal clinics	20
Health checks on children	14

new contract lays great emphasis on the performance of health promotion duties, the results show that much of the practice nurses' time is devoted to treatment-oriented services . . . A slightly slower proportion of practice nurses in the present sample than in Greenfield *Et al.*'s 1987 survey reported undertaking specific clinical duties. For example, suture removal was performed by 85 per cent of the present sample compared with 95 per cent of the 1987 sample . . .

Respondents were asked whether they contributed to practice meetings, and 70 per cent reported that they did so. The number of years that practice nurses had spent in the professions was proportionally linked to contributing at practice meetings, with 75 per cent of those who had spent more than ten years in the profession contributing at practice meetings, compared with 62 per cent of those who had been in practice nursing for less than a year.

Seventy-five per cent of practice nurses said they would like more health promotion or clinical training. There were no statistically significant differences between age groups or between practice nurses with different professional qualifications in terms of the proportion of respondents who said they would like further training . . . The training needs of respondents are predominantly in areas of health promotion rather than clinical.

Views about health promotion

Respondents were asked to rank five models of promoting health and to indicate which one they used in practice (Table 7.2). Two of the more

Table 7.2   *Rankings of models of promoting health*

	Percentage of respondents ranking model highest	*Percentage of respondents ranking model lowest*	
Educational[1]	36	8	(n = 50)
Social change[2]	22	64	(n = 50)
Behaviour change[3]	22	2	(n = 46)
Client directed[4]	13	17	(n = 47)
Medical[5]	9	20	(n = 46)

1 'Promoting an understanding of health issues enabling patients to make an informed choice.'
2 'Working to change political and social environments to make healthier choices easier choices.'
3 'Encouraging people to change to healthier lifestyles.'
4 'Working on health issues identified by the client.'
5 'Promoting medical intervention through persuasive methods, screening, vaccination etc.'

radical health promoting models, the social change and educational models, together were ranked highest by 58 per cent of respondents. However, the pattern of support for these models is complex (Table 7.2). For the social change model of promoting health respondents' views were polarised. Although 22 per cent of respondents rated the social change model highest, it was also ranked lowest by 64 per cent. One factor contributing to this polarised response may be respondents' use of the social change model in practice, because only one respondent indicated that she did so. Conversely, the medical model was ranked highest by only 9 per cent of respondents, but was reported to be the model used in practice by 37 per cent of respondents (Figure 7.1). The behaviour change model, which reflects a prescriptive approach to promoting health, was ranked highest or second highest by 50 per cent of respondents, while the client-directed model was only ranked highest by 13 per cent of respondents.

Younger practice nurses were more likely to support the radical models of promoting health. Twenty-nine per cent of the under 40 age group and 15 per cent of the over 40 group ranked the social change model of promoting health highest. The under 30 age group compared with all other age groups provided a starker differential with 43 per cent of the under 30 group and 17 per cent of the over 30 group ranking the social change model highest, although the difference is not statistically significant (Fisher's exact test, $p > 0.05$). The support of younger age groups for more radical models is underlined by the resistance of these groups to the most conservative model, the medical model. A total of 25 per cent of respondents aged under 40 rated the medical model lowest, compared with only 17 per cent of respondents aged over 40.

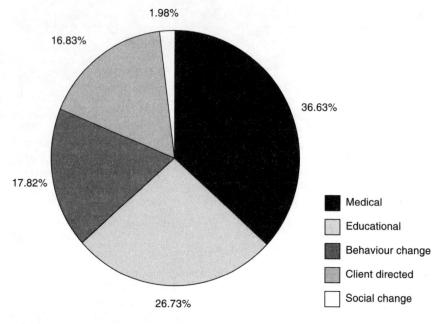

Figure 7.1   *Models used in practice*

Those respondents who ranked the social change or client-directed models highest were most likely to contribute at practice meetings, while those who ranked the medical model highest were least likely to contribute Table 7.3). Comparing respondents who rated the medical or behaviour change models highest with those who did not, the difference in participation at practice meetings is not statistically significant at the 0.05 level ($\chi^2 = 3.468$ with 1 d.f., $p < 0.10$).

There was little relationship between the number of years that respondents had spent in practice nursing and the rankings of the models

Table 7.3   *Association between rankings of models and contribution to practice meetings*

Model ranked highest	Percentage of respondents contributing at practice meetings (n = 49)
Social change	91
Educational model	61
Client directed	100
Behaviour change	60
Medical	25

of health promotion. Twenty-one per cent of respondents who had been in the profession for less than five years ranked the social change model highest, compared with 20 per cent of those who had more than five years practice nursing experience. Similar results were obtained for the other models, and these findings were replicated when the number of years in present post was analysed by rankings of models. Respondents also gave similar rankings of models regardless of professional qualification, and the model used in practice did not differ between qualification groups.

Using Likert response scales, respondents were asked to indicate the extent to which they agreed or disagreed with statements about the nature of health promotion (Table 7.4). Statements (b), (c) and (d) in Table 7.4 are linked to the most radical model of promoting health, the social change model, while statement (a) reflects the most conservative models, the medical and behaviour change models. Overall, respondents were more in agreement with the radical statements of health promotion and more than half of the respondents disagreed with the most conservative statement. The statement with which the largest proportion of respondents were in agreement (88 per cent) is, 'If I spend time educating people about their health they in turn will educate others'. Statement (c),

Table 7.4   *Views about health promotion statements (percentages)*

	Agree or strongly agree	Neutral	Disagree or strongly disagree	
(a) Patients are not concerned with issues beyond their own health status	23	23	54	(*n* = 65)
(b) If I spend time educating people about their health they in turn will educate others	88	6	6	(*n* = 65)
(c) Health promotion should enable individuals, families and communities to reach their own decisions about health issues	80	13	8	(*n* = 64)
(d) Health promotion should include meeting people to work together to change health policy	55	42	3	(*n* = 65)

which extends the concept of enablement beyond the individual, produced a slightly lower level of agreement (80 per cent), while there was a considerably lower level of agreement (55 per cent) with statement (d), 'Health promotion should include meeting people to work together to change health policy', and a large proportion of respondents (42 per cent) remained neutral to this statement.

A breakdown of responses by age shows some relationship between age and agreement with the more radical statements. Thus, for example, while 93 per cent of respondents aged under 40 agreed that the health information that they give will be passed on, only 81 per cent of respondents aged over 40 agreed with this. The differential is increased when the responses of the under 30 age group are compared with those of the over 50 group, where 100 per cent and 71 per cent respectively agreed that their patients would pass on health information. Similarly, whilst 80 per cent of the under 30 age group disagreed with statement (a), 'Patients are not concerned with issues beyond their own health status', only 35 per cent of the 50–9 age group disagreed. This result is statistically significant (Fisher's Exact Test, $p = 0.009$). Conversely, although almost one half of respondents in the over 50 age group were in agreement with this statement not one respondent in the under 30 group was in agreement. However, the relationship between age and views about health promotion is not a simple one. Eighty-seven per cent of respondents aged over 40 compared with only 70 per cent of respondents aged under 40, agreed with the statement, 'Health promotion should enable individuals, families and communities to reach their own decisions about health issues'. Furthermore, in response to the most radical statement, 'Health promotion should include meeting people to work together to change health policy', the over 40 and under 40 age groups produced similar results, with 53 per cent and 57 per cent in agreement respectively.

The number of years that respondents had spent in practice nursing had little association with their responses to the health promotion statements. Almost identical responses were recorded for all statements from those who had been in the profession for less than five years and those who had more than five years' experience.

Respondents who were in agreement with the more radical statements were found to be those who also ranked the more radical models of promoting health the highest. This demonstrates the consistency and value of these models as an investigative theory for health promotion.

Discussion

Practice nurses undertake a wide range of tasks, and most carry out both treatment-oriented and health promoting work. Thus, most practice nurses in this district are not employed solely to undertake the preventive work set out in the new contract. The high levels of activity reported for clinical tasks are to be expected, since these were well established duties of the practice nurse before the new contract. In terms of the health promotion workload resulting directly from the 1990 contract, the activity which the largest numbers of practice nurses undertake is health promotion clinics. Of these, diabetes and asthma are the two clinics most frequently undertaken by practice nurses. These could be seen as disease management rather than strictly primary health promotion, and despite the existence of FHSA protocols for these clinics their position as primary health promotion clinics is debatable.

Comparison of the results with those of Greenfield *et al.* (1987) provide some evidence that in addition to the new health promotion responsibilities assumed by practice nurses since 1990, there has been a slight shift in the other tasks undertaken, with more emphasis now on health promotion activities rather than treatment-oriented work. Some practice nurses do not have contracts, job descriptions or protocols (Stilwell, 1991), in which case the new emphasis on health promotion work could prove to be important in establishing a stronger role definition for the profession. Indeed, it may be that health promotion will provide an appropriate avenue for an extended role for the practice nurses since there is evidence that the scope for extension into medical areas is less certain (Greenfield *et al.*, 1987).

Given the developing nature of the role and professionalisation of the practice nurse it would seem important for practice nurses to be aware of current developments in their field and to incorporate these into their work. The importance of health promotion training is underlined in this investigation where training needs identified by practice nurses were centred around health promotion issues.

The pattern of views about health promotion among practice nurses is complex. While a majority of practice nurses expressed support for either the social change or the educational model of promoting health, almost two-thirds of respondents ranked the social change model lowest, suggesting a diversity of views within the profession about appropriate health promotion strategies. The high level of support for the educational model is reflected in the extent of agreement with the statement, 'If I spend time educating people about their health they in turn will educate others'. These results suggest that respondents believe that their patients will convey health messages which they themselves have imparted and recognise that the influence of the practice nurse extends beyond the individual. The level of agreement with this statement also suggests that practice nurses perceive themselves as having an educational role and are willing to spend time providing people with health information. The lower level of agreement with the statement 'Health promotion should enable individuals, families and communities to reach their own decisions about health issues' suggests that while educating the individual is widely accepted by practice nurses as a feature of health promotion, the concept of empowering groups is less so. Considerably fewer practice nurses agreed with the statement 'Health promotion should include meeting people to work together to change health policy', and a large proportion expressed a neutral position. The implication of this may be that while many practice nurses recognise that health promotion has socio-political implications, the concept appears to be far removed from their working practice. This relates to the finding that although 22 per cent ranked the social change model highest, only 2 per cent said that it was the model that they used in practice. Thus it seems that there is some agreement in principle with more radical approaches to health promotion, but their application in practice nursing is at present limited.

Further evidence of the interaction between working practice and views about health promotion is provided by the association between contributing to practice meetings and support for the more radical models of promoting health. Those who favour more radical models of promoting health are more likely to view health as the product of a wide range of physical, social, economic and political influences (Ewles *et al.*, 1988). Thus, it may be that those respondents who rank the more radical models highest believe that their participation in these forums can affect health care provision and policy. Conversely, those favouring the more individualistic medical or behaviour change models may be less likely to believe that health can be promoted in these ways, and therefore participate less.

The way in which practice nurses perform health promotion services, that is, the content and structure and context of health promotion clinics and health checks, will strongly influence the nature of health promotion in general practice. The prominence of the use of the medical model of promoting health amongst practice nurses and the types of health promotion clinics undertaken by respondents suggests that health promotion services are at present largely prescriptive and centred upon the individual, rather than providing a wider and social emphasis. Clearly, the attitudes of practice nurses towards health promotion and the factors which may influence these attitudes are key determinants of the way in which health promotion services are provided in general practice. The general empathy of the younger respondents with more radical models and statements of health promotion may be one factor which in the longer term will bring about changes in the nature of health promotion in general practice.

Conclusion

Provision of health promotion services is central to the role of the practice nurse in this district, but practice nurses are also responsible for a wide range of treatment-related duties. It could be that the diversity of the workload of practice nurses produces a degree of role conflict for them. Views about health promotion amongst practice nurses are diverse, but it is clear that for many there is a discrepancy between their views about health promotion and their working practice. However, there is also evidence that views about health promotion interact with working practice. Given that younger members of the profession are the most supportive of a radical approach to health promotion, it may be that over the next few years there will be a gradual change in the way in which health promotion services are provided.

References

Bechoffer, F. (1989). Individuals politics and society. In Martin, C. and McQueen, D. (eds), *Readings for a New Public Health*. Edinburgh: Edinburgh University

Department of Health (DHS) (1990). Department of Health statistics for general medical practitioners in England and Wales 1978–1988, *Statistical Bulletin*, *4* (6), 9.

Ewles, L. and Simnett, I. (1988). *Promoting Health: A practical guide to Health Education*. Chichester: Wiley.

Fry, J. (1991). The contract: is it working? *Update* (15 July), 71–72.

Greenfield, S., Stilwell, B. and Drury, M. (1987). Practice nurses: social and occupational characteristics, *Journal of the Royal College of General Practitioners*, *37*, 341–345.

Hannay, D., Usherwood, T. and Platts, M. (1992). Workload of general practitioners before and after the new contract, *British Medical Journal*, *304*, 615–618.

Muntz, A. (1988). Value judgements in health visiting, *Health Visitor*, *61*, 145–146.

Selby, A. (1992). More practice, *Health Service Journal* (19 March), 31.

Stilwell, B. (1991). The rise of practice nurse, *Nursing Times*, *87*, 26–28.

8 Innovation diffusion and health education in schools*

Gordon Macdonald

Introduction

The adoption and take up of new ideas and curricula in schools has been the subject of much research here in the United Kingdom, the United States and Canada (Bollam, 1982; Schools Council, 1980; Fullan and Pomfret, 1977; Parcel *et al.*, 1988; Counsins and Leithwood, 1993). This research has been primarily concerned with determining the extent and the reach of dissemination of new curricula materials and not with the application or testing of innovation diffusion theory.

The communication of innovations or innovation diffusion theory has been developed to help us understand the factors that affect the dissemination of new ideas, practices and products within a community over a period of time. Not many diffusion studies, at least until recently, have concentrated on schools as adaptors. They have tended to focus more on agricultural and health innovations in developing countries (Rogers, 1983).

However, with the emergence of health promotion as a discipline (Macdonald 1991; Bunton and Macdonald, 1992) the interest in health education developments in schools has waxed and studies in the take up of new health education curriculum materials and the application of innovation diffusion theory have mushroomed, (Leithwood, 1991; Orlandi *et al.*, 1990; Parcel *et al.*, 1990; Hansen, 1992). This interest in school curriculum development and adoption has not be confined to products but has also included ideas. The development and adoption of the idea of the 'health promoting school' for example, has received some attention on both sides of the Atlantic in the last decade (Stevens and Davis, 1988; Nutbeam *et al.*, 1990) and has become the subject of interest in innovation diffusion theory (Parcel *et al.*, 1990).

The theory of innovation diffusion

Innovation diffusion theory has four essential elements: the innovation

---

* Commissioned for this volume.

(invention) itself; the communication channel; the time lapse (from invention to adoption) and the community or social system identified as receiver of the innovation and often called the 'unit of adoption'.

The innovation can be an idea, practice or product that is perceived as new by the unit of adoption but may not actually be 'new'. The communication channel can be face to face dissemination, or local, national and international media (or indeed a combination of all four). The rate of diffusion is obviously affected by the nature of the communication channel. Mass media channels (radio, television and newspapers) are faster diffusion channels but appear limited to raising awareness of the innovation. Interpersonal channels appear more important to early adopters and to have more affect on adoption decision (Rogers, 1983).

Rogers and Shoemaker (1971) and Rogers (1983) have derived a set of 103 generalisations from analyses of hundreds of research programmes on innovation adoption and produced an adoption model based on four functional stages:

Stage One: Knowledge (of the innovation);
Stage Two: Persuasion (attitude towards innovation);
Stage Three: Decision (testing the acceptability of innovation);
Stage Four: Adoption (taking up new idea or practice).

The model relies heavily on the rational conceptualisation of decision making. That is that units of adoption (individuals, communities or organisations) are perceived as rational actors preoccupied with weighing up the consequences of certain courses of action relative to the goals they want to maximise (Rich, 1991). It is generally assumed that following the initial development of the innovation, adoption will automatically follow, and follow sequentially through the stages. Of course in reality an individual unit of adoption may act emotionally rather than rationally and lose interest at any stage and reject the innovation. The adoption or rejection of the innovation depends on two key attribution issues, each of which can be sub-divided.

The first key issue concerns the attributes of the innovation itself and may loosely be called the input side of innovation diffusion theory. Researchers in this area argue that the attributes of the innovation will affect the adoption, or adoption rate. Rogers (1983) summarises them as being:

- Relative advantage: of innovation over other ideas, practices or products;
- Compatibility: between the innovation and value system of adopter;
- Complexity: or difficulty in understanding or using the innovation;
- Trailability: or the ability to test the idea or material before adoption;
- Observability: or the visibility of the results of the innovation;

Others, such as Zaltman and Duncan (1977), have added other attributes of the innovation such as reversibility (can the potential adopter revert back to old ways?), communicability (is it easily passed on to others?) and uncertainty (how does the adopter know it is better?) to make the model more complete.

The second key issue, which may be identified as the output side of innovation diffusion theory, relates to the characteristics of the units of adoption. Researchers have identified patterns of adoption by different segments of the target population over time, which have been interpreted by Rogers (1983) as adopter categories. These are: innovators, early adopters, early majority, late majority and laggards. Innovators are thought of as being eager to try new ideas and to take risks. Early adopters may be prepared to take risks as well but are more respected and connected to their community. They are often perceived as making careful and wise decisions and therefore act as role models for the early majority. The early majority generally take more time to make decisions but in turn they reach, through personal and social relations, the majority of the community.

The late majority and laggards tend to be less open to new ideas and practices and innovation adoption may be determined by factors other than personal characteristics. However the rate of diffusion of an innovation can also be affected by the role and function (if any) of a change agent.

A change agent can be defined as an individual (or agency) who influences the decision of the recipient of the innovation, the unit of adoption. The influence is almost always in the direction deemed desirable by the innovator. The change agent seeks to promote the adoption of the ideas policies or practices perceived as innovatory on behalf of the innovation agency. The change agent may act as a link between the agency which developed the innovation and the recipient of the new idea or product.

Health education in schools

The 1960s witnessed a rapid and radical period of social change and, it has been argued, the dramatic expansion of education provision in the 1950s and early 1960s, precipitated that change (Arnot and Weiner, 1987). Investment in education was based on the premise that education establishments, in particular schools, were the most appropriate vehicle for innovatory thinking and change. Health education, in its more modern form was therefore placed firmly and deliberately within schools (Macdonald, 1992a). The view was that only through the process of curriculum development and innovation, and by employing various teaching methodologies and pupil centre learning could education, concerned with behaviour change, take place.

The role placed on schools to relate education to health behaviour was indicted by Kolbe (1987) who argues that schools can 'provide one of the most universal and efficient means of . . . protecting and improving the health of communities.' Further health education has been seen increasingly within a whole school context and given rise to the idea that the school should develop its role as a health promoting institution (Basch, 1984). In the last ten years or so a number of studies principally in the United States have looked at the ways in which schools have taken up new curriculum materials and ideas and used them within the classroom and the school as a whole (Basch, Eveland and Portnoy, 1986). These studies whilst using innovation diffusion as a theoretical prop, were principally concerned with describing how a particular topic based programme was disseminated to schools and its take up rate (Anderson and Portnoy, 1989; Rohrbach *et al.*, 1993). The studies recognise that good quality programmes are taken up by teachers sometimes despite and not because of structural obstacles. They cite organisation issues, change agents and liaison with outside agencies as key components in any diffusion programme.

However, as Whitehead (1989) has argued, there is a limit to what schools can be expected to achieve and they should not be expected to be more successful than other agents of social change. This is especially true if policies and innovations are concerned solely with classroom developments. However, in tandem with the curriculum changes in the 1980s, a new concept emerged that should have helped schools deal with broader issues associated with health and health education – the health promoting school.

The health promoting school

The concept of the health promoting school grew out of efforts in the early 1980s to build a bridge between health education and what was considered to be the broader umbrella of health promotion. In its earlier version the term was used to integrate, into a framework, the relationship between the health curriculum and the wider school ethos as an attempt to strengthen both (Farley, 1991).

The basis for this perspective rests on the belief that information, knowledge and skills gained within the classroom can be reinforced and supported, or undermined and contradicted by what might happen outside the classroom in the rest of the school. For example, smoking education programmes in school will have far less credibility if teachers are seen or allowed to smoke in school. There is a growing recognition that the health promoting school concept is concerned with all of its members, pupils, teaching and non-teaching staff. In the United States some schools are concentrating on promoting the health of staff before embarking on a health education programme for pupils (Stevens and Davis, 1988). This has been done by encouraging school administrators to make schools healthier places. Examples of the kind of work that was studied by Stevens and Davis included not only staff development but also social and organizational factors, school food and exercise regimes. In addition schools were expected to keep an inventory of the physical condition of the buildings as part of their wider health promoting institution role.

In the United Kingdom the concept of a health promoting school has been extended to include the school's physical environment, the encouragement of health enhancing policies and the involvement of school health staff in integrated health education programmes (Nutbeam *et al.*, 1990). Some local education authorities have co-operated with local authorities on a number of initiatives which have encouraged the growth of the health promoting school concept and which illustrates one of its principles, namely links between schools and the wider community (Lewis, 1993). One report provides a detailed case study on the process involved in setting up a health promoting school which has proved a useful guide to schools implementing the idea. In many local education authorities a ten point criteria health school award has been set up to encourage schools to think beyond the classroom and one LEA has recently directed all its schools to become non-smoking (Joyce and Binstead, 1989).

Some of the teaching packs disseminated over the last ten years or so have involved training activities designed to encourage staff to think about the health promoting features of their schools (SCHEP 13–18, 1981; Healthskills, 1983). In this sense the school has to be thought of in a similar context to any other organisation.

However, much of the research that has been undertaken in the area of innovation diffusion in organisations (principally in the United States) has been ignored in school health education projects in the United Kingdom. Orlandi's (1986) study of worksite health promotion innovations has largely gone unnoticed in UK research, even though he does indicate the need for organisations to assess the feasibility of implementing innovations in relation to organisational structures that don't compare with classical adoption unit characteristics. Other researchers in the United States have advocated refocusing attention away from adoption decisions towards the implementation process (Basch, 1984). This research is of crucial importance to school-based innovation diffusion programmes since an emphasis on the implementation of a programme in the organisation (school) could hinder an understanding of the process.

Within the United Kingdom, however, there is little evidence that schools have considered another aspect of the health promoting school concept, that of health promotion policy development. Whilst there is some evidence that schools may have topic specific policies that relate to smoking, drugs and nutrition very few seem to have adopted general statements or policies that promote the school as an agency for health (Nutbeam *et al.*, 1987).

The critical point of the health promoting school concept is that schools, as agents and organisations concerned with health, should be producing statements or policies that address wider issues relating to health. These should involve the notions of equality and equity and informed decision making. Anderson (1986) makes the point that unless schools actively discuss the ways staff and pupils can be empowered to make informed decisions then the whole idea of a health promoting school is illusory.

Within the whole curriculum some attention must be paid to integrating the health education syllabus with these wider equity issues and particularly within a multi-cultural context. The Schools Council went some way in helping schools develop this aspect of policy by issuing advisory statements and holding seminars throughout the 1970s and 1980s.

The health promoting school concept places emphasis on the curriculum being integrated within the whole school ethos and on strengthening links with parents and the surrounding community. Some of the teaching packs implemented in primary and secondary schools within Britain have addressed this. A dental health education programme (Natural Nashers) designed for integration within the biology syllabus included an element that involved parents, through a homework programme. In an evaluation of the impact it was found that families whose children took part in the programme (n = 35) improved their knowledge (22/35), and changed their behaviour (12/35) (Craft and Croucher, 1979).

In an evaluation of the My Body project (Wilcox *et al.*, 1981) researchers discovered that children took much of their classroom experiences home and discussed them with parents. A second study (Murray *et al.*, 1984) found that more parents of the children following the programme had stopped smoking compared to a control group. Nevertheless it is probably true to say that most health education projects for schools don't include parental and family involvement explicitly and little research has been carried out to find out their impact on family behaviour (Williams, 1986).

Examples of other aspects of involvement by the school in the community are even less although the development of the European Health Promoting School Network should encourage projects in this area (WHO, 1993). Already in Wales there is the kernel of innovatory work particularly in relation to environmental pollution (Curriculum Council for Wales/Health Promotion Wales, 1994). Sample schools have been encouraged to work with environmental health services and community voluntary groups to tackle the problem of local pollution. Schools can and do also get involved in local and national health promoting campaigns such as National No Smoking days but the possibility of many more links is great. In a very limited sense the health promoting school concept provides a more than suitable vehicle for a partnership between the school and health and other agencies in the locality. The promotion of the concept and practice as an innovatory approach to school health is a future challenge.

Diffusion in schools as organizations

Schools are complex organisations with both internal social networks and external liaison functions, and in this sense comply with the structure associated with hospitals also. Consequently the development and implementation of school health education curricula are affected by a multiplicity of factors. These factors include the organisation or setting itself: the users of the innovation, i.e. the teachers (in the main); the change agents, which could be the innovator or at least the individual or agency which brought the new scheme to the school's attention and the innovation itself (the new curriculum or teaching pack) (Green and Kreuter, 1991). Some work has been carried out in both the United Kingdom and the United States on curriculum innovation and its long term impact (Fullan and Pomfret, 1977; Hall and Loucks, 1978; Schools Council, 1980), but little research has concerned itself with an analysis of those factors which inhibit or facilitate curriculum innovation and development.

A school is an organisation and therefore subject to the same kind of parameters as any other institution when it comes to innovation diffusion. That is, the innovativeness of the organisation depends on such factors as the degree of centralisation (the amount of power and control in relatively few hands), complexity (relating to the level of professional expertise within the organisation), formalisation (the amount of rules and regulations), networking (informal staff links within the organisation) and finally organisational slack (relating to the amount of uncommitted resources within an organisation). The problem is that although some of these variables facilitate innovativeness at the initiation stage they handicap it at the implementation stage (Zaltman and Duncan, 1977).

The Rohrbach *et al.* study (1993) on the dissemination of a substance misuse prevention programme argues that even if the decision to adopt a particular package is made at institutional level it cannot guarantee continuance and maintenance with the new materials. The authors state that this will depend on the process within the school and particularly the characteristics of the classroom teacher.

Their research identified recent recruits who had undergone further teacher training. They were prepared to experiment with different teaching methods and were more likely to implement new programmes. The take up of new programmes was further enhanced if the principal or headteacher was instrumental in supporting the introduction of the new materials. However, this research, and many other studies on organisation innovativeness produced inconclusive results. There appears to be little correlation between the variables like centralisation, complexity, and formalisation with diffusion take up rates. Indeed organisations with low centralisation, low formalisation but high complexity seem to facilitate the early stages of innovation but militate against the implementation stage (Orlandi, 1986).

Schools as organisations facilitating change have been the focus of study and research (Schools Council, 1980; Fullan and Pomfret, 1977; Parcel, *et al.*, 1988, 1990; Bollam, 1982). Yet it appears that little is known even now on why some schools adopt new practices and others don't. This is principally because most research concentrates on the outcome, that is the actual use made of new ideas or practices rather than the way decisions were made on whether to adopt or not. Change is then to do with process and process involves time. Time is usually something researchers are short of. This means that process evaluation or action research is often lacking in work associated with innovation take up in schools. Fullan (1985) identifies three main phases of the change process in schools that could aid research. Firstly the initiation phase which includes the mobilisation of staff and resources, adoption of decision making processes, and early development of materials. Secondly, the implementation phase, which involves putting the change into practice. And thirdly the institutionalising phase, which broadly means maintaining the change by building it into the system.

Fullan (1985) points out that based on a number of studies guidelines emerge on the best way to implement change. These can be summarised into three main categories:

1. Good planning by school staff and outside advisers is indispensable as a first step. Mechanisms for testing and getting feedback, and then altering the plan (if necessary) are important, particularly if the school is unused to innovation.
2. Role clarification of staff within schools and outside advisory staff. Teaching staff need to be involved in all three phases (outlined above) if the innovation is to be successfully adopted and institutionalised. This second category should include support in terms of training and resources and critically psychological support for teaching staff expected to carry through the change.
3. Planning for continuation and dissemination. This should involve plans to introduce new staff to the change or innovation: identifying

resources each year for the new 'product'. The change should gradually involve all staff in the school and in time the innovation could be disseminated to other schools in the region. This may need outside help.

Several innovatory programmes in health education and health promotion particularly in the United States have tried to implement these stages and categories to try and overcome traditional problems associated with adoption of new curriculum materials. A school-based tobacco-use prevention programme developed some of Fullan's ideas and built on various smaller scale studies (Parcel *et al.*, 1989). The study identified four phases – Dissemination, Adoption, Implementation and Maintenance – and aimed to involve head teachers and teaching staff in all four phases. The theoretical basis for smoking prevention which included social learning theory, modelling and the health belief model formed part of the teacher training on the innovation. The researchers were also acutely aware that the teachers needed incentives to accept and adopt the intervention. These were offered in the form of a demonstration on how the programme would benefit the users and the professional benefit to teachers in using the material.

The dissemination phases provided school staff with information on the prevalence of tobacco use, but more importantly described the prevention education programme and ways in which to increase motivation of potential users to adopt the programme. These phases involved a great deal of outside agency help including the recruitment of local opinion leaders, network development and the involvement of the local media. These outside agencies involved education advisers and, in US terms, regional health education specialists promoting the innovation.

The adoption phase was characterised by a direct mailing of a newsletter to the target schools with details of how to enrol for the programme and savings to be made for early registration. This charging for curriculum development and advice pre-dated the radical changes now taking place within the school system in England and Wales following the 1988 Education Act.

The implementation phase in the Parcel study in Texas involved testing two methodologies for tobacco-use prevention in schools, a teacher-based workshop and a self-instructional video. Both were subjected to evaluation, the results of which are due to be published soon.

The maintenance phase must be seen as crucial and in the Texas study both the teachers and the students were included. Teachers joined focus groups to help determine maintenance strategies and learning outcomes were monitored.

Parcel concluded that whilst the receptivity of schools to a new tobacco-use prevention programme is high, the actual use of curriculum materials is relatively low. Parcel argues that the challenge is not in the development of educational interventions but in their comprehensive dissemination. The opposite may be the case in the United Kingdom. Schools are perhaps suffering from innovation fatigue although good dissemination of materials and projects usually means use and adoption.

The Parcel study and others (Basch, 1984; Gottleib, *et al.*, 1987) all emphasise the need to win school support for the innovation in the first place. This may increasingly involve incentives to increase recruitment. This is particularly the case in the United Kingdom with what is now commonly referred to as 'innovation overload' amongst teaching staff and within schools generally. Much of the work on curriculum development in the United Kingdom and United States have similar characteristics that tend, at least historically, not to allow for teacher value systems or behavioural traits. The reasons for this are twofold. Most research is funded by national or local governments, or other tax funded agencies, in order to find the most efficient cost-effective way of ensuring the successful dissemination and implementation of their 'products'. The implicit assumption is that all innovations are 'good' and therefore worth adopting and implementing.

Teacher attributes

The perspective adopted in most studies tends to be a top down one and most researchers adopt the so-called 'fidelity approach' (Bollam, 1982) in that they look for implementation that is true to the original innovation. The underlying assumption appears to be that men and women are rational creatures and will respond to rationally presented innovations. Subsequently they will behave rationally and systematically during the adoption, implementation and maintenance phases of the diffusion process. This ignores the increasing evidence (Parcel, *et al.*, 1988; Smith, *et al.*, 1992) that teachers, like many other professionals, tend not to use systematic planning techniques and methods, do not read research reports as a matter of course and tend to behave more intuitively.

There are, of course, signs that this is changing especially in the United Kingdom with the recent overhaul of state education. Nevertheless most research into innovation diffusion in schools assumes that teachers are able to act and respond in a planned and organised way when in fact they are under increasing pressure to take on an ever-increasing workload associated with the national curriculum, key stage assessment and performance indicators.

The standard approach ignores that fact that teachers operate within a complex organisation that allows very little time to plan, organise and reflect and that in many cases the teacher and the school could be dealing with more than one innovation at any one time. Innovation diffusion also has to take cognisance of the ever-changing staffing levels and memberships in schools. In the 1990s staff turnover in many schools has approached 20 per cent. From the dissemination or initiation stage through the adoption, implementation and maintenance stages, the staffing levels and membership in schools could change dramatically. This is bound to have a very important implications for the understanding and usage of the innovation.

A major study undertaken in the United Kingdom in the early 1980s (Schools Council, 1980) highlights a number of issues that constrain the dissemination and impact of an innovation. The study was designed to determine how best to disseminate Schools Council material to effect maximum impact and take up. The Council led the way in the production and dissemination of teacher materials and programmes in the 1970s, but it was concerned that some materials was used more than others and some not at all.

The study found that when teachers were asked what factors hindered the introduction of new ideas, methods or teaching materials in schools, 20 per cent mentioned cost, 18 per cent mentioned time, and 14 per cent identified staff attitudes. Other comments included external examination requirements, school structures and the lack of applicability of the innovation to their particular school. To some extent these findings are replicated in later work carried out in Wales (Smith *et al.*, 1992). Both mirror the concerns I have outlined above that innovation in schools has to acknowledge the organisational structure of the school, the processes that hinder or help adoption, the ability of the teacher to devote time to the programme and, importantly, the psychological map of the teacher. This means paying greater attention to the value system operating within the school and to the teacher's own beliefs, attitudes and behaviour.

Innovators would do well to gain an understanding of the relationship between these three psycho-social attributes, and apply them to teachers. It might be that only then will a real understanding emerge on the best methods for the diffusion of innovations to schools.

References

Anderson, J. (1986). *Health Skills Project training manual.* CCDU, University of Leeds.

Anderson, D. and Portnoy, B. (1989). Diffusion of cancer education into schools, *Journal of School Health*, 59(5).

Arnot, M. and Weiner, G. (1987). *Gender and the Politics of Schooling.* London: The Open University/Unwin Hyman.

Basch, C. (1984). Research on disseminating and implementing health education programmes in schools, *Journal of School Health*, 54.

Basch, C., Eveland, J. and Portnoy, B. (1986). Diffusion systems for education and learning about health, *Family and Community Health* 9(2).

Bollam, R. (1982). Research into dissemination and implementation of educational innovation, paper presented at the National Educational Conference. Bristol.

Bunton, R. and Macdonald, G. (eds) (1992). *Health Promotion: Disciplines and diversity.* London: Routledge.

Counsins, J. and Leithwood, K. (1993). Enhancing knowledge utilization as a strategy for school improvement, *Knowledge: Creation, Diffusion, Utilization, 14.*

Craft, M. and Croucher, R. (1979). Preventive dental health in adolescents: results of a controlled trial, *Royal Society of Health, 99(2).*

Curriculum Council for Wales/Health Promotion Wales (1994). The health promoting school in Wales. Cardiff: CCW.

Farley, P. (1991). From school to community. in Nutbeam, D., Haglund, B., Farley P. and Tillgren, P. (eds), *Youth Health Promotion.* London: Forbes.

Fullan, M. (1985). Change processes and strategies at the local level, *The Elementary School Journal, 85(3).*

Fullan, M. and Pomfret, A. (1977). Research on curriculum and instruction implementation, *Review of Educational Research, 47(2).*

Gottleib, N., Lloyd, L. and Bounds, J. (1987). The adoption of health education by state agencies, *Journal of Public Health Management, 16.*

Green, L. and Kreuter, M. (1991). Enhancing knowledge utilization as a strategy for school improvement, *Knowledge: Creation, Diffusion and Utilization, 14.*

Hall, G. and Loucks, S. (1978). Innovation configurations; analysing the adoption of innovations, Austin: University of Texas, Research and Development Centre.

Hansen, W. (1992). School based substance abuse prevention: a review of the state of the art of the curriculum 1980-1990, *Health Education Research, 7(3).*

Healthskills (1983). London: Health Education Council.

Joyce, R. and Binstead, M. (1989). *The health promoting school: A guide to its introduction.* Cambridge: Cambridgeshire Local Education Authority.

Kolbe, L. (1987). What can we expect from school health education?, *Journal of School Health, 52.*

Leithwood, K. (1991). Curriculum diffusion. in Lewy, A. (ed)., *The International Encyclopaedia of Curriculum.* New York: Macmillan.

Lewis, M. (1993). A review of the development of health education over 50 years, *Health Education Journal, 52(3).*

Macdonald, G. (1991). Has health promotion matured as a discipline?, *Health Promotion International, 6(2).*

Macdonald, G. (1992a). Health promotion and sustainable development, *Health Promotion International, 7(2).*

Macdonald, G. (1992b). Communication theory and health promotion. in Bunton, R. and Macdonald, G. (eds), *Health Promotion: Disciplines and Diversity,* London: Routledge.

Murray, M., Swan, A. and Clarke, G. (1984). Long term effects of school anti-smoking programme, *Journal of Epidemiology and Community Health, 38.*

Nutbeam, D., Farley, P. and Smith, C. (1990). England and Wales: perspectives in school health, *Journal of School Health, 60(7).*

Nutbeam, D., Clarkson, J., Phillips, K., Everett, V., Hill, A. and Catford, J. (1987). The health promoting school, organization and policy development in Welsh secondary schools, *Health Education Journal, 46(3).*

Orlandi, M. (1986). The diffusion and adoption of worksite health promotion innovations: an analysis of barriers, *Preventive Medicine, 15.*

Orlandi, M., Landers, C., Weston, R. and Haley, N. (1990). Diffusion of health promotion innovations. in Glanz, K., Lewis, F. and Rimer, F. (eds), *Health Behaviour and Health Education: Theory, research and practice.* San Francisco: Jossey-Bass.

Parcel, G., Perry, C. and Taylor, W. (1990). Beyond demonstration; diffusion of health promotion innovations. In N. Bracht (ed), *Health Promotion at the Community Level.* Newbury Park: Sage.

Parcel, G., Simons-Morton, G. and Kolbe, L. (1988). Health promotion: integrating organizational change and student learning strategies, *Health Education Quarterly, 15(4).*

Parcel, G., Erikson, M., Lovato, C., Gottleib, N., Brinks, S. and Green, L. (1989). The diffusion of school based tobacco use prevention programmes: project description and baseline data, *Health Education Research, 4(1)*.

Rich, R. (1991). Knowledge creation, diffusion and utilization, *Knowledge: Creation, Diffusion and Utilization, 12*.

Rogers, E. (1983). *Diffusion of Innovations*. New York: Free Press.

Rogers, E. and Shoemaker, F. (1971). *Communication of Innovations: A cross cultural approach*. New York: Free Press.

Rohrbach, A., Graham, J. and Hansen, W. (1993). Diffusion of a substance abuse prevention program. Predictions of program implementation, *Preventive Medicine, 22*.

Schools Council (1980). *Impact and Take Up Project*. London: Schools Council.

Schools Council (1981). *Health Education Project (SCHEP) (13–18)*. London, Forbes.

Smith, C., Nutbeam, D. and Macdonald, G. (1992). The health promoting school: progress and future challenges in Welsh secondary schools, *Health Promotion International, 7(3)*.

Stevens, N. and Davis, L. (1988). Exemplary school health education: a new charge for HOT districts, *Health Education Quarterly, 15*.

Whitehead, M. (1989). Swimming up-stream: trends and prospects in education for health, London: Kings Fund Institute.

World Health Organization (1993). *The European Network of Health Promoting Schools*. Copenhagen: WHO.

Wilcox, B., Gillies, P., Wilcox, J., Reid, D. (1981). Do children influence their parents' smoking?, *Health Education Journal, 40(2)*.

Williams, T. (1986). School health education 15 years on, *Health Education Journal, 45(4)*.

Zaltman, G. and Duncan, R. (1977). *Strategies for planned change*. New York: Wiley.

9 Counselling people affected by HIV and AIDS*

John Sketchley

Introduction

The title of this chapter embraces AIDS patients, the HIV-infected, people near to them, and the worried well, all of whom may become clients of the counsellor. Given the incurability of HIV infection, health education and counselling have assumed an importance hitherto denied them. The Scottish Health Education Group with the British Association for Counselling is in the process of producing a training manual for training counsellors to deal with clients affected by HIV. The House of Commons Select Committee has given a positive endorsement of counselling in this field. and the World Health Organization has appointed an international group of consultants to advise it about counselling people with AIDS and all people affected by HIV.

To understand the following principles and issues, a review of the medical background appears necessary. The human immunodeficiency virus (HIV) is transmitted through blood, semen, and cervical secretions, and from an infected pregnant mother to her unborn child. This means that precautions need to be taken during sexual activity and injections, the main protections being the use of condoms and not sharing needles. Everyday social activities, such as shaking hands, kissing, and using lavatories, do not constitute a risk. The World Health Organization's guidelines on HIV and breast-feeding continue to advocate it as breast milk is not regarded as a high risk.

Once HIV enters a person, a range of possibilities lies ahead. Within 3 months the immune system produces an antibody, which is almost powerless against the virus, but which can be detected by a blood test. It is important to note that a negative result of the antibody test does not mean the person is uninfected, because of the delay between infection and the production of the antibody. The antibody-positive person may remain in that state for years, perhaps without knowing, apparently healthy but able

---

* From Dryden, W., Charles-Edward, C. and Woolfe, R. (1989). *Handbook of Counselling in Britain*, Chapter 22, pp. 347–363. Published in association with the British Association for Counselling. London: Routledge.

to infect others. There is thus a difference between HIV infection and HIV-related diseases.

At any stage, the HIV-infected person may move along the spectrum into manifestations of HIV-related diseases. The first and least serious possibility is generalised lymphadenopathy, when the glands in the neck and armpits are persistently swollen. The second is AIDS-related complex (ARC), a collection of symptoms such as tiredness, constant fevers, loss of weight, diarrhoea, night sweats, and sometimes shingles, herpes, and thrush in the mouth. These are profound changes, and not just an occasional sleepless night or attack of diarrhoea. These two conditions may be episodic, with periods of remission. The third possibility is dementia, similar to that in the elderly, and results from the virus attacking the central nervous system.

Lastly, there is AIDS itself, which can appear at any time after infection by HIV, or after episodes of other manifestations. The HIV virus causes a severe defect in certain cells which are critical in the body's defence system. The virus incapacitates the immune system so drastically that illnesses normally repelled by the body seize their opportunity and take hold. The main ones are Kaposi's sarcoma (a skin cancer) and pneumocystis carinii (a type of pneumonia). Virtually unchecked by the immune system, they can kill, though the patient may be able to lead a reasonably normal life at home for some of the time.

There is no way of telling when a person with HIV will progress to ARC, AIDS, or any other manifestation; but it is thought that in time all HIV-infected people will die of HIV-related diseases. Infection by HIV is for life, and the infected person may unwittingly transmit the virus to others, while appearing to be healthy. HIV and AIDS, furthermore, are no chooser of persons, and can infect men, women, or children who are exposed to them. It is therefore more helpful to think of risk activities rather than risk groups, though numerically homosexual men and drug-addicts have suffered most in Britain.

Principles

Before HIV antibody test

Counsellors and most health professionals in the field agree that all people seeking or advised to be tested for HIV antibodies should be properly counselled before the test. The counselling should provide information about what the test can and cannot do, with a clear explanation of the difference between HIV infection and AIDS, and the main means of transmission of HIV. During this process it may become obvious that the client has been involved in risk activities, such as sex with an infected person, sharing a needle, or a transfusion of infected blood. Alternatively, the client may reveal that he or she has not engaged in high-risk activities, in which case it would be relevant to help them examine more closely why they wish to be tested, as it may be unnecessary.

The information in effect consists of explaining modes of transmission of HIV and how to prevent it, and looking at the advantages and disadvantages of the test. The advantages are that some people want to be certain one way or the other, available treatment can be applied, decisions can be taken about behaviours and relationships, and decisions made about healthy living and about pregnancy. The disadvantages include possible depression if the result is positive, rejection by family, friends, and employers, and problems about insurance if others learn of the positive result or even about the request for the test. A negative result leaves a person still uncertain, either because it may be a false negative or because the antibody is not yet detectable. In this case, a person engaging in high-risk activities may need to consider having a further test after 3 months.

The main focus of pre-test counselling will be on the psycho-social issues, arising from known and unknown factors. A positive result cannot be received neutrally, and will have serious implications for the person's life, loved ones, family and work. The counsellor should explore the feelings that a positive result will arouse in the client, and the effects in other quarters. At this stage it is worth trying to understand more fully the motives behind the request to have the test. If the motive is to discover whether the client needs to change his or her behaviour, it is necessary to underline that whether a person has the test or not, whether the test is positive or not, the client should develop safer behaviour. The reason is that the ways to avoid being infected and the way to avoid transmitting HIV to others are the same. i.e. using a condom and not sharing needles. The illumination of motives may reveal tears, guilt, and apprehensions: fears of possible or probable infection, guilt about behaviour and the likelihood of having infected others, apprehension about the results of the test and its implications for living and relationships. As in all counselling, the counsellor has to elicit these feelings in a non-judgemental way and probe them further to enable the client to resolve them and to give permission to the clients to be the persons they are. Feelings, it may be pointed out, naturally arise in us. In the author's view, we are not responsible for their presence, but we are responsible for what we do with them.

The aspects of responsibility can cover: whom to protect, organising one's life to ensure protective measures are available at the right time, leading a healthy life, reviewing one's system of values and beliefs, and taking a realistic decision about having the test or not. It is easy, to take on an air of moralising when addressing these points, and the counsellor must guard carefully against such an eventuality.

Some clients who have engaged in known high-risk activities resist the idea of possible infection. This denial needs confronting by the counsellor, as it is an unrealistic response. Behind it may lie a deep fear of dying, being 'found out', guilt over a casual sexual experience or a one-off homosexual encounter, belief that he or she is being punished, worry that certain freedoms or behaviours will have to be given up, concern for actual or desired children, and anger with the person who transmitted the virus to them. The inability to accept these feelings may lead to denial, and thus the counsellor must enable the client to bring them to the surface. Once the feelings are acknowledged and owned, the range of decisions that may help to resolve them must be examined and a realistic choice made by the client. The counsellor may need to provide support during the implementation of any decisions.

At the end of the counselling session a decision has to be considered. The client, whether referred by others or by self, must be the one to decide whether to go ahead with the test. This decision will embrace also the responsibility for dealing with the consequences of the result, such as making changes in behaviour and relationships, and living with an uncertain future.

After the HIV antibody test

Negative result

The relief afforded by a negative result has to be tempered by other considerations. A sexually active person or drug-addict must consider changes in life-style and sexual behaviour to avoid infection, and to avoid possible transmission since a negative result is never conclusive, for the reasons given in the introduction to this chapter. The uncertainty and fear outlined when describing counselling before the test may therefore still remain, and the counsellor may need to help the client review many of the issues again, as a negative result may be perceived as 'no progress'. A further consideration here is that the partners of the client may also experience a sense of relief, but uncertainty and mistrust may return as they wonder why the test was requested in the first place. The counsellor may need to be available for future sessions to enable the client to cope with the uncertain situation. The background of risk may help the client to decide whether to ask for a repeat test after 3 months.

Positive result (Miller, 1987a)

The test is conducted by health professionals, but the counsellor may be asked to give the result. There are bad ways of doing this: over the phone, by letter, in a hurry, just before the weekend (Richards,1986), without the possibility of immediate counselling and further information. There is no easy way of giving a positive result, but it should be direct, face to face, simple, and brief, so as to avoid confusion and misunderstanding. Whether the news is imparted by the health personnel or by a counsellor, there must be time immediately available for the counsellor to deal with the client's reactions.

The first reaction in the client is deep shock (Grimshaw, 1987), described by one health adviser like this:

> It is as if the patient is suddenly reduced to an impotent point. The will or ability to talk may vanish. Thought processes and feelings seem suddenly to shut down. The person feels a completely powerless victim who can do nothing to avoid the inevitable, having lost all control, being a victim and not an agent. This is the reversal of the usual state of mind, producing despondency and anger, while thoughts of illness and death fill the mind. (Palmer, personal communication 1987)

How can the counsellor proceed? The first aim will be to enable the client to talk and discharge the feelings verbally; the second will be to help restore the feeling of being in control; the third will be to take stock of the implications; and lastly, to make realistic decisions for the future based on meaningful motives.

The first aim is to enable the client to talk and discharge the feelings. As a first step the counsellor must respond to feelings with feelings. The only possibility may be non-verbal, perhaps holding the client's hand, or embracing the person, and sitting together in silence, allowing the client to weep and show despair, or simply being there and available, and sharing the distress. Gradually it may be possible to encourage the client to put into words what information has been received. He or she may believe they have been told they have AIDS, or that they are going to die, or that they must be hospitalised immediately. The counsellor should not condemn any misunderstandings, but will need to repeat many times the difference between HIV infection and AIDS. Questions such as: 'Try and tell me in your own words what you have understood', 'What did the doctor (or other informant) tell you?', 'What did the doctor say you had to do?' may be ignored by some clients. An alternative is to ask closed questions, where the client can signal assent or disagreement by movements: 'Did they give you the result?', 'Was it positive?': 'Did you understand it?', 'Is anyone (friend, spouse) waiting for you?'; 'Do you remember what we discussed before the test?' From general questions the counsellor can move into specific ones: 'Can you remember the difference between HIV and the illnesses it can cause?', 'Do you remember that condoms are a good form of protection?' The counsellor will need also to provide a great deal of feedback to the client: 'I see you are very distressed', 'You are obviously worried about yourself; 'I understand how concerned you are about partners/children'; 'I see how confused you are.' The effect of this feedback is to give a sense of reality to the client.

As speech returns, the understanding of the information needs to be checked, since misunderstandings can provoke extra anxieties and are not a basis for decision-making Many of the educational issues reviewed before the test will need revisiting. At the same time the feelings will be verbalised, probably in a random, poorly articulated fashion. Guilt, fear, anger, isolation, rejection, and, most importantly, lack of control, are commonly experienced. Suicidal thoughts can be serious and should be addressed if present (Miller, 1987b).

The second aim of counselling the antibody-positive client is to help the client regain a sense of control, the key to dealing with the other feelings. The lack of control should be explored: 'What is uncontrollable?'; 'Who is uncontrollable?'; 'There's nothing I can do' is a statement that must be analysed so as to undermine its universality. Can the client continue to work? Go to the cinema, a football match? Take exercise, eat well, avoid stress? The stark truth that HIV infection is for life must be acknowledged, but in its turn it can be a motive for doing other things such as deciding whom to inform of the news, how to protect others, how to avoid illness, and how to lead a satisfactory life amid the uncertainty. Clients who are blood donors should inform the transfusion service, so that appropriate action can be taken to protect others.

A further decision to consider is whether to join a support group, such as Body Positive (an offshoot of the Terrence Higgins Trust), where hope is maintained, solutions to practical problems may emerge, new social skills can be practised, friends can be found, and knowledge about HIV infection is updated.

There are other areas where control can be taken. It is known that prolonged anxiety reduces the effectiveness of the immune system (Coates *et al.*, 1984), and thus stressful situations should be avoided where possible. This can be enhanced by eating properly, taking regular exercise, proper rest and recreation, treating any infections promptly, and having regular health checks every 3 months. Yet again, it may help clients to put their affairs in order and perhaps write a will, do things that have been put off, such as patching up a family relationship, and generally dealing with what is called unfinished business.

During the few weeks following the imparting of the positive result, the client may want access to further counselling. The counsellor, therefore, will need to agree with the client how this can be done: by appointment, by phone, at what times. This is yet another matter where the client must have the feeling of control, initiating the contacts when necessary. Alternatively, the client may wish to find another counsellor, or another sympathetic person with whom he or she can share feelings. In any case, this person is likely to be outside the immediate circle of friends and family. Time made available in this way can take on a symbolic value, indicating the person's worth and acceptability to others.

Third, the client needs to take stock of the implications. While everyday social life and work may continue, the antibody-positive person has to consider how to protect others, and the implications for life insurance, medical and dental care, family planning, and pregnancy (perhaps even abortion).

Finally, after the review of all the feelings, issues, and implications, the client has to make realistic decisions for the future. The counsellor has to keep two issues to the forefront: first. that the client may need support in implementing the decisions, and, indeed, some homework to practise the implementation (for example, buying condoms, exchanging needles, rehearsing how to tell someone of the antibody status); and second, that the decisions have to be based on the values and beliefs of the client, so that they can be incorporated into an operational system of personal motives. Religious, social, moral, and family considerations may be important in providing the motives to underpin the decisions. How have important decisions (such as leaving home, settling down with a partner, changing jobs) been taken before? On what principles? How have uncertainty, bad news, and events been dealt with in the past? Can the same principles help now?

It is interesting to note from this description that counselling has a contribution to make to encouraging individual growth and personal development in a positive way: it is not just for helping to resolve problems and crises.

Some counsellors working with HIV-infected people have noticed paradoxical behaviour in some clients, with an increase of risk behaviour once the positive status is confirmed. Often this arises out of the unconscious use of denial as a coping mechanism. It is however usually found to be temporary, and the counsellor needs to be particularly accepting during this time, while encouraging the client to face up to the reality and implications of the infection.

Counselling people with AIDS

Learning that one has AIDS is traumatic. The counsellor will probably need to deal with it as already described for the counselling of a person with HIV. In other words, the initial counselling will concentrate on opening up communication with the client. All the feelings of guilt, anger, and denial may be resurrected. It is vital that they be expressed and acknowledged rather than challenged by the counsellor at the outset.

It will probably be necessary to review the information about HIV and its various effects, relating what is known to this particular client's state of health, and giving some idea of what may be expected. Issues of control, leading a normal life, and work have to be addressed and decisions made.

The psycho-social issues are considerable, and the need for counselling may increase as medical care looms larger and normal life diminishes. Different emotions emerge as new developments appear, and the client may need repeated counselling to adjust.

The first stage is crisis, manifested in shock, fear, and denial. The counsellor's role will be to establish effective communication without challenging the denial.

The second stage is one of adjustment to the news, although denial will probably continue intermittently, associated with anger, anxiety, depression (Burton, 1987), and guilt. Thoughts of suicide are less common in people with AIDS than those who are antibody positive, who seem to be in greater uncertainty (Miller, 1987b). During this stage, social disruption and withdrawal is common. Clients may abandon their jobs, refuse to see family and friends, hide away, and even leave their present accommodation, as an expression of guilt, shame, and fear. They may ask the health carers and the counsellor to collude with them in telling lies to family and employers. The counsellor's response will need to help them ventilate the feelings that prompt these actions, to own them, and decide how to deal with them. The counsellor can help clients restructure relationships with family, friends. and employers by examining with them their system of values and beliefs, so as to uncover deep personal reasons for realistic action. The counsellor may need to rehearse with the client coping strategies for dealing with the reactions of others. The client may want the counsellor to be present when family and friends come visiting and this can be helpful if the client and others know what is happening.

During this time of social adjustment, the counsellor can encourage the client to participate in a peer group where more support becomes available. This may be particularly necessary if the client is receiving psychiatric and medical treatment, which can arouse feelings of anxiety and isolation. The counsellor, of course, will probably deal with these feelings during counselling sessions, but a peer group can also help. The counsellor may need to have the client's permission to liaise with the health professionals about the progress of the illness, so as to adjust the counselling more closely to the client's needs.

The third stage is one of acceptance. The client takes on a new sense of self within the limitations imposed by the illness. This is a positive achievement, and the counsellor's response is to encourage and reinforce it by reflecting back to the person this new perception of self. Some clients will take on an altruistic outlook at this stage, and may wish to become involved in helping others with HIV-related conditions, in the belief and hope that some good can come out of the situation They will also begin to return to activities and relationships that existed before, rebuilding bridges and connections. The support of the counsellor can be expressed in helping to review options, within the constraints of the illness, and to make realistic decisions for implementation.

The fourth and last stage is preparation for death. Predominant issues are fear of dependence, pain, being abandoned, isolation, and death itself. However the counsellor's response will be to encourage the client to complete any unfinished business, to employ a constructive approach to any legal or family matters (Miller,1987c), and to talk about the feelings.

This sequential account of four stages sounds more logical than is the case in reality The client may regress from one stage to another. The uncertain progress of the disease can engender new fears. There may be apprehension about the disease's future effects. The gradual loss of physical strength and appearance, sexual activity, social life, status, and privacy can increase the feeling of being dependent. The counsellor may need to encourage family, friends, and health-care staff to allow clients to make their own decisions. They must be further encouraged to touch and embrace the clients, for whom physical closeness and contact are as great a need as ever. Without such contact the person's feeling of loss of self-esteem, personal identity, and isolation are increased, leading clients to stigmatise themselves yet further as immoral people, deserving of punishment (Boyd, 1987). The client remains a sexual being with sexual needs, but fear of infecting others or of being infected may undermine sexual identity and worth, leading perhaps to sexual dysfunctions . . .

Other concerns may be brought to the counsellor because of health-related issues and treatment. A morbid fear of everyday infections like influenza may develop, and the client may be bewildered by the claims for experimental drugs or alternative therapies, unsure of what to do. Dementia, anticipated or actual, can be one of the greatest concerns of a client. How can the counsellor respond to these issues? By enabling clients to distinguish the real from the imaginary, by encouraging them to focus on being alive and on what is possible, and by helping them to plan future activities, especially enjoyable ones. A meal out with friends, a visit to the cinema, choosing some new clothes, going to a football match, reading a book – each client will have a different list. By capitalising on the moment when they wish to help others, clients may see themselves anew as a positive resource, and this can be reflected back to them.

Throughout, the counsellor may find the client's family and friends themselves seeking counselling, as they struggle to accept the person with the illness and with possibly a newly revealed nature as a drug-user, homosexual, or a person with many sexual partners. Some will exhibit considerably more worry, and perhaps depression, than the client: they feel helpless as they see the decline, while the client may be reconciled to the truth. Counselling will address the same issues as hitherto described . . .

Counselling, education and advice, and changing behaviour

In considering the need for behaviour change, the issue of non-directive counselling arises and its relationship to education and advice. The educational aspect is perhaps the easiest to accept: it covers the modes of transmission and infection of HIV, the consequences of HIV infection, safer-sex techniques.

In turning to advice, the situation is less clear. It could conceivably cover matters like: dealing with vomit, blood, menstrual flow. whether to work, whether to send a child with HIV to school. But what about: whether to have sex, whether to use safer-sex techniques, whether to tell one's sex partners. There emerges a higher order of consideration: the balance between the social responsibility of both client and counsellor, and the freedom of the individual, and the rights of other parties. Counsellors already have experience of dealing with clients who wish to find a way of fulfilling their own needs while respecting the needs of others, but the presence of a potentially fatal virus brings the dilemma into the counsellor's own conscience, to affect not only his or her relationship with the client but also the commitment to confidentiality. Does counselling of HIV clients therefore involve advice? The counsellor will try to help clients to consider their social responsibilities at a moment when their personal needs are most demanding, and to help clients think through the implications of behavioural change, not simply as an option for personal growth, but as a responsibility (a duty?, a moral obligation?) towards other people, whose safety has to be taken into account.

I would like to propose a different counselling response, to be called

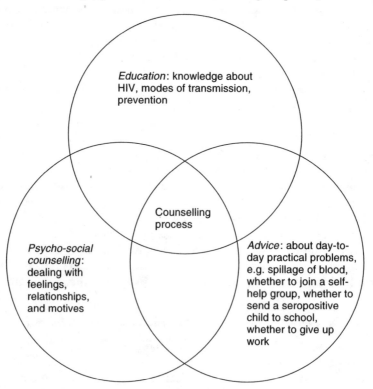

Figure 9.1 *A model of prevention counselling*

prevention counselling,[1] which could legitimately include education and advice. Figure 9.1 illustrates this. The education circle covers information about HIV, modes of transmission, methods of prevention, and techniques of safer sex. The advice circle deals with, for example, how to deal with vomit and blood, whether to send an HIV-positive child to school, whether a reasonably independent person with AIDS should continue to work, and how to use a condom. The psycho-social circle deals with the feelings and motivation of a person with HIV or AIDs, but also with his or her relationships to others who may be potentially and mortally threatened by that person's HIV-positive status. The counselling process is the place where the three overlap. In the process, one way forward is to invite clients to elicit their own reasons for change and to put them into their own words, thus feeling they are in control of their own life. Using existing values and beliefs, the counsellor can help them gradually build up a sense of social responsibility to others. Since change will need to be incorporated into an existing lifestyle, the counsellor will need to assist the client to construct a programme of implementation, differentiating perhaps between decisions with immediate effect, such as using a condom, and long-term decisions like informing other people, or joining a self-help group.

The implementation will take time to incorporate into the client's own belief and value system, which covers such basic questions as: Where do I come from?, Why am I here?, What will become of me? In other words they refer not just to reasons for doing things, but one's very existence, self-worth, and the symbolism between action and being. If, for example, a man thinks (or more likely, feels) that condoms render him less manly, he will find them difficult to use. If a person feels marginalised living in an industrial, uncaring society, sexual intercourse may be one of the few moments when he or she feels fully human: any attempt to interfere with the number of sexual partners or to introduce condoms may be resisted.

The programme of change will therefore need careful consideration of feelings, relationships, and motives, as well as information and advice. The gradual implementation of change can be helped by homework. At first it would include fairly undemanding actions like finding out some information, reading, writing a letter, talking to someone; but it can move on to more difficult things like informing someone of the positive status, buying condoms, learning to use condoms, trying out new (but safer) forms of sexual pleasure. The programme of change and related homework needs working out according to the unique needs, opportunities, and personal strengths of the client. As in other areas of counselling, progress needs evaluating by clients themselves with the help of the counsellor, who can reinforce success with praise and avoid blame for failures or shortcomings. In this way, supportive counselling leaves clients feeling they are in charge . . .

What is certain is that, in the absence of cure, counselling will have a new importance. It will help people not only to deal with their feelings. but also to make important decisions about their behaviour and relationships. Counselling thus will assume a social as well as an individual significance.

Notes

1. This term was invented by Dr G. Lloyd of Tulane University, New Orleans, who, with the present author, is writing The World Health Organization training materials on HIV/AIDS and counselling.

References

Boyd, K. M.(1987). The moral challenge of AIDS, *Journal of the Royal Society of Medicine*, *80*, 281–284.

Burton, S. W. (1987). The psychiatry of HIV infection, *British Medical Journal*, *295*, 228–289.

Coates, T. J., Temoshok, L. and Mandel, J. (1984) Psychosocial research is essential to understanding and treating AIDS, *American Psychologist*, *39*, 1309.

Grimshaw, J. (1987). Being HIV antibody positive, *British Medical Journal*, *295*, 256–257.

Miller, D. (1986). How to counsel patients about HIV disease – those who have it and those who fear it, *Maternal and Child Health*, *11(10)*, 322–330.

Miller, D. 1987a). ABC of AIDS: Counselling, *British Medical Journal*, *294*, 1671.

Miller, D. (1987b). HIV counselling: some practical problems and issues, *Journal of the Royal Society of Medicine*, *80*, 278–281.

Miller, D.(1987c). *Living with AIDS and HIV*, London: Macmillan.

Miller, D., Jeffries, D. J., Green, J., Willie Harris, J. R. and Pinching, A. J. (1986). HTLV-III: should testing ever be routine?, *British Medical Journal*, *292*, 941–943.

Parry, A. and Seymour, H. (1987). AIDS and female prostitution, *Health Education Journal*, *46(2)*, 71–73.

Richards, T. (1986). Don't tell me on a Friday, *British Medical Journal* , *292*, 943.

10 *Communicating across cultural boundaries** *

Alyson Peberdy

Consultations by the Commission for Racial Equality amongst Black and
minority ethnic groups in Britain reveal considerable dissatisfaction with
primary health care services especially with regard to lack of sensitivity to
the full range of cultural, religious and linguistic diversity. In recent years,
attempts have been made at a number of levels to improve this situation,
but it remains the case that far too often cultural , linguistic and religious
difference is regarded simply as a problem in relation to health care and
health promotion. The following account by a British nurse who describes
herself as Asian sums this up only too well:

> When I was training we had an outside speaker who came in to talk
> about 'Asian patients'. He talked mainly about the difficulties that
> Asian people caused in hospital: eating different food, showering
> instead of bathing, wanting their families to visit, causing all kinds of
> problems. There was also a feeling about how long would we have to
> put up with all this kind of thing, when we could expect them to be
> completely westernised. The whole feeling was that Asians were a
> problem. (Asian SRN, quoted in Mares *et al.*, 1985)

Clearly when cultural difference is simply regarded as an obstacle to the
efficient delivery of health care or health promotion there seems little
point in spending time learning about the culture and experience of ethnic
minorities. Thankfully many health workers have a more positive
approach towards diversity but find they do not have time to develop a
detailed knowledge of the language, beliefs, values and experience of each
of the many ethnic groups with whom they might, one day, come into
contact. It is possible, however, for health workers to develop an
awareness of some key areas of difference and to learn more about ways of
communicating across cultural boundaries.

Some cultural boundaries are highly visible and marked by a distinctive
form of clothing such as the Sikh turban (or medical white coat and
stethoscope), whilst others only become apparent through particular forms

---

* Commissioned for this volume.

of behaviour or use of language. Often it is unexpected problems in communication that first point to the existence of a cultural boundary. As communicating across cultural boundaries is never entirely straight-forward it is important to find ways of identifying and analysing where the relevant differences lie and and how they may be overcome.This forms the main task of this article.

First,we need to explore briefly what is meant by 'culture' and why it is relevant in the field of health and health promotion. One way of looking at culture is to regard it as a web of meaning that provides a framework for understanding and action. Such a framework provides an 'intersubjective world of common understandings' (Geertz, 1966) learned and taken for granted by those who share them. Cecil Helman's description of culture as a set of implicit and explicit guide-lines which tell members how to view the world, how to experience it emotionally and how to behave in it (Helman 1990) provides an adequate definition for our present purpose.

Focusing on culture and difference is sometimes criticised on the grounds that it distracts attention away from the more fundamental issue of racism. But, I would argue, encouraging professionals to recognise ways in which their communication is culture-specific and helping them to explore alternatives is one important element in the wider movement to reduce racism. Reflecting on the nature and process of communication across cultural boundaries, appreciating the interdependence of language, culture, meaning and identity all serve to 'bring home' to dominant groups ways in which verbal and non-verbal communication may function as a means of indirect discrimination.

Britain is one of the most ethnically diverse countries in Europe. The 1991 census indicated that about 3 million people in England and Wales (approximately 6 per cent of the population) regard themselves as belonging to Black and minority ethnic groups. This gives a fairly reliable picture of the numbers of people belonging to minority ethnic groups but masks some important internal differences *within* this population. The census asked people to classify themselves in terms of the following, broad, ethnic categories: White, Black Caribbean, Black African, Black other, Indian, Pakistani, Bangladeshi, Chinese, other Asian or other ethnic group. Yet within each of these categories there are major differences in written and spoken language, religion, lifestyle, and family structure as well as place of origin, present geographical location and access to education and employment in Britain. For instance, Black Africans living in the United Kingdom have their origins in a large number of different African countries and within each of these countries come from very different language and tribal groups. So for example people from Nigeria may be Moslem or Christian and be native speakers of Yoruba, Ibo, Hausa, Twi or another indigenous language. Such cultural and religious differences are often overlooked in Britain because many Nigerians are fluent in English.

One way of appreciating the extent to which general categories may hide important differences is to look closely at the term 'South Asian', so often assumed by white British people to represent a single group. McKeigue and Seval identify several distinct groupings based on place of origin and also distinguished by language, religion, family and caste structures and current settlement areas. Gujarati Hindus migrated from East Africa and West India and have settled mainly in North West London and Leicester. Gujarati is the spoken and written language. Sikhs came from the Punjab in India and in Britain now live mainly in West London and the Midlands. Their spoken language is Punjabi but their written language is in the Gurmukhi script. Pakistani Muslims have settled in the West Midlands, West Yorkshire and Waltham Forest, London. Urdu is their main spoken and written language. Bangladeshis come from the province of Sylhet and have settled largely in East London and Birmingham. They are mostly Muslims, their spoken language is Sylheti and written language Bengali (McKeigue and Seval, 1994).

Each of these 'South Asian' groupings differs from the others on a number of dimensions in ways that are likely to have major implications for their beliefs and values, their sense of identity and social structure, their understanding and experience of health, their access to employment, housing, health services and their degree of familiarity with spoken and written English. Yet to an outsider they may appear homogeneous and be treated as such.

When difficulties are experienced in communicating about health across cultural boundaries these may stem from differences in one or more of a number of dimensions. The main ones we shall consider here are: the meaning and value attached to health; structures of authority and rules of conduct; and finally language and language use.

Concepts, beliefs and values

Our understanding of the nature of health, what contributes to health, the interpretations we draw on and the responses we make to disturbances in health depend heavily on cultural assumptions and values. This is just as true for professional health workers in the late twentieth century as for anyone else. Historical studies reveal ways in which concepts of health and illness have changed, sometimes quite dramatically. An even greater diversity becomes apparent if we look closely at the experience of cultures rooted in histories and environments very different from our own. The western medical model with its distinction between mind and body and between medical, religious and social dimensions of life is clearly only one of a whole spectrum of possibilities.

In many African contexts, for instance, good health (both mental and physical) is seen as an aspect or expression of 'right relationships'.

According to a Zulu woman, 'good health means the harmonious working and coordination of the universe' (Ngubane, 1977, p.27) Neglect of obligations towards ancestors and disharmony within the social group, are regarded as major causes of illness.Similarly, writing of the Maya people of South America, Fabrega and Silver note, 'The individual himself [sic], his worldly contemporaries and the gods are linked in a triple web of relationships, and a frequent expression of disarticulation in this set of relationships is illness.' (Fabrega and Silver, 1973, p.80). For peoples using this kind of framework, health promotion, in so far as it lies in human hands, is likely to be primarily a matter of behaving correctly towards other people as well as towards ancestors, spirits and so on.

Here in Britain this theme of correct behaviour and the fulfilment of obligations is echoed in Caroline Currer's study of Pathan women living in Bradford. The emphasis here is not on trying to secure health through correct behaviour but rather to behave correctly in the face of illness. Apart from issues of health maintenance relating to taking precautions against temperature change and ensuring a diet balancing 'hot' and 'cold' foods, these women felt little responsibility for the occurrence of illness (Currer, 1986). Health and illness are simply viewed as part of the way things are. Health was not seen as an aim or ideal and the most important concern of the women was to be able to function in their role and maintain their value in caring for their families and managing their homes.

It is important not to use an intensive, local, study such as this to make general statements about 'Asians in Britain' or to conclude, for instance, that Asians have a fundamentally passive and fatalistic approach to health and illness. The picture is far more complex and generalisations need to be grounded in careful, detailed, research such as the Health Education Authority's survey of Black and minority ethnic groups in England (HEA, 1994). Concepts, beliefs and values relating to health are intimately linked with social and economic structures. The role people play in any given society understandably influences both the value others attach to them and their own sense of who they are and how to gain approval and respect. So, for instance, where people's main value is derived from their ability to work and 'keep going', as is the case with the Pathan women, this will fundamentally shape the meaning and value they attach to health. Similarly, in cultures where children have for generations provided the most reliable form of insurance for old age, high fertility and large families will be continue to be valued as sources of security (Bradley and Peberdy, 1988).

Those health workers who fail to see the internal logic of such perspectives are likely to regard groups and individuals who do not share their own preference for small families, 'healthy lifestyles' and individual responsibility for health as desperately in need of education and change. Meanwhile on the other side of the cultural boundary there may be no desire for change and, perhaps, no sense that health workers speak with any special authority on such matters.

Structures of authority and rules of conduct

The question of by what right health workers may try to change people is something of an old chestnut. Less frequently encountered are questions about authority structures *within* the groups with whom health promoters seek to work. Yet notions of authority, of who may decide what and who may mix with whom vary enormously between cultures. Some societies and groups operate with clearly defined hierarchies in the form of caste or class systems whilst others have less obvious distinctions, though even the most 'egalitarian' of structures is likely to have rules and expectations based on age and gender. Its important that health workers should find out what these rules are in order to avoid causing offence and to see which communication strategies stand a chance of success .

For instance in cultures that afford more importance and authority to religious leaders than to professional health workers it may sometimes be possible to use religious organisations and their leaders to mediate health concerns. One successful example has been the use of ulamas (Islamic religious leaders) and Koranic (scripture) reading clubs in Indonesia to encourage people to boil all drinking water (Prihartono *et al.*, 1994).

In a study of organ donation Randall (1991) notes that for Hispanic families it is women who make decisions relating to health although they are certainly not regarded as head of household. In order to ask consent for a dead child to donate organs the grandmother or mother is the person to approach. In many other cultures the situation is very different which means that health workers need to actively find out the patterns of decision making that operate in each particular context. For instance, amongst many Moroccan women living in the Netherlands participation in meetings at community centres is dependent on permission of the husband (Van Wersch and Uniken Venema, 1994).

The extent to which it is acceptable for women to participate in the public sphere is a key question to be considered when working across cultures. A Dutch strategy of providing health education for ethnic minority women in their first language at local community centres had to be revised when it was discovered that many Moroccan women never visit these centres. Alternative strategies suggested by Van Wersch and Uniken Venema include seeking a husband's permission for his wife to attend or instigating individual home visits.

In all cultures there are rules and expectations restricting or prohibiting discussion of some subjects. Such prohibitions most often relate to sex but may also refer to kinds of behaviour such as smoking, especially amongst Sikhs or, amongst Moslems, drinking alcohol. Some prohibitions are total whilst others govern relations between particular categories of people. So, for example, it might be acceptable for women to talk about sex or reproduction with women but not with men and children. This has repercussions for the choice of health workers or interpreters. So, for instance, when a health worker expects a child to interpret for a mother regarding some gynaecological matter there are likely to be problems in communication and possibly a great deal of embarrassment.

Language and use of English

Where English is not a person's first language, there will always be some words and concepts that are extremely difficult for them to understand or express because of fundamental gaps between languages. An illustration of this can be seen from the experience of translating and using the Health Education Authority's health and lifestyle survey questionnaire in several Asian languages.

> A wide range of terms were not understood in some communities: these included 'stress', lack of personal space', 'environmental pollution', 'healthy foods', and many medical terms such as 'diabetes', 'gangrene', 'degenerative illness'. We found that in some cases it was the concepts which were untranslatable, and that where respondents were familiar with the concepts, they tended to use English words for them. (HEA 1994, p. 13)

Similarly there are terms, concepts and distinctions drawn in other languages that cannot be translated directly into English and for which people sometimes have to use their indigenous language. For instance, in a number of languages speakers cannot refer to themselves without taking into account how they fit into society, with as many as ten different pronouns equivalent to the English 'you and I' (we) depending on generation level, kin relation, and other factors (Romaine, 1994, p. 28).

A further area in which there may be fundamental differences is in the general style and tone of communication. Although it is often difficult to analyse the nature of such differences its existence is undeniable and in some instances it becomes a major obstacle. An observation of counselling interviews in an Asian Resources Centre and a housing advice centre found that encounters between Asian counsellors and clients and white counsellors and clients were qualitatively different. In the Asian encounters, clients routinely gave little information; the counsellor asked questions, and inferred from factual responses what the difficulty was. In the white encounters clients tended to explain their position with a mixture of facts and evaluative comment.Where the counsellor was Asian and the client white, or vice versa, differences in interactive style led to more protracted negotiations, a greater sense of discomfort and less clear outcomes (Gumperz and Roberts in Roberts *et al.*, 1992, p. 128)

The oft-repeated advice to speak slowly and be polite begs the question of what counts as politeness in different cultures. Roberts *et al.*, (1992) gives an example of an employee for whom English was a second language, attempting to express criticism as indirectly and politely as possible by using metaphors and proverbs translated directly from his first language rather than using the system of modality in found in English (at least in middle class usage) to express indirectness, such as 'I think it might be possible that . . . '. His intention was completely misinterpreted.

In an attempt to identify the various levels at which people with different cultural backgrounds may fail to communicate, Roberts *et al.* identifies three dimensions which should be looked at. One is the accumulated knowledge, beliefs, values and structured experience people bring with them. This he terms *schema* and includes much that we have described as culture. The second, which he terms the *frame*, tells us how to behave and what to expect and is comprised of the strategies for interpreting what is going on in the interaction. The third relates directly to *language* use. The three form part of a single process and any one of them can be the basis for misunderstanding. The worst case is where there are major differences at all three levels and this is most likely to occur where two speakers do not have a common language.

The extent to which ethnic groups are fluent in English varies between groups and within them. As the following data shows familiarity with English has grown within the last ten or so. The Black and White Britain survey (Brown, 1984) showed that 76 per cent of Bangladeshi women, 70 per cent of Pakistani women, 50 per cent of Bangladeshi men and 42 per cent of Indian women in the United Kingdom spoke little or no English. A more recent survey (HEA, 1994) based on respondents self-assessment indicates that 66 per cent of Bangladeshi women and 29 per cent of Bangladeshi men do not speak English, though amongst those under 30 years of age English is much more common with 68 per cent of females and 92 per cent of males in this age group speaking English. According to the same survey 72 per cent of Pakistanis speak English and 85 per cent of Indian people. In all three groups the frequency is greater among young than old and among men than women.

This means that written material for these ethnic groups needs to be bilingual and the critical languages in which they should be provided in addition to English are Urdu, Bengali, Gujerati and Punjabi (HEA, 1994, p. 116). It also means that the provision of professional interpreters is of great importance. Their role may be not only to provide a direct translation of what is being said but also to ease the communication at every level where there is sufficient time and trust for this to happen.

A white British midwife, writing of her use of a Bengali interpreter in a research project, welcomed the way in which the interpreter adopted a role of partnership rather than aiming at 'invisibility'. A short extract from an interview illustrates the way the interpreter, discerning that the interviewee was not expressing her thoughts, prompted her to do so:

Researcher: How was the delivery and time in hospital?

Interviewee: They looked after me well.

Interpreter: Why not tell the truth? This is confidential, no one will tell anything against you.

Interviewee: When the first baby was born they cared a little bit. This time not at all. I had to come back home the next day . . . I was very anaemic and very tired. (Hennings *et al.*, 1996)

Considering how to communicate across cultural boundaries presses us to think hard about what we mean by 'communication'. To a great extent the difficulties that arise may be present in any communication. Concepts, beliefs and values; structures of authority and rules of conduct; language and language use are simultaneously both bridges and obstacles to communication. Where things go wrong attempts at repair and bridge building at each of these three levels may need to be considered. Asking the person on the other side of the 'cultural boundary' what s/he feels is going wrong and what would be most helpful is probably the best place to begin.

References:

Bradley, C. and Peberdy, A. (1988). 'Reproductive Decision-Making and the Value of Children: the Tolai of East New Britain' in McDowell, N. (ed.), *Reproductive Decision Making and the Value of Children in Rural Papua New Guinea* Papua New Guinea: Institute of Applied Social and Economic Research.

Brown, C. (1984). *Black and White Britain: the Third PSI Survey*. London: Heinemann Educational.

Currer, C. (1986). *Concepts of mental well and ill-being: the case of Pathan mothers in Britain*. In Currer, C., and Stacey, M. (eds), *Concepts of Health and Illness and Disease. A comparative prespective*. Oxford: Berg.

Fabrega, H. and Silver, D. (1973). *Illness and Shamanistic Curing in Zinacantan*. Stanford, CA: Stanford University Press.

Geertz, C. (1966). 'Religion as a cultural system'. In Banton, M. (ed.), *Anthropological Approaches to Religion*. London: Tavistock.

Helman, C. (1990). *Culture, Health and Illness. London:* Butterworth-Heinemann.

Health Education Authority (HEA) (1994). *Black and Minority Ethnic Groups in England*. London: HEA.

Hennings, J., Williams, J. and Haque, B. N. (1996). Exploring the health needs of Bangladeshi women: a case study in using qualitative research methods. *Health Education Journal*, 55, 11–23.

Mares, P., Henley, A. and Baxter, C. (1985). *Health Care in Multi-Racial Britain*. London: Health Education Council and National Extension College.

McKeigue, P. and Seval, L. (1994). *Coronary Heart Disease in South Asian Communities*.

London: Health Education Authority.

Ngubane, H. (1977). *Body and Mind in Zulu Medicine*. London: Academic Press.

Prihartono, M., Damayanti, R., Adisamita, A. and Tarigani, L. (1994). A community trial involving religious leaders to improve water preparation hygiene as part of diarrheal disease prevention in South Kalimantan, Indonesia *International Quarterly of Community Health Education, 14* (4), 391–402. London: Baywood Publishing.

Randall, T. (1991). Key to organ donation may be cultual awareness *Journal of the American Medical Association, 285:2*, 170–8.

Roberts, C., Davies E., and Jupp, T. (1992). *Language and Discrimination. A Study of Communication in Multi-ethnic Workplaces*. London: Longmans.

Romaine, S. (1994). *Language in Society: an introduction to socio-linguistics*. Oxford: Oxford University Press.

Van Wersch, S.and Uniken Venema, H. (1994). *Qualitative research supports health education for ethnic minority women: how to reach 'inaccessible' women, International Quarterly of Community health Education, 14*, (4), 379–389. London: Baywood Publishing

11 The social marketing imbroglio in health promotion

Ralph C. Lefebvre

The article, by Hastings and Haywood (1991), coupled with conversations with a number of attendees at the recent WHO Seminar on Leadership Training in Health Promotion and the International Summer School on Health Promotion held in Cardiff in September 1991, caused me concern over how health promotion professionals think about, and use, social marketing in their work. Some of the key concerns I have about the present state of affairs, and what appear to be topics not being considered adequately by all of us, are presented to broaden the discussion, and roles, of social marketing in health promotion.

Concerns

Social marketing = health promotion

Because much of the focus of work and publications about social marketing occur within a 'health problem' context, there are, at times, interchangeable use of the terms (one 'socially markets' nutrition to patients with cardiovascular disease). At other times, the discussions of social marketing become so focused on individual health behaviours, or lifestyles, that professionals concerned with environmental and other social issues wonder if they are in the right conference room. We need to understand that social marketing is a tool that can be used for health promotion, but is not the exclusive province of health promoters. This brings me to a second issue.

Social marketing is a theory for health promotion

Without delving into the epistemological aspects of this concern, the recurring questions I receive about the 'theory of social marketing' give me pause. Often, it is University faculty and students who are 'exploring the theory' and advance these questions. What they are finding is that there 'is not much theory' to social marketing. Other groups, particularly those who fund research, are asking 'Does social marketing work?' as if it's

* From *Health Promotion International*, 7 (1) (1992), pp.61–64. Oxford: Oxford University Press. © Oxford University Press 1992.

different from other theoretical approaches to health promotion. What is clear to me is that social marketing is a framework, or structure (perhaps a paradigm?) in which to approach social and health problems. It is the theory of change which imbues this general approach and gives it a chance to succeed. Failures of social marketing programmes are failures to theory or implementation. Attributing lack of success with a programme to social marketing is, to me, akin to attributing failure of a group to solve a problem to an inherent problem with Robert's Rules of Order (which also highlights that just as some groups have never read Robert, some health promoters do not understand social marketing to effectively use it).

Social marketing targets people

I have become increasingly concerned that social marketing programmes continue to be presented in only an individual behaviour change context. In an early article, June Flora and I discussed the use of social marketing to target social institutions and structures (Lefebvre and Flora, 1988). While such efforts are being launched by various special interests and advocacy groups, we need to remind ourselves in health promotion that social marketing programmes not only have to be sensitive to their environment, but also be directed towards creating a healthier one.

Social marketing = mass communication

Perhaps the most difficult issue for me to understand is how social marketing has become equated with mass communication approaches to health promotion *only*. This issue arises for me when people ask 'How can we do social marketing programmes when community development approaches are what we are supposed to be doing?' Indeed, I have spent entire days working with health promotion offices to 'try to integrate the two'. For me, there is no reason why a 'social marketing programme' cannot *exclusively* take a community development approach to solving a problem. If programme *strategy* is based on identifying consumer needs, identifying priority audiences, knowing how to best reach these audiences, and structuring the project as a 'marketing mix' (though the terms may be different), then selecting the *tactics* of community development or mass communication is secondary. A marketing programme is constructed to target a social concern and reach certain objectives. Going back to the 'theory' concern, social marketing is a framework in which to address problems. It is not exclusive of any theoretical approach to solving problems. The interesting research question would be: Using a social marketing model, is community development theory or mass communications theory more effective in creating an intervention that leads to healthier lifestyles and environments?

Challenges

Environmental scanning

As noted by Hastings and Haywood (1991), health promoters need to be aware of their internal and external environments as they plan strategies and tactics. On-going SWOT analysis (strengths, weaknesses, opportunities, threats) is imperative for effective marketing efforts. A SWOT analysis can be used both within the organisation and throughout the environment.

When doing this scanning key themes include (i) demographic and lifestyle trends, (ii) economic forecasts, (iii) business/industry activities, (iv) legislative/regulatory initiatives, and (v) potential partners, collaborators and intermediary groups for programme involvement. My scanning process includes reading marketing and business magazines, financial sections of newspapers, and professional newsletters. I also talk with many different types of people in order to 'take the pulse' of what people are thinking about, planning to do, or about to embark upon. It minimises surprises, and can often lead to unique opportunities for programme expansion and increased activity. More focus needs to be given to analysing the context of our marketing efforts, and identifying how the context, and our response to it, shapes the intervention strategy and tactics.

Audiences

The central concern of social marketing is the consumer: we must stay in touch with them or risk creating programmes that are not responsive to their needs, issues and unique situations. An over-riding and continuing interest in the consumer is what differentiates social marketing from health information or health education campaigns. Empowering people, advocating for them, and using community development approaches (as already noted) should be included as part of the marketing planning and implementation process. Social marketing is often portrayed as a 'top-down' approach; yet, when we keep consumers in the centre of the programme, and have a continuing dialogue with them, a 'bottom-up' effect is inevitable. Modern marketing practice is looking to 'build relationships with consumers': it's a goal we in health promotion should set for ourselves as well.

Channel

How to reach our key audiences with our messages, products and services should be a constant question for us. Intersectoral action can be viewed as a way to open up numerous channels for health promotion. However the nagging issue of so-called 'hard-to-reach' audiences is one that occupies much of our attention. We each have our particular 'hard-to-reach' groups. What I have noticed is that we can often characterise these groups quite well – down to the brand of cigarettes they smoke and the alcoholic beverage they consume. My question is, 'Why can tobacco and alcohol advertisers reach these people and we can't?' I do not believe the answer is simply they have more money and resources than we do! I think that health promotion professionals need to get smarter. We have to spend more time studying what these people do, learn from them and then use it to our advantage.

Process tracking

Many health promotion programmes are plagued by a lack of information on what they do and how effectively they do it. I do not mean by this that more programmes need outcome evaluation, but rather that *all* programmes need to understand whether they are reaching their intended audiences, whether these audiences understand that we are trying to communicate to them, and whether this understanding leads to attitudinal, and more importantly, behavioural change. Without process tracking systems, programme managers have little idea of how well they are progressing towards their objectives. It's somewhat akin to showing a person on a map a rather long, complicated and tortuous route to getting somewhere, and then sending them on their way without the map. Health promoters need to have their maps – not just to know where they are going, but to continually refer back so that they stay on the right path.

Exchanges

Marketing is a process of facilitating mutually rewarding exchanges between two or more parties – often referred to as 'creating win–win situations.' Making such exchanges tangible to consumers and health promoters occupies much of our time because, by virtue of our business, we are not always asking people for something tangible (e.g. money) in exchange for tangible goods (e.g. food, automobiles). What we do not understand very well is what I call the 'economics of health behaviour', that is, how and why people make decisions to adopt more healthful practices. In business marketing, consumer behaviour is an area of study in its own right. While health promoters have many theories from which to draw in developing their programmes, a critical part of the equation is missing. We need a good motivational theory for health behaviours, not just more rational ideas on how things should be. My question is always 'How do we motivate people?' The answer, when we stumble upon it, then defines how we structure the exchange process so we are successful (win) in improving the public's health (win).

Institutionalisation

Another shortcoming of many health promotion programmes is their transitory existence. As long as funding is available (usually from a single source), the programme thrives and is successful. Yet, as soon as funding is reduced, or cut altogether, the programme withers and dies. I have outlined elsewhere how institutionalisation or the long-term maintenance, of health promotion programmes can be approached within a social marketing context (Lefebvre. 1990). What are important issues to consider include:

- Planning for institutionalisation from the beginning of a programme or new initiative, not during its demise.
- Developing indigenous resources or secondary resources, to support the initiative.
- Demonstrating success to both grass-roots opinion and the policy-makers.

These issues need to be continually revisited by health promotion leaders if *our* long-term goals are to be met.

Management

The most critical variable for successful social marketing programmes is the management of the process. Among the issues I have touched upon, this is, to me, the weakest link in health promotion practice. We have to recognise that we will always be operating in a changing set of circumstances and, indeed, a changing world. The title of Tom Peter's book, *Thriving on Chaos*, needs to become our battle-cry – not our lament. Health promotion professionals must learn to manage change, not just in our sphere of health, but across the economic. social, business and political sectors of our world. This reticence to do so may be our Achilles heel. As Bill Novelli noted in a recent presentation, it is our unwillingness to earn our 'black belts' in marketing that limit the scope of what we can achieve.

Among the ideas touched upon by Peters that resonate with my view of health promotion management are the following:

- We need to *push* responsibility for programmes and initiatives *down* in our bureaucracies. We have to expect, and facilitate, excellence from our staffs.
- We need to 'fail forwards fast', to not be afraid of failure, but to encourage in our staffs an exhilaration for innovation. Failure needs to be viewed in the organisation as an opportunity to learn, not to point fingers. But we also need to learn fast, and get on with it!

Finally, to be leaders in health promotion, we have to stop asking ourselves, our supervisors, and our staffs 'Why?' Rather, to end with a quote form George Bernard Shaw, we need to set the vision:

You see things; and you say, 'Why?' but I dream things that never were; and I say, 'Why not?'

References

Hastings, G. and Haywood, A. (1991). Social marketing and communication in health promotion; *Health Promotion International*, 6, 135–145.

Lefebvre, R. C. (1990) Strategies to maintain and institutionalise successful programmes: a marketing framework. In Bracht, N. (ed.) *Health Promotion at the Community Level*. California: Newburg Press, 209–228.

Lefebvre, R. C. and Flora, J. A. (1988). Social marketing and public health intervention, *Health Education Quarterly*, 15, 299–315.

Robert, S. C. (1990). The Scott, Foresman Roberts's Rule of Order (new revised). Glenview, IL: Scott, Foresman.

Peter, T. (1987). *Thriving on Chaos: Handbook for the management revolution*. New York: Knopf.

Novelli, W. D. (1990). Getting a 'black-belt' in social marketing. Presentation at the American Marketing Association (Washington, DC Chapter) Social Marketing Conference.

12 *A case study of ethical issues in health promotion – mammography screening: the nurse's position* *

Alison Dines

Introduction

All nurses in the United Kingdom may be called upon to play a part in the national mammography screening programme. This may involve anything from working in a screening centre to simply being ready to inform members of the public about breast cancer screening should their professional knowledge be called upon. The programme, which forms an important part of the government's health promotion strategy, poses complex ethical issues. No work has so far examined how nurses and other health promoters might respond to these. This chapter explores the nurse's position in the light of these moral dilemmas.

Background to mammography screening

Early detection of disease through screening is generally held to be one component of health promotion (see for example Tannahill, 1985). The United Kingdom now has a national mammography screening programme for the early detection of breast cancer as part of its health promotion strategy (Department of Health, 1992). This was originally recommended by the Forrest Report in 1986 (Department of Health and Social Security, 1986). Now women between 50 and 64 years are invited to be screened every three years. The rationale for this is that successful screening will detect the disease at a stage when there is scope for effective treatment, thereby reducing the overall mortality rate.

Mammography, however, is a contentious issue. Internationally, opinion differs considerably about its benefit. Thus Sir Patrick Forrest (1990, p. 104) concluded, 'There can be no doubt that screening by mammography benefits women who develop breast cancer'. In contrast,

* From Wilson-Barnett, J. and Macleod Clark (eds) (1994) *Research in Health Promotion and Nursing*, Chapter 6, pp. 43–50. London: Macmillan.

Schmidt (1990, p. 223), an authority writing from Switzerland, believes, 'Breast cancer screening does likely more harm than good . . . to women of the 50–75 age group'. The uncertainty surrounding mammography is further complicated by the fact that the first reports from the UK trial (UK Trial of Early Detection of Breast Cancer Group, 1988), whilst demonstrating that the mortality rate *is* lower in the screened population by 15 per cent, did *not show this to be statistically significant*. The reasons for the absence of *statistical* benefit are complex, but it may be due to low attendance for mammography.

Mammography therefore raises complex ethical issues. This chapter explores the nurse's position in the light of these moral dilemmas. Two specific questions will be addressed. What position should a nurse take in a position of such uncertainty? In addition, if as health promoters we are interested in participation and enablement, how can we offer women health education in this situation?

The nurse's position

The question 'what is an ethical response in a situation of such uncertainty?' may be approached by thinking about four positions a nurse might adopt. These are outlined below.

Position I
The nurse might assess the evidence and decide mammography is of benefit and therefore be fully involved with the programme.

Position II
The nurse might assess the evidence, decide mammography is harmful, have no involvement with the programme and endeavour to have it stopped.

Position III
The nurse might decide it is best not to be involved with a programme that is not proven and wait until the evidence is conclusive.

Position IV
The nurse might decide to maintain a 'healthy scepticism' about the programme, be involved with it, whilst at the same time observing the continued evaluation of the effectiveness of the programme and informing women about the uncertain situation.

Let us now examine these positions in greater depth. Each 'position' has been given a name to help capture something of the flavour of the ethical stance being adopted.

Position I 'Nurse committed'

A nurse of this persuasion might say:

> The negative findings of various research reports into mammography screening can all be explained in terms of various methodological issues. Breast cancer is a huge problem and we must do something about it. I think time will show it to work.

It is interesting when examining each of these 'positions' to look at some of the assumptions being made. Nurse Committed assumes that 'doing something' in the face of a problem is better than doing nothing. This is an approach almost 'reinforced' at times by nursing itself. It has been challenged by some in recent years as not always appropriate. The advantages of Nurse Committed's approach is that women have a chance of being helped in the fight against breast cancer. In addition, mammography has the best chance of being tested as a new procedure because of high uptake. The disadvantages of her stance are that if mammography is subsequently found not to benefit women the public may be harmed through the perceived misuse of resources, a loss of confidence in health promoters and what may be viewed as an unnecessary intrusion into people's lives. The moral duties which are pertinent here are the duty of beneficence or doing good, the duty of veracity or truth telling and the duty of non-maleficence or not causing harm.

Position II 'Nurse agin'

A nurse of this persuasion might say:

> There is enough evidence from the international trials to show that mammography is not working. We are raising false expectations to allow it to continue. It was only introduced because it was politically useful in an election year.

The advantage of Nurse Agin's position is that it avoids the possibility of harming the public, at least in the short term. The disadvantage, however, is that mammography remains untested and women continue to die with breast cancer. The same moral duties of non-maleficence, veracity and beneficence mentioned with Nurse Committed are also relevant here.

Position III 'Nurse sidelines'

This nurse might say:

> It is unethical to offer untested remedies to members of the public. Until there is sufficient evidence to prove mammography works I cannot be involved.

Nurse Sidelines makes some interesting assumptions. First, that it is possible to 'prove' something. Many thinkers concerned with the philosophy of science would question this view of scientific knowledge. She also assumes it is possible to 'not be involved' and that inaction is a morally neutral position. Once again, many people would challenge this, seeing inaction as equivalent to a decision not to act and therefore not as neutral as we might first think. The advantage of Nurse Sidelines position is that she does not personally risk causing harm to members of the public through a new procedure. The disadvantage of the view is that if everyone adopted this position no advances in research would ever be made and in this case women would continue to die of breast cancer. Similar moral duties appear to be important here to those identified with Nurse Committed and Nurse Agin, in particular the tension between present and future beneficence.

Position IV 'Nurse fence-sitter'

This nurse might say:

> The only way to behave in such uncertainty is to try mammography out and see, but keeping a 'weather eye' on the programme monitoring and evaluation and keeping women aware of the uncertain position.

The advantages of Nurse Fence-Sitter's position are that she is being honest with the women thereby enhancing their autonomy and the women have a chance of being helped through the early diagnosis of breast cancer. The disadvantages are that the women she encounters may be confused and worried, they may not attend for breast screening and therefore have no opportunity of benefit. In addition, the programme is less likely to work due to poor attendance. There may also be a personal cost to the health promoter arising from her involvement with a programme that may not be working. The moral duties involved include veracity, respect for persons and non-maleficence.

Having looked more closely at the four Nurses views, the intriguing question is, who is behaving in the most ethical fashion? Is it

Nurse Committed, Nurse Agin, Nurse Sidelines or Nurse Fence-Sitter?

Health education about mammography

Let us now leave this as food for thought for a moment and consider the question, how can we as health promoters educate women in this situation? Once again we shall examine how the various 'Nurses' above would approach this.

Nurse Committed might say to the women she is working with, 'Finding breast cancer early gives the best chance of cure, do go when invited'.[1] Alternatively, she might suggest, 'The benefit of being screened for breast cancer far outweighs any risk of harm, make sure you take advantage of the service'.[2]

Nurse Agin might say in her work as a health promoter, 'Mammography does not offer women any benefit, I recommend you do not bother to go'. In a stronger fashion she might say, 'Mammography is harmful, it should be stopped'.

Nurse Sidelines might remain silent or say, 'I have no comment I cannot advise you about breast cancer screening'.

Nurse Fence-Sitter might say, 'Mammography has possible benefits and drawbacks, it is very complex'. She could then ask the woman what she wishes to know about mammography and drawing upon her communication skills she may try to convey some background facts in a manner appropriate to the individual woman. Nurse Fence-Sitter might draw upon some of the following information for this discussion.

- Every year your chances of dying from breast cancer are 1 in 2400, after screening they may be about 1 in 2900 (Rodgers, 1990).
- Breast cancer screening offers the possibility of less radical treatment for breast cancer (Austoker, 1990).
- The woman's breast will need to be compressed to 4.5 cm (Forrest, 1990).
- 14 000 women will need to be screened to save one life (Rodgers, 1990).
- 142 000 women will be recalled with some false positives and some overdiagnosis (Rodgers, 1990).
- For every seven women found to have breast cancer, six will not live any longer as a result of early diagnosis (Rodgers, 1990)
- Some breast cancers will be missed at mammography (Rodgers, 1990;

Skrabanek, 1989; Woods, 1991).
- Some cancers will develop in the three-year interval (Forrest, 1990).
- The cost of saving one life from screening is £80 000 (Rees, 1986).
- Treatment of breast cancer may include lumpectomy, mastectomy, radiotherapy, chemotherapy, hormone treatment.
- *Individual* benefit cannot be guaranteed (Skrabanek, 1989).

Having considered how the various 'Nurses' above would approach health education, it is interesting to ask, what are the strengths and weaknesses of these various ways of informing women?

Nurse Committed's information is clear, simple and persuasive. It is based on a professional's paternalistic judgement about what is of benefit to women and advises on that basis. Women are given clear simple guidance about their health and are spared the burden of assessing complicated evidence for themselves. At the same time, however, they receive little information about which to make their own judgements and remain dependent upon the health promoter. The women are therefore denied the opportunity to assess mammography for themselves and make a free choice on that basis. They may be harmed if the paternalistic judgement of the health promoter proves to have been incorrect or differs from the judgement that the women themselves would have made had they been given the opportunity.

Nurse Agin's information is clear, simple and persuasive. It too is based upon a professional's paternalistic judgement about what is of benefit to women and advises on that basis. The strengths and weaknesses of Nurse Agin's stance are very similar to those of Nurse Committed, as once again women are given clear, simple guidance about their health but little information upon which to make their own judgements.

Nurse Sidelines' information is straightforward and non-committal, it provides little information and does not advise. Women are given an honest response by the professional but receive no guidance about their health and no information about which to make their own judgements. This approach might be harmful if adopted by all health promoters.

Nurse Fence-Sitter's information depends to some extent upon her communication skills and her ability to respond to and convey a message appropriate to the individual women whose health she is concerned to promote. The information at her disposal is detailed, somewhat complicated and non-committal. Attempting to share this knowledge is based upon a belief in the need to respect a person's autonomy through informed consent. The women are given no advice and may be confused or alarmed, in addition they may be less likely to attend for breast screening. The women do, however, have a lot of information about which to make their own judgements. In addition, the health promoter has been honest with the women.

Which then is the most ethically sound approach in health promotion? Is the paternalism of Nurse Committed and Nurse Agin most appropriate, the 'neutrality' of Nurse Sidelines or the respect for autonomy through informed consent of Nurse Fence-Sitter?

The answer to this question is complex, it is worth considering some other questions which might help us as we think about our own view. In health promotion we are concerned with encouraging people to work with us as partners in safeguarding their health, enhancing and regaining control over their health. Two interesting questions are therefore, which of these approaches allows the woman to *participate* in her own health to the greatest degree? Which of these approaches *enables* the woman to increase control over her health? In addition, we might note that we accept both paternalistic judgements and those respecting autonomy through informed consent in caring for *patients*. Does the fact that *healthy people* are involved in breast cancer screening make any difference? What if we view women attending for mammography screening as *research subjects* how might this influence our health education as either paternalistic or respecting autonomy through informed consent? What if we view the women as *potential patients*, does this make any difference to health education? Does the question of whether the duty of the nurse is to the *individual* before her or to *society* as a whole have any relevance?

Conclusion

The ethical issues in mammography screening are paralleled in many other areas of health promotion. The evidence in this chapter suggests that nurses and other health promoters are placed in a difficult position in situations of such uncertainty. We need to debate the best way forward to be certain we are behaving in an ethical fashion.

This chapter has raised many questions and begun to answer only a few. These ideas are left as continuing food for thought and debate amongst nurses in their work as health promoters.

Acknowledgements

This chapter draws upon research being undertaken for Ph.D. studies. The research is being jointly supervised by Professor Jennifer Wilson-Barnett, Department of Nursing Studies, Kings College, University of London and Dr Alan Cribb, Lecturer in Ethics and Education, Centre for Educational Studies, Kings College, University of London.

Notes

1. The phrases used here are adapted from the Women's National Cancer Control Campaign (1989) leaflet entitled, 'Breast screening by mammography.Your questions answered', and the poster entitled, 'Have you heard about free breast screening?'
2. The phrases used here are adapted from the Women's National Cancer Control

Campaign (1989) 1eaflet entitled, 'Breast screening by mammography. Your questions answered', and a Cancer Research Campaign (1991) leaflet entitled, 'Be breast aware'.

References

Austoker, J. (1990 Rev. Ed) *Breast Cancer Screening: a practical guide for primary care teams.* NHSBSP (National Health Breast Screening Programme), Oxford.

Department of Health and Social Security (1986). *Breast Cancer Screening.* Report to the Health Ministers of England, Wales, Scotland and Northern Ireland, by a working group chaired by Professor Sir Patrick Forrest. London: HMSO.

Department of Health (1992). The Health of the Nation. London: HMSO.

Forrest, P. (1990). *Breast Cancer: the Decision to Screen.* London: Nuffield Provincial Hospitals Trust.

Rees, G. (1986) Cost benefits of cancer services. *The Health Service Journal* (10 April), 490–491.

Rodgers. A. (1990). The UK breast cancer screening programme: an expensive mistake, *Journal of Public Health Medicine, 12,* (3–4), 197–204.

Schmidt, J. G. (1990). The epidemiology of mass breast cancer screening – a plea for a valid measure of benefit, *Journal of Clinical Epidemiology, 43(3),* 215–225.

Skrabanek, P. (1989). Mass mammography: the time for reappraisal, *International Journal of Technology Assessment in Health Care,* 5, 423–430.

Tannahill, A. (1985). What is health promotion?, *Health Education Journal, 44,* 167–168.

UK Trial of Early Detection of Breast Cancer Group (1988). First results on mortality reduction in the UK trial of early detection of breast cancer, *Lancet, ii,* 411–416.

Woods, M. (1991). Behind a screen, *Nursing Times, 87,* (27 November), 48.

Questioning the evidence base of health promotion

Health promotion has sometimes been criticised for basing interventions on what might be viewed as insubstantial evidence and for a less than robust approach to evaluation. To justify its place in the purchaser–provider market, it is argued, health promotion must become more rigorous, self-critical and outcome focused. This links to a broader endorsement of the concept of evidence-based health care, with the implication that much health practice hitherto was not based on research data but on clinical judgement. However, even when there is information which appears to be reliable, it may prove to be contradictory and provide more questions than answers. This Section seeks to lay out these issues and particularly unravel the question of what counts as evidence in health promotion. At a practical level answering this question is important for clients who want advice about healthy choices and for purchasers and policy makers seeking to use public money wisely At a more philosophical level it relates to wider debates about the nature of evidence and whose views count.

In 'Explaining the French Paradox', Michael Burr (Chapter 13) refers to the comparatively low incidence of and mortality rates from ischaemic heart disease in France. These rates seem to be unexpectedly low given the high French intake of saturated fat and the fact that serum cholesterol, blood pressure and smoking prevalence rates in France are similar to other countries. The role of wine drinking with meals is examined to ascertain whether this confers protection against some of the effects of food. This 'paradox' is illustrative of the ways in which information is sometimes misconceived and presented; there is clearly something different happening in France and maybe wine plays a role but we cannot therefore assume that wine drinking with food is necessarily a protective measure. Sustaining the French example, Desenclos *et al.* in Chapter 14 look at one possible health danger encountered by French eating habits, that of contracting salmonella from eating goats' milk cheese. This study illustrates the importance of conducting a study of carefully matched cases and controls before making assumptions about causality, though how far this is in practice possible remains open to debate.

Taking up the theme that it is important to understand the methods used in collecting data before making assumptions about the relevance and reliability of conclusions reached, Joe Abramson argues in Chapter 15 that epidemiological studies need to be scrutinised in relation to a number of factors before using these results as the basis for interventions. He argues that despite methodological drawbacks, well conducted epidemiological research can collate evidence sufficiently reliably to enable informed decision making. However, conflicting evidence, as seen during the BSE debacles, are as much part of epidemiological enquiry as is the replacing of old knowledge by new. Hence 'Epidemiology should be taken with care'.

Two studies illustrate the particular usefulness of epidemiological data for health promotion. Beale and Nethercott in Chapter 16 looked at GP consultation rates comparing employees of a factory threatened with closure and other local residents. This study demonstrates that drawing conclusions about relationships between the threat of unemployment and consultation rates is rife with difficulties, but still can indicate certain patterns. Andrew Tannahill in Chapter 17 supports the view that reliable evidence is an essential prerequisite before embarking on interventions. He argues for carefully scrutinised planning in health promotion and more resources to be channelled into acquiring reliable research evidence to facilitate an integrated and positive approach to health education and health promotion.

Dey and her colleagues in Chapter 18 use the gold standard of epidemiological enquiry, a randomised controlled trial to measure the effectiveness of using health education leaflets in reducing the incidence of sunburn. They argue that when embarking on interventions that 'seem' to make sense, it is essential to use such epidemiological methods to measure whether these interventions are indeed effective. Their study demonstrated that leaving health warning leaflets readily accessible for would-be travellers was, indeed, of little use and possibly a waste of resources.

But what is to count as evidence, and who should decide? In an increasingly market-based health system, purchasers are expected to ground their decisions in evidence of effectiveness and value for money. Yet such evidence is hard to come by and evaluations and reviews of evaluation studies have, for the most part, failed to produce the kind of practical guidance called for by purchasers and policy makers. Does this indicate an urgent need for more and better research or does it, perhaps, suggest that the expectation is unrealistic?

In response to this question, Godfrey's Chapter 19, 'Is prevention better than cure?' takes a largely optimistic and pragmatic view. Recognising that much work remains to be done, she teases out the kinds of comparisons that can be drawn and the tools that will help. Models such as PREVENT help predict health gain though most available models are limited to mortality measures and she also calls for ways of measuring changes in morbidity.

Echoing Godfrey's carefully analytic tone, but pointing to a very different conclusion, Robin Bunton and his colleagues argue in Chapter 20 that the hope of providing guidance for purchasers about the cost-effectiveness of health promotion initiatives is primarily a mirage. The project is essentially misconceived, they maintain, because health promotion does not lend itself to the kind of evaluation that has proved fruitful in biomedical research. Biomedicine and health promotion belong to different worlds (characterised respectively as modern and post-modern) and so require different kinds of evaluation. The object of study in the evaluation of health promotion (human interaction and behaviour) is an 'open system' subject to very complex patterns of determination at a number of levels. In short, no amount of technical and methodological refinement will provide solid evidence of cost-effectiveness in health promotion and it is pointless to keep trying.

What other forms of evaluation exist? Writing primarily from experience of the evaluation of social work, Everitt and Hardicker in Chapter 21 sketch out an alternative 'critical' framework which, unlike rational–technical evaluation, acknowledges the significance of subjectivity, values and power. In so doing they provide a powerful challenge to both medical and managerial assumptions about the nature of evidence and the meaning of success. It is important to be reminded that debates about the evidence base of health promotion need to be understood in the context of wider philosophical debates.

13 *Explaining the French paradox**

Michael L. Burr

The French paradox

In many Western countries, including Britain, the biggest single cause of death is ischaemic heart disease (IHD). There are, however, some European countries where IHD mortality is much lower, and one of them is France, which has the second lowest IHD death-rate among developed countries, just above that of Japan. The differences are not trivial: the mean age-standardised IHD death rates for men and women in Austria, Germany and the Netherlands are twice the French rate, and those in the United Kingdom and Denmark are three times as high (Renaud and de Lorgeril, 1992). The question arises as to why the French are so fortunate.

Differences in fat intake are not the explanation: the average consumption of dairy fat is similar in all the above countries, although it is substantially lower in other Mediterranean countries that share France's low IHD mortality. The three classical IHD risk factors – blood pressure, serum cholesterol and cigarette smoking – are no lower in France than in other industrialised countries. These observations led Renaud and de Lorgeril (1992) to draw attention to 'the French paradox' of a low IHD mortality associated with a high intake of saturated fat and with other risk factors. A recent paper in the *Lancet* (Criqui and Ringel, 1994) examined data from 21 developed countries in an effort to resolve this paradox.

Is it an artefact?

Before we turn our attention to the various peculiarities of the French lifestyle as possible solutions, we should first ask whether the differences in death rates are real. Whenever the data from one country are markedly out of line with those from other areas, the possibility must be considered that there is some artefact of nomenclature or classification. Diagnosis is at best an inexact science, and when causes of death are entered on death certificates the wording may vary according to the certifying doctor's training, presuppositions and language as well as the actual pathology.

* From *Journal of the Royal Society of Health* (August 1995), pp. 217–219.

Many deaths involve more than one disease process, and the doctor has to decide which to select as the underlying cause of death; if several are mentioned on the death certificate the order in which they appear will determine how the death is ultimately classified. Fashions in terminology and certification are known to vary from one country to another, so that differences in disease-specific death races should not necessarily be taken at face value.

The MONICA project set up by the World Health Organisation has provided some information about the comparability of mortality and morbidity statistics from different countries. The results suggested that death certificate diagnoses are not the same in all populations, as there may be differential reporting of potential coronary deaths.

Three areas of France that participated in the study appeared to have very low IHD death rates, but on investigation it transpired that some deaths that elsewhere would be attributed to IHD were in France described in some other (usually vaguer) way. This appears to contribute to the French paradox, but it does not wholly explain it, since even when the French death rates were corrected for this low bias they still remained relatively low (Tunstall-Pedoe *et al.*, 1994).

Is it the wine?

It seems, then, that the French really do have lower IHD death rates than might be expected from their fat intake, serum cholesterol levels, blood pressures and smoking habits. Something about the French way of life must give them some protection from this disease.

France is famous for its wines, and the hypothesis that wine is the protective agent seems to have gained wide acceptance among the public at large. It certainly is an attractive idea. It also has some support from the evidence, particularly when different countries are compared with respect to their wine intakes and IHD death rates. St Leger *et al* (1979) examined various data from 18 developed countries and found that IHD mortality was related positively to intakes of total and saturated fats, and negatively to alcohol consumption. When alcohol intake was classified as wine, beers and spirits, the alcohol effect appeared to be entirely accounted for by the wine intake. The wine effect was undiminished whatever other variables (such as gross national product, cigarettes, or diet) were taken into account. The analysis was repeated with France excluded (because of the possibility that France under-reports IHD deaths), but the results were not substantially altered. The authors concluded that a protective effect of wine is likely to be due to constituents other than alcohol. They regretted that they were unable co advise their friends about the relative advantages of red, white or rosé wine.

Some evidence on this latter point has been supplied by work on the anti-oxidant properties of red wine. There are certain phenolic compounds in red wine with properties that powerfully counteract the oxidation of low-density lipoprotein (LDL) in the blood, a process which contributes to the arterial damage underlying IHD (Frankel *et al.* 1993). The authors considered that their results provided a plausible explanation of the French paradox. Furthermore, a study in healthy volunteers showed that the consumption of red (but not white) wine with meals reduces the susceptibility of plasma and LDL to lipid peroxidation (Fuhrman *et al.*, 1995).

Is it the alcohol?

The evidence pointing specifically to wine as the protective agent is largely drawn from comparisons between countries, in terms of their IHD death rates and *per capita* wine consumption. Another approach is to record the drinking habits of a large number of individuals, follow them up over time, and relate their initial intakes to their subsequent development of (or death from) IHD. There have been numerous studies of this kind, in different countries. and the results have been remarkably consistent in showing that the incidence and mortality of IHD are higher among moderate drinkers than among, non-drinkers (Burr. 1994). A follow-up of British doctors confirmed previous studies in this regard (Doll *et al.*, 1994). The relationship between alcohol consumption, and all-cause mortality is U-shaped – i.e. the protection afforded by a moderate intake against IHD is not offset by increased deaths from other causes, although at higher intakes this is certainly the case. Two recent studies suggest that alcohol may protect against non-insulin-dependent diabetes, a condition related to IHD (Rimm *et al.*, 1995; Perry *et al.*, 1995).

In most of these studies of individuals (as distinct from between-country comparisons) any alcoholic drinks appear to be protective. In an American study wine and beer appeared to be similarly protective, but 'liquor' (spirits) was not associated with any reduction in risk (Klatsky and Armstrong, 1993). Preference for red wine did not confer any advantage – indeed, those who preferred other types of wine had a marginally lower risk. A recent Danish study found that mortality from cardiovascular and cerebrovascular disease appeared to be reduced by beer-drinking and (especially) wine-drinking, but not by drinking spirits; wine-drinkers had the further advantage of a lower all-cause mortality (Grønbaek *et al.*, 1995). People who chose different types of alcohol may differ in other ways, however; those who drink spirits tend to have unfavourable characteristics that may outweigh any protection derived from the alcohol.

Some of the physiological effects of alcohol could account for its apparent effect on IHD. It raises the blood concentration of high-density lipoprotein, which is negatively associated with IHD risk (Burr *et al.*,

1986). A negative (favourable) association with plasma insulin has been reported in women (Razay *et al.*, 1992). Alcohol has favourable associations with plasma fibrinogen (negative) and blood fibrinolytic activity (positive), which affect the formation of blood clots (Meade *et al.*, 1979). The French custom of drinking, wine with the meal may confer extra benefit in that the alcohol is absorbed slowly and thus has a prolonged effect on clotting factors at a time when they are adversely affected by dietary fat: this protection has been detected experimentally 13 hours later (Hendriks *et al.*, 1994). Alcohol reduces platelet aggregation, another component of the clotting mechanism that operates in heart attacks, and this action presumably accounts for the observation that platelet aggregation was 55 per cent lower in French farmers than in Scottish farmers (Renaud and de Lorgeril, 1992). These observations have led to the conclusion that the French paradox is soluble – it can be explained by the fact that the French have the highest intake of alcohol in the world (Criqui and Ringel, 1994).

Is it the diet?

The authors just quoted considered the possibility of a dietary explanation, but dismissed it because of inconsistencies when data from different years were compared. A more detailed analysis examined the consumption of various nutrients in 17 European countries (Bellizzi *et al.*, l994). This analysis showed that IHD mortality was positively related to dairy products and their characteristic fatty acids, and negatively related to wine, vegetables, vegetable oils, vitamin C, β-carotene. and α-tocopherol (a component of vitamin E): the strongest relationships were with α-tocopherol, wine and vegetables. Mean blood levels of α-tocopherol, vitamin C and carotene show a similar inverse association with national IHD death rates, the α-tocopherol being the most important (Gey *et al.*, 1993). Each of these nutrients has antioxidant properties that may be relevant to IHD risk

A randomised trial of a 'Mediterranean diet' has been conducted in France and showed a significant reduction in IHD mortality in men who had recently recovered from a heart attack (de Lorgeril *et al.*, 1994). Although the authors laid special emphasis on the fatty acid composition of the diet it involved a higher intake of fruit and vegetables and produced higher blood levels of vitamins C and E. Follow-up studies of individuals showed that people with a higher vitamin E intake had a lower risk of IHD death (Rimm *et al.*, 1993: Stampfer *et al.*, 1993). These and other considerations led Bellizi *et al.* (1994) to conclude that the 'European paradox' (as they prefer to call it) is explained by vitamin E, derived from various sources of which wine is only one.

What can we conclude?

The French paradox is exaggerated by under-reporting of IHD deaths but not entirely explained by it. Something about the French (and southern European) lifestyle seems to protect against IHD, despite unfavourable factors such as fat intake, blood cholesterol, blood pressure and smoking habit.

Two main explanations have emerged: alcohol and anti-oxidants. Both are known to affect physiological processes in ways that could reduce IHD risk. Both are characteristic of France, being found together in wine though not restricted to it. It is perhaps noteworthy that Criqui and Ringel (1994) found the negative association between IHD and wine ethanol to be stronger than the associations with total ethanol (as would be expected if alcohol were the only factor) or with wine volume (as would occur if something specific to wine were responsible). Maybe the French habit of drinking with the meal rather than at some later time confers additional benefit.

What are the practical implications? Criqui and Ringel point out that the cardioprotective effect of alcohol in France is cancelled out by increases in other causes of death. The U-shaped curve relating alcohol to all-cause mortality suggests that a moderate intake (say two drinks daily) may confer benefits which are not outweighed by other risks. Maybe if we eat more fruit and vegetables and drink wine with our meals we can be less worried about our blood cholesterol and so share the benefits of the French paradox.

References

Bellizzi, M. C., Franklin, D. E., Duthie, G. G. and James, W. P. T. (1994). Vitamin E and coronary heart disease: the European paradox, *European Journal of Clinical Nutrition, 48*, 822–831

Burr, M. L. (1994). Alcohol and ischaemic heart disease, *Journal of the Royal Society of Health, 114*, 216-218

Burr, M. L. Fehily, A. M., Butland B. K., Bolton, C. H. and Eastham, R. D. (1986). Alcohol and high density lipoprotein cholesterol: a randomised controlled trial. *British Journal of Nutrition, 56*, pp. 81–86

Criqui, M. H. and Ringel, B. L. (1994). Does diet or alcohol explain the French paradox? *Lancet, 344.* pp. 1719-1723

De Lorgeril, M., Renaud, S., Mamelle, N., Salen, P., Martin, J-L., Manjaud, I., Guidollet, J., Touboul, P. and Delaye, J. (1994). Mediterranean alpha-linolenic acid-rich diet in secondary prevention of coronary heart disease. *Lancet, 343*, pp. 1454-1459

Doll, R., Peto, R., Hall, E., Wheatley, K. and Gray, R. (1994). Mortality in relation to consumption of alcohol: 13 years observations on male British doctors. *British Medical Journal, 309.* pp. 911-918

Frankel, E. N., Kanner, J., German, J. B., Parks, E. and Kinsella, J. E. (1993). Inhibition of oxidation of human low-density lipoprotein by phenolic substances in red wine. *Lancet, 341.* pp. 454-457

Fuhrman, B., Lavy, A. and Aviram, M. (1995). Consumption of red wine with meals reduces the susceptibilities of human plasma and low-density lipoprotein to lipid peroxidation. *American Journal of Clinical Nutrition, 61*. pp. 549–554

Gey, K. F., Moser, U. K., Jordan, P., Stahelin, H. B., Eichholzer, M. and Lüdin, E. (1993). Increased risk of cardio-vascular disease at suboptimal plasma concentrations of essential antioxidants: an epidemiological update with special attention to carotene and vitamin C. *American Journal of Clinical Nutrition, 57*. pp. 7875–7975

Grønbaek, M., Deis, A., Sorensen, T. I. A., Becker, U, Schnohr, P. and Jensen, G. (1995). Mortality associated with moderate intakes of wine, beer and spirits. *British Medical Journal, 310*. pp. 1163–1169

Hendriks, H. F. J., Veenstra, J., Wierik, E. J. M. V-te., Schaafsma, G. and Kluft, C. (1994). Effect of moderate dose of alcohol with evening meal on fibrinolytic factors. *British Medical Journal, 308*. pp. 1003–1006

Klatsky, A. L. and Armstrong, M. A. (1993) Alcoholic beverage choice and risk of coronary artery disease mortality: do red wine drinkers fare best? *American Journal of Cardiology, 71*. pp. 467–469

Meade, T. W., Chakrebarti, R., Haines, A. P., North, W. R. S. and Stirling, Y. (1979) Characteristics affecting fibrinolytic activity and plasma fibrinogen concentrations. *British Medical Journal, 1*. pp. 153–156

Perry, I. J., Wannamethee, S. G., Walker, M. K., Thomson, A. G., Whincup, P. H. and Shaper, A. G. (1995). Prospective study of risk factors for development of non-insulin dependent diabetes in middle aged British men. *British Medical Journal, 310*. pp. 560–564

Razay, G., Heaton, K. W., Bolton, C. H. and Hughes, A. O. (1992) Alcohol consumption and its relation to cardiovascular risk factors in British women. *British Medical Journal, 304*. pp. 80–83

Renaud, S. and De Lorgeril, M. (1992).Wine, alcohol, platelets, and the French paradox for coronary heart disease. *Lancet, 339*. 1523–1526

Rimm, E. B., Chan, J., Stampfer, M. J., Colditz, G. A. and Willett, W. C. (1995). Prospective study of cigarette smoking, alcohol use, and the risk of diabetes in men. *British Medical Journal, 310*. pp. 555–559

Rimm, E. B., Stampfer, M. J., Ascherio, A., Giovannucci, E., Colditz, A. and Willett, W. C. (1993). Vitamin E consumption and the risk of coronary heart disease in men. *New England Journal of Medicine, 328*. pp. 1450–1456

St Leger, A. S., Cochrane, A. L. and Moore, F. (1979). Factors associated with cardiac mortality in developed countries with particular reference to the consumption of wine. *Lancet, 1*. pp. 1017–1020

Stampfer, M. J., Hennekens, C. H., Manson, J. E., Colditz, G. A., Rosner, B. and Willett, W. C. (1993). Vitamin E consumption and the risk of coronary disease in women. *New England Journal of Medicine, 328*. pp. 1444–1449

Tunstall-Pedoe, H., Kuulasmaa, K., Amouyel, P., Arveiler, D., Rajakangas, A-m. and Pajak, A. (1994). Myocardial infarction and coronary deaths in the World Health Organization MONICA Project. Registration procedures, event rates, and case fatality rates in 38 populations from 21 countries in four continents. *Circulation, 90*. pp. 583–612

14 Large outbreak of Salmonella enterica serotype paratyphi B infection caused by goats' milk cheese, France, 1993: a case finding epidemiological study*

Jean-Claude Desenclos, Philippe Bouvet,
Elizabeth Benz-Lemoine, Francine Grimont,
Hélène Desqueyroux, Isabelle Rebière and
Patrick A. Grimont

Introduction

Salmonella enterica serotype *paratyphi B* causes sporadic gastroenteritis and, less frequently, paratyphoid fever (Benenson, 1990). Few foodborne outbreaks of *S paratyphi B* infection have been reported. In France two or more outbreaks have occurred in the past 10 years (Potelon *et al.*, 1989; Grimont and Bouvet, 1991). An outbreak in 1990 (277 cases) was possibly related to contaminated goats' milk cheese (Grimont and Bouvet, 1991). Unpasteurised dairy products have caused outbreaks of salmonellosis, campylobacteriosis, listeriosis, and the haemolytic-uraemic syndrome (Benenson, 1990). In France large amounts of many different types of raw milk cheeses are consumed, yet raw milk cheese has only rarely been incriminated in foodborne outbreaks.

We describe a large nationwide outbreak of *S paratyphi B* infection caused by unpasteurised goats' milk cheese.

Subjects and methods

Salmonella surveillance

In France surveillance for salmonellosis is carried out by the National Reference Centre for Salmonella and Shigella, which receives isolates for

* *British Medical Journal, 312* (13 January 1996), pp. 91–94.

serotyping from one third of the 4000 microbiology laboratories. For the past 12 years monthly trends have been computed for each serotype of *Salmonella* isolated. During the third week of October 1993 a nationwide increase in the number of *S paratyphi B* isolates submitted for typing was observed.

Epidemiological investigation

A case was defined as a resident of France from whom a specimen (stools, blood, or other body tissue) had been culture positive for *S paratyphi B* between 1 August and 30 November 1993. Cases were identified by reviewing isolates received by the National Reference Centre. Multiple isolates from the same patient were excluded. Additional cases were sought by district public health officers from local laboratories. For each case identified, the patient's sex and age (<1, 1–5, 6–14, 15–64, and ⩾65 years) and the date, site, region, and laboratory were recorded. Missing data were obtained by contacting the relevant laboratory.

After the outbreak was recognised a food questionnaire given to a few patients indicated that most had consumed brand A medium size round goats' milk cheese. Because a relation whith a similar cheese had been suggesed in the 1990 outbreak we hypothesised that this cheese was the vehicle of infection in the present outbreak. To test this hypothesis we conducted a case-control study. Patients were included as cases if they had *S paratyphi B* gastroenteritis)more than three loose stools daily) or septicaemia. For each case investigated a community control matched for age (within the ranges <1, 1–4, 5–14, 15–34, 35–44, 45–54, 55–64, and ⩾65 years), sex (for cases >5 only), and city of residence was sought from the telephone directory. People whose names (different spelling from the case name) came after the case name in the directory were called alphabetically until one was located who met the matching criteria. Potential controls who reported diarrhoea (more than three loose stools daily) in the previous three months were excluded.

Cases and matched controls (or their mothers if under 18) were interviewed by telephone by district public health physicians or a medical epidemiologist from the National Public Health Network using a standardised questionnaire. This was mainly targeted at milk products, particularly cow and goats' milk cheeses, and included questions on names and types of cheeses. Cases and controls were interviewed two to 12 weeks after the illness. Hence rather than ask them to try to recall the foods actually eaten during the three days before the illness we aimed at ascertaining their food preferences. Interviewers were not blinded to the subjects' case or control status.

Environmental investigation

In early November the processing plant (plant A) that produced the suspect cheese was inspected by a district veterinarian from the Ministry of Agriculture and one of us (EBL). Goats' milk sources, cheese production and storage, and the microbiological monitoring of milk and cheese produced at the plant between June and November 1993 were reviewed. In addition, stool specimens were obtained from goats, cows, dogs, a cat, and workers from a farm that had supplied plant A with milk found to be contaminated by *Salmonella*.

Laboratory investigations

Salmonella serotype *paratyphi B* isolates (human, milk, and cheese) were phage typed at the National Reference Centre for Enteric Molecular Typing by using Felix and Callow's (1951) international system. Human and food isolates were also subjected to genotypic IS 200 typing (Ezquerra *et al.*, 1993).

Statistical analysis

Isolation groups were calculated by age group and administrative region by using data from the 1990 French census as denominators (Institut National de la Statistique, 1991). Data from the case-control study were analysed by calculating univariate matched odds ratios and 95% confidence intervals (Schlesselman, 1982).

Results

Epidemiology

Two hundred and seventy three cases (4.3/million residents) were recorded (259 by the National Reference Centre, 14 by other laboratories). In 240 cases (88 per cent) *S paratyphi B* was isolated from stools, in 15 (5.5 per cent) it was isolated from blood, and in 14 (5 per cent) it was isolated from other tissue (site unknown for four isolates). Clinical details were obtained for 97 (36 per cent) patients by telephone interview. Thirty six (37 per cent) had been admitted to hospital and one died. Gastroenteritis was characterised by diarrhoea (three to over 20 stools daily, median 6) that lasted from three to 27 days (median 5 days), fever (>38°C; 80 cases), abdominal cramp (76 cases), nausea (33 cases), and vomiting (30 cases). Of the 259 isolates phage typed, 203 (78 per cent) belonged to phage type 1 var 3.

The outbreak began during the second week of August 1993 and continued till the second week of November (Figure 14.1). Most of the

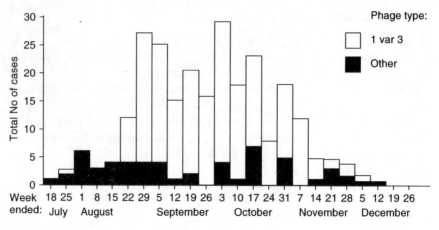

Figure 14.1   *Numbers of cases of* salmonella enterica *serotype* paratyphi B *infection, by week of isolation and phagetype, France, 1993*

infections were due to phage type 1 var 3. Cases were distributed nationally, however, the incidence was greatest in Poitou–Charentes (a traditional area of goats' milk cheese production) and the surrounding regions (Figure14.2). The isolation rate was highest among infants and children aged 1 to 5 years (Table 14.1).

Food questionnaires were completed for 72 pairs of cases and controls. Because most of the infections in the outbreak were attributed to phage type 1 var 3 the analysis was restricted to the 59 (82 per cent) pairs in which that phage type was isolated. The 59 cases did not differ from the total series of 203 patients infected with phage type 1 var 3 in age ($P = 0.9$), sex ($P = 0.9$), or region of isolation ($P = 0.2$). There was a trend towards an increased risk in the presence of an underlying illness (for example, diabetes, malignancy, treatment with corticosteroids, chemotherapy; odds ratio 2.0 (95 per cent confidence interval 0.6 to 6.7)).

Table 14.1   *Cases of Salmonella enterica serotype paratyphi B infection by age, France, August – November 1993*

Age (years)	No (%) of cases[a]	Rate per million population
<1	16 (6.0)	21.0
1–5	77 (29.1)	20.3
6–14	53 (20.0)	7.7
15–64	94 (35.5)	2.5
≥65	25 (9.4)	3.0

Note:
a Age missing for eight patients.

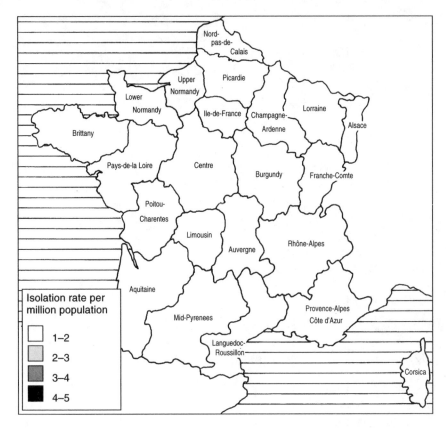

Figure 14.2 Salmonella enterica *serotype* paratyphi B *isolation rate per million poulation, by region, France, August – November 1993*

Analysis of the consumption of milk products showed a 3.8-fold greater risk of illness among people who ate goats' milk cheese (Table 14.2). For the subsequent analysis cheeses were categorised as brand A goats' milk cheese (a medium size round cheese), medium size round goats' milk cheese of unspecified brand, other types of goats' milk cheese, and non-goats' milk cheese. Compared with the risk of illness among people who did not eat goats' milk cheese, there was a 12-fold greater risk among those who ate brand A and a six-fold greater risk among those who ate medium size round goats' milk cheese of unspecified brand. There was no substantially increased risk of illness among people who ate other goats' milk cheeses (Table 14.2).

Environmental and microbiological investigations

Cheese A is made from raw goats' milk at a single plant and distributed to food stores and supermarkets nationally. Every other day two batches of cheese A are made (11,000 to 15,000 cheeses (200 g each) per batch),

Table 14.2   Cases of Salmonella enterica serotype paratyphi B infection (phage type 1 var 3) and controls by dairy food and type of goats' milk cheeses eaten, France, August – November 1993

Dairy food	No (%) of cases (total = 59)	No (%) of controls (total = 59)	Matched Odds ratio	95% confidence Interval
Milk	45 (76.3)	53 (89.8)	0.2	0.04 to 0.9
Cream	25 (42.4)	33 (55.9)	0.6	0.3 to 1.2
Cheese (any)	57 (96.6)	55 (93.2)	2.0	0.4 to 10.9
White cheese [a]	31 (52.5)	29 (50.9)	1.2	0.6 to 2.4
Cows' milk cheese	49 (83.1)	53 (89.8)	0.6	0.2 to 1.7
Goats' milk cheese	46 (78.0)	29 (49.2)	3.8	1.6 to 9.4
Types of goats' milk cheese [b, c]				
Brand A	32 (54.2)	10 (17.2)	12.0	1.6 to 92.3
Medium size round of unspecified brand	9 (15.3)	8 (13.8)	6.0	0.7 to 49.8
Other	5 (8.5)	10 (17.2)	1.7	0.4 to 7.0
None	13 (22.0)	30 (51.7)	1.0 (reference)	Reference

a   Data mising for two controls.
b   Matched odds ratios refer to no goats' milk cheese.
c   Data missing for one control.

each corresponding to a pool of 40 farms supplying goats' milk. Cheeses are stored for 11 days at the plant for maturation before distribution. The 'use by' date is 45 days after the cheeses leave the plant.

Before October 1993 internal control for *Salmonella* at the plant consisted of a weekly culture on five cheeses picked from a single batch. Then, on 6 October, one brand A cheese grew *Salmonella*, later typed as *paratyphi B*. Subsequently, from 7 October, all batches of cheese stored at the plant, milk pools, and milk from all the farms that supplied each pool were sampled daily for *Salmonella*. The district public health authorities remained unaware of these matters until 8 November, when the district public health physician contacted the district veterinarian's office about a possible link of the outbreak with cheese A. The milk pool corresponding to the batch that grew *S paratyphi B* on 6 October was also positive for *S paratyphi B* on 9 October but negative on the 7, 11, and 13 [October].

S paratyphi B was recovered from the milk of only one of the 40 suppliers. No salmonella was found in stool specimens from workers, cows, goats, and pets at the farm. Cheese A and goats' milk isolates belonged to the epidemic phage type (1 var 3). IS 200 genotypic typing was done on three human and four cheese A 1 var 3 isolates. All seven strains exhibited a common IS 200 pattern (profile 2.7).

Around 30 tonnes of cheese, corresponding to the batches stored at the plant between 21 September and 6 October, were destroyed after the isolation of *S paratyphi B* from cheese A, and cheese production from the relevant milk pool was pasteurised until daily *Salmonella* control of each batch was implemented. Subsequently all batches produced have been tested for *Salmonella* on day 1 (milk pool), on days 2 and 6 of the maturation process, and on days 9 and 12 (packaging and distribution, respectively).

Discussion

This large nationwide outbreak of salmonellosis was caused by unpasteurised goats' milk cheese made in a single plant. Evidence comes from the results of the case control study and the isolation from cheese A and goats' milk of an *S paratyphi B* strain of the same phage type and IS 200 pattern as the epidemic strain. The increased risk suggested in the case-control study for medium size round goats' milk cheese of unspecified brand may reflect consumption of cheese A, because this exposure category may have included people who ate cheese A but could not recall the brand name.

Contamination of the milk pool from which one of the two batches was made originated from a single farm. However, the precise source of infection (human, animal, or environmental) was not identified. The duration of the outbreak (three months) indicated that cheese A had been contaminated for a similar period, probably from mid-June (date of onset of the epidemic minus three days for the incubation period, 11 days for cheese maturation, and 45 days before the use by date). The outbreak was detected during the third week of October, when contamination had gone unnoticed for almost three months. Detection of contamination at the plant in early October was not notified to the authorities and so did not contribute to faster recognition of the outbreak. (Routine micro-biological control programmes in food processing plants are carried out voluntarily by producers to reduce the risk of foodborne infections; however, the results are not required to be notified to public health authorities.) Routine daily control of each batch for *Salmonella* would have detected the contamination much earlier.

In France only one third of laboratories send isolates of *Salmonella* for typing. Furthermore, only about 6 per cent of patients with diarrhoea have a stool culture (Chauvin *et al.*, 1993) and some patients with diarrhoea do not see a doctor at all. Hence the true size of the epidemic was probably much underestimated. Several thousands of cases may have occurred because of contamination of the cheese.

Despite the amount of raw milk cheese consumed daily in France outbreaks of infection remain comparatively rare (Grimont and Bouvet, 1991; Casenove *et al.*, 1993). In France pasteurisation of raw milk cheeses is not feasible for cultural, social, and economic reasons. Strategies for preventing infection by raw milk cheeses should therefore be aimed at both producers and consumers. Strict and carefully planned hazard analysis critical control point procedures should be developed and implemented for unpasteurised dairy products (Commission of the Codex Alimentarius, 1993). As part of this procedure any batch of cheese made from raw milk should be closely monitored for *Salmonella* and not be distributed until known to be clear. Producers should also report positive results of end production internal sampling to public health authorities. Consumers – particularly those susceptible to infectious diseases (for example, infants, elderly people, immunocompromised patients) – should also be warned that a nil risk cannot be warranted for raw milk products.

Key messages

- Contaminated raw goats' milk cheese produced by a single processing plant caused a three month nationwide outbreak of *Salmonella paratyphi B* infection in France in 1993
- Though the cheese was probably contaminated for more than two months, the outbreak continued undetected for a further two months
- The source of the infection was goats' milk from one of the 40 farms that supplied the cheese processing plant
- Internal microbiological monitoring at the plant was not sensitive

enough to detect the salmonella contamination initially

- Any batch of unpasteurised cheese or milk product should be closely monitored for *Salmonella* and should not be distributed until known to be clear

Notes

We thank the following public health physicians who participated: M. Andrillon, A Armangaud, C Barbier, F Belingard, D Bousquet, E Boutin, V Bleuzè, B Cabo, C Cazenave, F Charlet, M Charron, M J Communal, M Cunnac, M Desvaux, M C Dubois, M L Ferial, M Feltin, J Y Goarant, L Gossel, A Hetru, M Juge, A Meunier, J Patureau, C Piau, E Pons, F Quittançon, and P Rogez (Directions Départementales de l'Action Sanitaire et Sociale); V Goulet, B Hubert, N Lacan, E Laurent, I Mehl-Augier, R Pinget, and E Sariot (Réseau National de Santé Publique); A Lepoutre and C Moyse (Direction Générale de la Santé). We also thank public health veterinarian F Peyre (Direction des Services Vétérinaires des Deux-Sevres).

Funding This study was conducted as part of routine activities in the institutions concerned. The Réseau National de Santé Publique is funded by the Ministère de la Santé et de l'Assurance Maladie; the Centre National de Référence des Salmonella-Shigella and the Centre National de Référence de Typage Moléculaire Entérique are funded by the Ministère de la Santé et de l'Assurance Maladie and the Pasteur Institute; the Direction Départementale des Affaires Sanitaires et Sociales des Deux-Sèvres is funded by the Ministère de la Santé et de l'Assurance Maladie.

Conflict of interest: None.

References

Benenson, A. S. (1990). *Control of Communicable Diseases in Man*. Washington, DC: American Public Health Association.

Bille, J. (1990). Epidemiology of human listeriosis in Europe with special reference to the Swiss outbreak. In: Miller, A. J., Smith, J. L. and Somkuti, G. A. (eds) (1990). *Foodborne listeriosis*. Amsterdam: Elsevier, 71–4.

Cazenave, Desenclos, J. C., Maillot, E., Benoit, S., Deschenes, G. and Baron, S. (1993). Eclosion de syndrome hémolytique et urémique (SHU) dans une communauté rurale du Cher. *Bulletin Epidémiologique Hebdomadaire*, 48, 222–4

Chauvin, P., Diaz, C., Garnerin, P., Guiget, M., Massari, V. and Saidi, Y. *et al*. Réseau National Télé-informatique de surveillance et d'information sur les maladies transmissibles: bilan de la surveillance épidémiologique des médecins sentinelles en 1992. (1993). *Bulletin Epidémiologique Hebdomadaire*, 21, 93–6.

Commission of the Codex Alimentarius. (1993). *Guidelines for the application of the hazard analysis critical control point (HACCP) system*. Rome: Food and Agricultural Organisation (United Nations), World Health Organisation, (Codex alimentarius, alinorm 93/13A, appendix II.).

Ezquerre, E., Burnens, A., Jones, C. and Stanley, J. (1993). Genotypic typing and phylogenetic analysis of Salmonella paratyphi B and S java with IS 200. *Journal of General Microbiology*, 139, 2409–12.

Felix, A., Callow, B. R. (1951) Paratyphoid.B-Vi phage-typing. *Lancet*, ii, 10–4.

Grimont, P. A. D. and Bouvet, P. (1991). Les salmonelloses et les shigelloses en 1990 en France. *Bulletin Epidémiologique Hebdomadaire*, 25, 102.

Institut National de la Statistique (1991). *Recensement général de la population de 1990: logement, population, emploi; évolutions 1975–1990*. Paris: Ministère de l'Economie, des

Finances et du Budget, INS.

Linnan, M. J., Mascola, L., Lou, X. D., Goulet, V., May, S. and Salminen, C. *et al.* (1985). Epidemic listerosis associated with Mexican-style cheese. *New England Journal of Medicine, 319*, 823–9.

Potelon, J. L. , Ferley, J. P., Zmirou, D. and Entressangle, S. (1989). Epidémie de Salmonella paratyphi java dans une commune de l'Isère, en octobre 1988. *Bulletin Epidémiologique Hebdomadaire, 24*, 98–9.

Robinson, D. A., Edgar, W. J., Gibson, G. L., Matchett, A. A. and Robertson, L. (1979). Campylobacter enteridis associated with consumption of unpasteurised milk. *British Medical Journal, i,* 1171–3.

Robinson, D. A. and Jones, D. M. (1981). *British Medical Journal, 282*, 1374–6.

Schlesselman, J. J. (1982). *Case-control studies: design, conduct and analysis.* New York: Oxford University Press.

Talbot, J. C. Wancob, D. W., Robertson, L. and Parrell, I. D. (1967). A milk-borne outbreak of food poisoning due to Salmonella paratyphi B var java. *Public Health, 81,* 191–7.

Wright, E. P., Tillett, H. E., Hague, J. T., Clegg, F. G., Darnell, R. and Culshaw, J. A., *et al.* (1983).Milk-borne Campylobacter enteridis in a rural area. *Journal of Hygiene (Cambridge), 91,* 227–33.

15 *Epidemiology - to be taken with care*[*]

Joe H. Abramson

Epidemiology embraces not only the study of the distribution and determinants of health-related states and events in groups and populations, but also, according to the *Dictionary of Epidemiology* (Last, 1995), the application of this study to the control of health problems.

Epidemiological studies are not limited to diseases, deaths, disabilities, and other disorders. They encompass healthy growth and development, physical fitness, and other dimensions of positive health, as well as social, behavioural, environmental and other factors (including health attitudes and practices and the provision and use of health services) that influence health. This broad scope of interest and the wide range of methods (observational and experimental, quantitative and qualitative) available for the study of groups and populations enable epidemiology to supply much of the information required for the planning, implementation, monitoring and evaluation of health care, including health education and other intervention programmes aimed at enhancing the health status of a population or population sector. Epidemiology is the foundation science of public health (Detels, 1991).

But there is a need for caution – all that glitters is not gold. The results of epidemiological studies may sometimes be unhelpful or even misleading, and should never be utilised uncritically. Problems of various kinds may arise, singly or in combination. Ways of minimising these problems when doing epidemiological studies, and of recognising and handling them when interpreting findings, are central topics of all epidemiology teaching.

The main questions to be asked before using epidemiological results are:

1. Are the results accurately known?
2. How valid are the findings?
3. How valid are the inferences drawn from the findings?
4. How relevant is the information?
5. Is the information sufficient?

---

[*] Commissioned for this volume.

1 Accurate knowledge of the results

An obvious precaution is that decisions should not be based on inaccurate reports or impressions. Press, radio and television reports, in particular, may be misleading. 'Journalism is an activity with no scientific methodology' (de Semir, 1996). In the hunt for 'news', prominence may be given not only to weak studies, but to 'the one positive result in a sea of negative data' (Mann, 1995). The blame for these distortions sometimes lies with investigators or research institutions, who may make exaggerated claims that go beyond what is said in the published study report (Pini, 1995, Mann, 1995). Where possible, reliance should be placed only on original study reports or experts who have read them.

Selective reporting or use of results is especially hazardous when vested interests or political issues are involved, as at the start of the furore concerning bovine spongiform encephalopathy ('mad cow disease') in Britain in 1996; the borderline between selective reporting and deliberate misinformation may then become tenuous. If (rather presumptuously) we refer to epidemiological results as 'the truth', the aim should be to know the truth, the whole truth, and nothing but the truth.

It is unwise to rely on a single study if others are available. 'What medical journals publish is not received wisdom, but rather working papers . . . Each study becomes a piece of a puzzle that, when assembled, will help either to confirm or to refute a hypothesis' (Angell and Kassirer, 1994). Different studies of the same topic often produce different information, as a result of chance variation or differences in study methods or circumstances or between study populations. Examples of contradictory findings abound (Angell and Kassirer, 1994; Taubes, 1995). But each new study is reported in isolation, as a new breakthrough, provoking the question:

> Why can't researchers get it straight the first time?' (Angell and Kassirer, 1994)

A single study should not be relied on, but obtaining a fuller picture is not always easy. If meta-analyses have been done, they are thus particularly useful. These are overviews of research on a specific topic, in which studies are systematically sought, methods are appraised, findings are compared, the reasons for differences are explored, and an endeavour is made (using appropriate statistical methods) to reach balanced overall conclusions. An important recent advance in this area is the development of the Cochrane Collaboration, an international network of individuals and institutions committed to preparing, maintaining, and disseminating systematic reviews of the effects of health care (Chalmers, 1993).

Validity of findings

No epidemiological study is perfect, and a critical appraisal of the design and methods is always advisable before deciding whether to use the findings.

The main consideration is the possibility that the findings may be biased, that is, that they may deviate from the truth. Ostensible findings may be artefacts. Bias is usually caused by shortcomings either in the selection of individuals or groups for study (selection bias) or in the collection, recording, coding or analysis of data (information bias). Both forms of bias may come about in many ways, some avoidable and some unavoidable, and it may or may not be possible to appraise their direction and magnitude, and compensate for their effects. The problems are generally methodological ones, although bias may also (rarely) result from conscious fraud or (more often) from lesser misdemeanours by scientists:

> Inventing data would clearly be wrong; suppression of inconvenient results would be less than honest. Yet they need not think too badly of themselves if they gloss over the study's methodological shortcomings, optimise the statistical analysis, cite published work selectively. (Lancet, 1995)

There may also be unconscious subjective processes whereby the investigator's preconceived opinions and preferences result in choices that lead to one-sided findings. Particular caution may be advisable with studies financed by tobacco firms or other manufacturers, or political or other bodies with vested interests; it is then prudent to be especially insistent on seeking confirmatory evidence elsewhere. A health worker with a grounding in basic epidemiological methods should have no difficulty in recognising a study's main weak points with respect to sampling, selection of control groups, operational definitions of variables, methods of data-collection, etc. Checklists are available, e.g. for appraising case-control studies (Stolley and Schlesselman, 1982, Lichtenstein *et al.*, 1987) and trials (Chalmers *et al.*, 1990). Study methods and their impact on the validity of information are considered in more detail by (*inter alia*) Abramson (1990, 1991), Berkelman and Buehler (1991), Feinleib *et al.* (1991), Greenberg and Ibrahim (1991), Hulley and Cummings (1988), Puska (1991), Schlesselman (1982) and Vaughan and Morrow (1989).

A critical appraisal of study methods requires basic epidemiological know-how – which is of course one of the reasons why it is so important for all health workers to have some training in epidemiology. Lacking this, an assessment by someone more knowledgeable should be sought. Unfortunately there are no simple short-cuts. Reliance on the reputation of the researchers, the sponsoring agency, or the journal in which the results are published, for example, may be misleading. Nor is it enough to know what techniques were used, without considering the details of their use. Sampling that is random in name only, badly-chosen controls, unnecessary matching, injudicious statistical testing, confidence interval estimation in the absence of random processes or in the presence of bias or confounding variables and other abuses may yield deceptive findings.

Validity of inferences drawn from the findings

However valid the factual findings may be, the conclusions drawn from them may be questionable, particularly in analytic studies that try to explain associations between variables, where interpretation may require considerable skill and experience. It is obviously incorrect to conclude that there is a cause–effect relationship, just because an association has been found. A study of dog-bites showed that dogs kept chained were much likelier than unchained dogs to bite non-household members, but the conclusion that:

> owners may be able to . . . modify risk by . . . not keeping them chained. (Gershman, 1992)

was questionable, and was later toned down to:

> A dog may be chained as the result of having exhibited aggressive behavior which itself may be a risk factor for biting, rather than chaining somehow causing a dog to bite. (Gershman *et al.*, 1994)

Sometimes it is enough to know that a characteristic is associated with a disease, whatever the explanation. This may permit use of the characteristic as a screening test that identifies individuals or groups especially likely to have the disease, or as a risk marker that identifies those especially likely to contract the disease in the future. These uses do not require a causal relationship. As an example, a 10-year follow-up study of 90 000 American women showed that the risk of a hip fracture was more than twice as high for women at least 5'8" tall than for women under 5'2", after allowing for effects connected with age, obesity and other variables. This led to the suggestion that 'taller elderly women should be advised to consider preventive measures' (Hemenway *et al.*, 1995). This recommendation is based solely on the presence of the association; tallness is used as a risk marker, and whether or not it is a contributory cause (maybe because taller women fall from a greater height) is irrelevant.

But data interpretation becomes much more difficult if etiologic explanations are wanted. As an example, a study of 994 men and women born in Hertfordshire, UK, in 1920–30 showed that those who had sucked a dummy (pacifier) in their first year of life, according to health records maintained at that time, had a lower average IQ score as adults (Gale and Martyn, 1996). About 69 per cent of them had a lower score than the mean score of those who had not used dummies. This might mean that dummy-sucking impairs cognitive development (maybe because of drowsiness or because the baby is more placid and therefore receives less attention). In other words, the dummy may be a true risk factor (i.e. a *maker*, rather than only a *marker*, of risk). But other explanations must be explored and rejected before an etiologic inference can be accepted. First, the association may be a chance one; a significance test showed this to be very improbable ($P < 0.0001$). Also, a relationship may occur between variables even if they are not causally linked, if they share associations with other (confounding) variables. Appropriate analyses yielded no evidence that the dummy–IQ connection could be attributed in this way to links with mother's age, father's occupation, birth rank, method of feeding, or weight in infancy. But other possible explanations could not be tested; for example, maybe parents who used dummies had weaker parenting skills or were less intelligent (Feldman and Feldman, 1996) or less interested in their children's health, since dummies were at that time regarded as health hazards by child-care experts, and health workers in Hertfordshire specifically advised against their use. Nor was consideration given to differences in the presence or strength of the dummy–IQ association in different subgroups (e.g. males and females), reflecting possible modifying effects of other variables on the association; interactions of this sort often throw light on causal processes. Also, there might be a causal association in the other direction – 'perhaps babies who are willing to accept a dummy . . . are slightly less intelligent'. The association thus remained unexplained.

Even had there been findings pointing to the unlikeliness of all these other explanations, most epidemiologists would be inclined to consider the dummy–IQ association as causal only if there was additional positive evidence (Hill, 1965; Susser, 1973, 1986), such as a correlation with the time spent dummy-sucking (a dose–response relationship) and, especially, consistency of the finding in different studies.

The validity of inferences about causation can thus not be taken for granted. It depends on whether they are grounded on valid data, analytical procedures that allow for possible confounding and modifying effects, and a proper approach and sound judgement in data interpretation. The interpretation of evidence is a matter of judgement, and unfortunately judges may disagree. Usually no major problem arises; but sometimes the conclusions are debatable, or obviously flawed.

Weak associations are especially likely to be due to chance, bias or con-founding variables (American Health Foundation, 1982), and unless the association has been confirmed repeatedly many epidemiologists demand at least a doubling (some say trebling or quadrupling) of risk before they will consider a cause-and-effect relationship, saying that 'it is so easy to be fooled that it is impossible to believe less-than-stunning results' (Taubes, 1995). But factors that increase risk only slightly can have a huge effect on the public's health if they are sufficiently widespread. This has been called 'the Catch-22 of modern epidemiology' (Taubes, 1995).

There is an extreme view, which most epidemiologists do not share, that epidemiological evidence alone, without laboratory and clinical studies that support and explain a causal relationship, can never be conclusive enough to warrant a preventive programme (Charlton, 1995). In this view, a preventive strategy at the population level is justified only if the 'black box' concealing the mysteries of causal mechanisms (Skrabenek, 1994) has been opened. Historical examples that refute this view include: the link between a dearth of fresh fruit and scurvy, demonstrated in 1753, long before vitamins were thought of (Lind, 1753); between exposure to soot and scrotal cancer, in 1775, when the carcinogenic role of polycyclic aromatic hydrocarbons was undreamt of (Pott, 1775); between polluted water and cholera, in 1855, before bacteria had been discovered (Snow, 1855); between a poor diet and pellagra in the second decade of the 20th century, when this was thought to be a communicable disease (Terris, 1964); and between smoking and lung cancer and other diseases before the pathogenetic mechanisms were understood (Doll and Hill, 1964; Hammond, 1966; Kahn, 1966). The link between smoking and cancer aroused a productive controversy (Gail, 1996), which culminated in the formulation of the criteria for drawing causal conclusions (Hill, 1965; Susser, 1973, 1986) – the 'rules of evidence' – now used by most epidemiologists.

A recent example is the finding that babies put to sleep on their stomachs have a higher risk of cot deaths (sudden infant death syndrome [SIDS]). Although the reasons for this association are as yet unclear, the recommendation that healthy infants should be put to sleep on their backs or sides (Kattwinkel *et al.*, 1992) has been applied in 'Back-to-Sleep' campaigns in the United Kingdom, New Zealand, Holland and other countries. These have been followed by appreciable reductions in cot deaths, without apparent decreases in other known risk factors (Court, 1995; Hunt, 1994; Wigfield *et al.*, 1994; Willinger, 1995). Interactions discovered in epidemiological studies, such as an increase in the risk attached to prone sleeping if no adult sleeps in the room (Scragg et al. 1996) or if the baby has very warm clothes or covers (Williams *et al.*, 1996) may, if confirmed, lead to a better understanding of the causal mechanisms.

There is often a need to decide whether to accept a specific causal explanation (knowing that this may later turn out to be incorrect) as a basis for action, whether to design a programme that caters for alternative etiologic possibilities, or whether to defer action.

Data interpretation and its problems are considered in more detail by (*inter alia*) Abramson (1994), Greenland (1991) and Susser (1973), symposia edited by Greenland (1987) and Rothman (1988), and most epidemiology textbooks. For statistical methods for use in analysing epidemiological findings, see Gahlinger and Abramson (1995), Kahn and Sempos (1989) and Selvin (1996).

How relevant is the information?

In a health care context, the epidemiological findings and inferences in question may not be very relevant to the specific group or population under consideration.

This problem does not arise if this group or population is the one that was studied, which is of course why emphasis is placed on local epidemiological studies (community diagnosis, needs assessment) in community-oriented primary health care (Kark, 1981; Abramson, 1988), health care in schools and work-places, district health care (Vaughan and Morrow, 1989), and other settings.

But the validity of generalisations from a study sample or population to another population (the 'external validity' of the study) always requires consideration. Populations differ in their health problems and in the occurrence of risk and protective factors; causal processes that are important in one population may be unimportant in another; and there is wide variation in circumstances that may influence the effectiveness of interventions. In planning a health promotion programme in a specific community, can use be made of information derived from a neighbouring or similar community, or of information collected at a national level? When planning a new programme, to what extent is it justifiable to use the results of evaluative studies conducted elsewhere? Are the results of studies of men applicable to women? Are results applicable across ethnic or age categories? Such questions may be hard to answer.

Is the information sufficient?

However valid and relevant, the information may not suffice for the purpose for which it is required, and there may be a need for more information about the population whose care is under consideration (i.e. a fuller community diagnosis) or for information from epidemiological studies elsewhere, as well as for information (e.g. on costs) from non-epidemiological sources.

The adequacy of the information will depend on the purpose for which it is required. For example, to decide whether there is a sufficiently strong case to warrant intervention, it is not enough to know that a problem exists, or even to have a quantitative measure of its occurrence. Three other main categories of information may be needed:

1. *Information about the importance of the problem* – e.g. its impact on mortality or the quality of life, and its relative importance compared with other problems competing for the same resources. A measure of impact may be more informative than a risk ratio; it is more helpful to know that 26–43 per cent of various asthma-like symptoms in young women in towns in East Anglia are attributable to the use of gas for cooking (Jarvis *et al.*, 1996; Brauer and Kennedy, 1996) than to know that the risk of these symptoms is elevated slightly in homes that use gas stoves.
2. *Facts relevant to the feasibility of intervention.* In the specific context, appraisal of feasibility may require information not only about costs and the availability of economic, professional and other resources, but about the community's felt needs and demands, its readiness and capacity to participate, prevalent attitudes and health practices, the nature and extent of the care presently available and given, the readiness of educational, welfare and other agencies to play their part, and so on.
3. *Information with a bearing on the predicted effectiveness and possible harmful effects of interventions*, taking account of biological, social, cultural and economic characteristics of the population (perceptions of the problem, probable compliance, etc.) and the results of evaluative studies elsewhere.

If it is intended to single out high-risk groups for special attention in a preventive programme, it is not enough to know that the probability that the disease or other problem will occur is higher – even many times so – when a given risk marker is present. Consideration must also be given to such features as the marker's estimated sensitivity and predictive value. The marker cannot be very helpful if it identifies only a small fraction of prospective cases; and if it identifies very many people who are not prospective cases this will impair the programme's cost-effectiveness and ethical justification. It may be helpful to know how many people must avoid exposure to a risk factor in order to prevent one case.

Similar considerations arise if screening tests are to be used to identify people with a high probability of currently having a particular disorder. Decisions may require such information as that 4000 women had to be screened to prevent each death from breast cancer, and about 400 000 tests and 200 biopsies are required to prevent one case of cervical cancer (Wall, 1995).

If it is proposed to communicate information to members of the public, community leaders, or decision-makers in order to modify individual behaviour or public policy, it is important to have the right facts for this purpose, expressed in language (or pictures) that non-professionals will easily understand. Information about smoking hazards, for example, might include estimates of the percentages of deaths, cases and hospital admissions that are attributable to smoking, and the effect on average life expectancy. As a final illustration, when appraising the value of a programme it may not be enough to know that the objective e.g. a reduction in the prevalence of hypertension – has been achieved. However 'encouraging this may be, the outcome cannot (except in a well-controlled programme trial) be attributed to the programme unless other possible explanations have been explored and there is also supportive evidence from a process evaluation (a look into the 'black box' concealing the programme's mechanism) providing information on coverage, the performance of programme activities, utilisation of services, compliance with treatment, etc.

Conclusion

Information alone cannot modify health. Health educators have long abandoned the simplistic idea that the transfer of information will itself produce changes in individual health behaviour. At a public policy level, decision-makers are influenced by powerful factors other than the information at their disposal, which they sometimes reject or ignore.

But there is no doubt that if health care is to be planned rationally and provided effectively, appropriate information – especially from epidemiological sources – is essential; or that the communication of information is one of the tools that, used in unison, can modify behaviour and policy.

The availability of suitable information depends, ultimately, on epidemiologists' perception of their role in health promotion and on the development of epidemiological theory and methods to fulfil this function (Wall, 1995). The agenda for epidemiologists interested in applications to health promotion includes the following requirements:

1. A macrosocial view (Susser, 1987) – more attention to societal factors, such as economic, political and ideological processes and their interrelationships with health and health care.
2. Improved methods of community diagnosis and surveillance, and methods of monitoring health programmes in local communities, schools and work-places.
3. Development of methods of measuring and predicting the outcomes of interventions, in terms relevant to the interests of decision-makers and the public.
4. Development of rapid epidemiological methods (Smith, 1989; Scrimshaw and Hurtado, 1987) that can provide real-time answers to practical questions.

5. Improved techniques of meta-analysis for nonexperimental studies, especially the exploration of reasons for heterogeneous findings (Petitti, 1994).
6. Improved methods of communication with users of epidemiological information – health workers, decision-makers, mass media, and the public. Epidemiologists should make recommendations on whether and how their results should be applied in practice, and not just 'light the touch paper and then stand back' (Pharaoh, 1996).

The importance of epidemiology in health promotion is unquestioned. Even critics who say that epidemiology relies heavily on judgement, that 'epidemiological attribution of causation is not a science but an activity more akin to the arguing of a case in law: based on evidence but not dictated by the evidence', and that it cannot at present produce predictions as reliable as those produced by some other scientific disciplines (Charlton, 1996), do not question that it can bring together evidence in a way that permits decision-making in situations where there is no completely valid answer.

But the available information in a given study or at a given time may be defective, judgement may be variable or faulty, and external validity may be limited, so that it is not surprising that conflicting conclusions are often reached, or that reversals sometimes occur as new knowledge replaces old. Every review of controlled trials published by the Cochrane Collaboration is accompanied by a quotation from Xenophan (570–475 BC): 'Through seeking we may learn and know things better. But as for certain truth, no man hath known it, for all is but a woven web of guesses' (Chalmers, 1995).

Epidemiological information should never be accepted with undue haste or blind trust.

References

Abramson, J. H. (1988). Community-oriented primary care – strategy, approaches, and practice: A review, *Public Health Reviews*, 16, 35–98.

Abramson, J. H. (1990). *Survey Methods in Community Medicine: Epidemiological studies, programme evaluation, clinical trials*, 4th edn. Edinburgh: Churchill Livingstone.

Abramson, J. H. (1991). Cross-sectional studies. In Holland, W. W., Detels, R. and Knox, G. (eds), *Oxford Textbook of Public Health*, 2nd edn, 2. *Methods of Public Health*. Oxford: Oxford University Press, 107–120.

Abramson, J. H. (1994). *Making Sense of Data: A self-instruction manual on the interpretation of epidemiologic data*, 2nd edn, New York: Oxford University Press.

American Health Foundation (1982). Conference report: weak associations in epidemiology and their interpretation, *Preventive Medicine, 11*, 464–476.

Angell, M. and Kassirer, J. P. (1994). Clinical research – what should the public believe?, *New England Journal of Medicine, 331*, 189–190.

Berkelman, R. L. and Buehler, J. W. (1991). Surveillance. In Holland, W. W., Detels, R. and Knox, G. (eds), *Oxford Textbook of Public Health*, 2nd edn, 2, *Methods of Public Health*. Oxford: Oxford University Press, 161–176.

Brauer, M. and Kennedy, S. M. (1996). Gas stoves and respiratory health, *Lancet, 347*, 412.

Chalmers, I. (1993). The Cochrane Collaboration: preparing, maintaining and disseminating systematic reviews of the effects of health care, *Annals of the New York Academy of Sciences, 703*, 156–63.

Chalmers, I. (1995). What would Archie Cochrane have said? *Lancet, 346*, 1300.

Chalmers, I., Adams, M., Dickersin, K., Hetherington, J., Tarnow- Mordi, W., Meinert, C., Tonascia, S. and Chalmers, T. C. (1990). A cohort study of summary reports of clinical trials, *JAMA, 263*, 1401–1405.

Charlton, B. G. (1995). A critique of Geoffrey Rose's 'population strategy' for preventive medicine, *Journal of the Royal Society of Medicine, 88*, 607–610.

Charlton, B. G. (1996). Attribution of causation in epidemiology: chain or mosaic?, *Journal of Clinical Epidemiology, 49*, 105–107.

Court, C. (1995). Britain: Incidence reduced by two thirds in five years, *British Medical Journal, 310*, 7–8.

De Semir, V. (1996). What is newsworthy?, *Lancet, 347*, 1163–1166.

Detels, R. (1991). Epidemiology: the foundation of public health. In Holland, W. W., Detels, R. and Knox, G., (eds), *Oxford Textbook of Public Health*, 2nd edn, 2, *Methods of Public Health*. Oxford: Oxford University Press, 285–291.

Doll, R. and Hill, A. B. (1964). Mortality in relation to smoking: ten years' observations of British doctors, *British Medical Journal, 1*, 1399–1410, 1460–1467.

Feinleib, M., Breslow, N. E. and Detels, R. (1991). Cohort studies. In Holland, W. W., Detels, R. and Knox, G. (eds), *Oxford Textbook of Public Health*, 2nd edn, 2, *Methods of Public Health*. Oxford: Oxford University Press, 145–159.

Feldman, W. and Feldman, M. E. (1996). The intelligence on infant feeding, *Lancet, 347*, 1057.

Gahlinger, P. M. and Abramson, J. H. (1995). *Computer Programs for Epidemiologic Analysis: PEPI Version 2*. Stone Mountain, Georgia: USD, Inc.

Gail, M. H. (1996). Statistics in action, *Journal of the American Statistical Association, 91*, 1–13.

Gale, C. R. and Martyn, C.N. (1996). Breastfeeding, dummy use, and adult intelligence, *Lancet, 347*, 1072–1075.

Gershman, K. (1992). Case-control study of which dogs bite (abstract), *American Journal of Epidemiology, 138*, 593.

Gershman, K. A., Sacks, J. J. and Wright, J. C. (1994). Which dogs bite? A case-control study of risk factors, *Pediatrics, 93*, 913–917.

Greenberg, R. S. and Ibrahim, M. A. (1991). The case-control study. In Holland, W. W., Detels, R. and Knox, G. (eds), *Oxford Textbook of Public Health*, 2nd edn, 2, *Methods of Public Health*. Oxford: Oxford University Press, 121–143.

Greenland, S. (1991). Concepts of validity in epidemiological research. In Holland, W. W., Detels, R. and Knox, G. (eds.) *Oxford Textbook of Public Health*, 2nd edn, 2, *Methods of Public Health*. Oxford: Oxford University Press, 254–270.

Greenland, S., (ed.) (1987). *Evolution of Epidemiologic Ideas: Annotated readings on concepts and methods*, Chestnut Hill, MA.: Epidemiology Resources Inc.

Hammond, E. C. (1966). Smoking in relation to the death rates on one million men and women. In Haenszel, W. (ed.), *Epidemiological Approaches to the Study of Cancer and Other Chronic Diseases*. Bethesda, M.: Public Health Service, US Department of Health, Education and Welfare, *National Cancer Institute Monograph, 19*, 127–204.

Hemenway, D., Feskanich, D. and Colditz, D. A. (1995). Body height and risk fracture: a cohort study of 90,000 women, *International Journal of Epidemiology, 24*, 783–786.

Hill, A. B. (1965). The environment and disease: association or causation?, *Proceedings of the Royal Society of Medicine, 58*, 295–300, reprinted in Greenland, S. (ed.) (1987) *Evolution of Epidemiologic Ideas: Annotated readings on concepts and methods*. Chestnut Hill, MA: Epidemiology Resources Inc.

Hulley, S.P. and Cummings, S. R. (eds) (1988). *Designing Clinical Research.* Baltimore: Williams & Wilkins.

Hunt, C. E. (1994). Infant sleep position and sudden infant death syndrome risk: a time for change, *Pediatrics, 94,* 105–107.

Jarvis, D., Chinn, S., Luczynska, C. and Burney, P. (1996). Association of respiratory symptoms and lung function in young adults with use of domestic gas appliances, *Lancet, 347,* 426–431.

Kahn, H. A. (1966). The Dorn study of smoking and mortality among US veterans: report on eight and one-half years of observation. In Haenszel, W. (ed.) *Epidemiological Approaches to the Study of Cancer and Other Chronic Diseases.* Bethesda, M.: Public Health Service, US Department of Health, Education and Welfare, *National Cancer Institute Monograph, 19,* 1–125.

Kahn, H. A. and Sempos, C. T. (1989). *Statistical Methods in Epidemiology.* New York: Oxford University Press.

Kark, S. L. (1981). *The Practice of Community-Oriented Primary Health Care.* New York: Appleton-Century-Crofts, reprinted (1989), Jerusalem: Akademon (Hebrew University).

Kattwinkel, J., Brooks, J. and Myerberg, D. (1992). Positioning and SIDS: AAP task force on infant positioning and SIDS, *Pediatrics, 89,* 1120–1126.

Lancet (1995). Editorial: *Shall we nim a horse?, Lancet, 345,* 1585–1586.

Last, J. M. (ed.), (1995). *A Dictionary of Epidemiology,* 3rd edn. New York: Oxford University Press.

Lichtenstein, M.J., Mulrow, C. D. and Elwood, P. C. (1987). Guidelines for reading case-control studies, *Journal of Chronic Diseases, 40,* 893–903.

Lind, J. (1753). *A Treatise of the Scurvy.* Edinburgh: Sands, Murray & Cochrane, reprinted (1953), Edinburgh: Edinburgh University Press.

Mann, C. C. (1995). Press coverage: leaving out the big picture, *Science, 269,* 166.

Petitti, D. B. (1994). *Meta-Analysis, Decision Analysis and Cost-Effectiveness Analysis: Methods for quantitative synthesis in medicine.* New York: Oxford University Press.

Pharaoh, P. (1996). Bed-sharing and sudden infant death, *Lancet, 347,* 2.

Pini, P. (1995). Media wars, *Lancet, 346,* 1681–1683.

Pott, P. (1775). Reproduced in Potter, M. (1963). *Percival Pott's Contribution to Cancer Research.* Washington, DC: *National Cancer Institute Monograph,* 10.

Puska, P. (1991). Intervention and experimental studies. In Holland, W. W., Detels, R. and Knox, G. (eds.) *Oxford Textbook of Public Health,* 2nd edn, 2, *Methods of Public Health.* Oxford: Oxford University Press, 177–187.

Rothman, K.J., (ed) (1988). *Causal Inference.* Chestnut Hill, MA.: Epidemiology Resources Inc.

Schlesselman, J. J. (1982). *Case-control studies: Design, conduct, analysis.* New York: Oxford University Press.

Scragg, R. K. R., Mitchell, E. A., Stewart, A. W., Ford, R. P. K., Taylor, B. J., Hassall, I. B., Williams, S. M. and Thompson, J. M. D. (1996). Infant room-sharing and prone sleep position in sudden infant death syndrome, *Lancet, 347,* 7–11.

Scrimshaw, S. C. M. and Hurtado, E. (1987). *Rapid Assessment Procedures for Nutrition and Primary Health Care: Anthropological approaches to improving programme effectiveness.* Los Angeles: UCLA Latin American Center Publications.

Selvin, S. (1996). *Statistical Analysis of Epidemiologic Data,* 2nd edn. New York: Oxford University Press.

Skrabanek, P. (1994). The emptiness of the black box, *Epidemiology, 5,* 553–555.

Smith, G. S. (1989). Development of rapid epidemiologic assessment methods to evaluate health status and delivery of health services, *International Journal of Epidemiology, 18,* (Supp. 2), S1.

Snow, J. (1855). *On the Mode of Communication of Cholera,* 2nd edn, London: Churchill, reprinted in Frost, W. H. (ed.) (1936). *Snow on Cholera.* New York: Commonwealth Fund (reprinted 1965, New York: Hafner).

Stolley, P. D. and Schlesselman, J. J. (1982). Planning and conducting a study. In Schlesselman, J. J., *Case-Control Studies: Design, conduct, analysis*. New York: Oxford University Press, 101–104.

Susser, M. (1973). *Causal Thinking in the Health Sciences*. New York: Oxford University Press.

Susser, M. (1986). The logic of Sir Karl Popper and the practice of epidemiology, *American Journal of Epidemiology*, *124*, 711–718).

Susser, M. (1987). *Epidemiology, Health, & Society: Selected papers*. New York: Oxford University Press, 171–232.

Swan, A. V. (1991). Statistical methods. In Holland, W. W., Detels, R. and Knox, G. (eds.), *Oxford Textbook of Public Health*, 2nd edn, 2, *Methods of Public Health*. Oxford: Oxford University Press, 189–223.

Taubes, G. (1995). Epidemiology faces its limits, *Science*, *269*, 164–169.

Terris, M. (ed.) (1964). *Goldberger on Pellagra*. Baton Rouge: Louisiana State University Press.

Vaughan, J. P. and Morrow, R. H. (eds.) (1989). *Manual of Epidemiology for District Health Management*. Geneva: World Health Organization.

Wall, S. (1995). Epidemiology for prevention, *International Journal of Epidemiology*, *24*, 655–664.

Wigfield, R., Gilbert, R. and Fleming, P. J. (1994). SIDS: risk reduction measures, *Early Human Development*, *38*, 161–164.

Williams, S. M., Taylor, B. J., Mitchell, E. A. and other members of the National Cot Death Study Group (1996). 'Sudden infant death syndrome: Insulation from bedding and clothing and its effect modifiers', *International Journal of Epidemiology*, *25*, 366–375.

Willinger, M. (1995). SIDS Prevention, *Pediatric Annals*, *24*, 358–364.

16 Job-loss and family morbidity: a study of a factory closure*

Norman Beale and Susan Nethercott

Introduction

There can be little doubt that losing one's job is likely to be a traumatic experience. However,, work itself is often stressful – many people are paid poorly for jobs which are tedious, grimy and sometimes dangerous. Nevertheless, despite the economic support provided by social security, most unemployed people repeatedly look for a job, at least while there remains any prospect of obtaining one. Clearly there must be incentives to work over and above any financial gain. These 'latent functions' of work were first described in the 1930s (Johada *et al.*, 1973) and later classified by Johada (1979) as follows:

- the imposition of a time structure on the day;
- regularly shared experiences;
- the linking of an individual to goals and purposes which transcend his own;
- the donation of personal status and identity;
- the enforcement of activity;

If work can gratify so many needs, the effects on the individual losing his job must be substantial. Childbirth, marriage and retirement are other examples of important psycho-social transitions (Murray Parkes, 1971) but the event for which increases in morbidity and even mortality have been most clearly demonstrated is bereavement (Dewi-Rees and Lutkins, 1967). The psychopathology of job-loss has been staged chronologically (as with bereavement); shock, optimism, pessimism, fatalism and eventual adaptation (Harrison, 1976). However, in the case of unemployment, there is little real evidence that these emotional upheavals result in increased psychiatric and/or physical morbidity. Watkins has summarised the problem of studying the health of the unemployed:

Comparisons of the health of employed people with that of the

* From *Journal of the Royal College of General Practitioners*, 35 (November 1985), pp. 510–514.

unemployed are confounded by the fact that unemployment falls disproportionately on groups who would be expected to have worse health, such as the lower social classes, people who live in deprived areas, people who work in declining industries, and people whose ability to work has been affected by their health. (Watkins, 1984)

It is possible to overcome this problem by studying a group of workers who have stable work records and subsequently lose their jobs because of the closure of their place of work. This type of investigation can demonstrate a causal relationship between unemployment and health; for example, that job-loss results in a decline in health.

Few studies of this type have been performed. Of the five studies reported in the literature (Jacobsen, 1972) none studied families and none were carried out by British general practitioners. Comparative review of these studies is difficult since all the groups used different criteria to measure morbidity. The longest (three and a half years) study was carried out by Iversen and Klausen (1981). Fisher (1965) and Westin and Norum (1977) studied women as well as men but did not distinguish between them. The only large, controlled study was that of Kasl and colleagues who examined 105 men before and after job-loss in two factories in the USA in the early 1960s (Kasl *et al.*, 1968; Kasl and Cobb, 1975). This particular study and also that of Jacobsen (1972) detected an increase in morbidity on anticipation of unemployment.

None of these workers was able to use sequential long-term records, such as are available in general practices in this country, to establish a baseline of morbidity for their study subjects. Moreover, as Kasl has reported (1983), many of the findings may not now be applicable with the increase in unemployment rates in the last decade. If unemployment does influence health this is likely to be of increasing significance, particularly for general practice as family doctors in Britain manage over 90 per cent of all reported illness without referral to specialist facilities.

Redundancies in Calne

In the first six months of 1982, the unemployment rate in the Calne area was 8.1 per cent – 9.3 per cent for men and 6.4 per cent for women (local Department of Employment statistics). Then, on 1 July 1982, the factory of C. and T. Harris (Calne) Ltd (manufacturers of bacon, sausages and pies) established in Calne in 1770, finally closed. For over two centuries the factory had been the most important work-place in the town and, until the mid-1960s, the only significant industrial concern.

The slaughterhouse and bacon-curing departments had closed, with little warning, in June 1979 – 86 men had lost their jobs leaving a workforce of approximately 800 in the factory. In January 1980, a further mass redundancy of 411 employees was announced. The workforce remaining after March 1980 were then given to understand that the company had a year in which to 'break even' and this veiled threat of complete closure took two years to realise.

Health care in Calne

Calne is a small market town with a population of 11,000. It is surrounded by numerous sparsely populated rural communities with a further 4000 people. The main employment within the town is now light industry.

Primary care in Calne is provided by two long-established practices. One group of four doctors (on which this study is based) works from a purpose-built heath centre which was opened in 1970; 11,500 patients are registered there. The other practice is two handed and serves the remainder of the population. There have been no substantial changes in the characteristics of the population for the last 10 years and patient turnover is below the national average.

The nearest district general hospital is 17 miles away and there is no community hospital in the town. Therefore, even when patients are emergencies or casualties, virtually all would first contact their own general practitioner or one of his partners.

Aims

This longitudinal study aimed to examine consultations, episodes of illness, referrals to hospital, and attendances at hospital out-patient departments in the families of workers made compulsorily redundant and in their control counterparts – families of other industrial workers who remained stably employed. As with other factory closure studies the null hypothesis for testing was that there would be no significant differences in these indices of morbidity in relation to job-loss. It was also hoped that the general practice records for these families (the only source of the data) would indicate our professional awareness of the employees' present occupational status.

Method

Subjects

A list of the names and addresses of all 302 employees made redundant from C. and T. Harris (Calne) Ltd between 18 June and 16 July 1982 was obtained from the personnel department of the firm. The company also supplied the following information for each employee: date of entry into the factory; hours of work; type of occupation – productive, clerical and so on; and department in the factory.

Identification of those employees who were registered with the practice proved to be quite simple using this information. Cross-reference with practice records and the local electoral roll allowed identification of dependent relatives – defined as spouses and, as at 30 June 1982, children aged 16 years and under who live at home.

The employees and their dependent relatives were incorporated into the study if:

1. The family were registered with the practice for the entire study period.
2. The employees were engaged by the company continuously for the entire study period (prior to redundancy).
3. The employees were engaged full-time, that is, 37 hours or more per week (there were insufficient part-time employees to form a separate group).
4. The employees were engaged in a productive or clerical capacity; that is, in Registrar General's social classes 3, 4 and 5 (there were insufficient managerial staff to examine separately).

After applying these criteria, men aged 61 years or over and women aged 56 years or over were omitted from the study as, in effect, they were experiencing early retirement.

C. and T. Harris (Calne) Ltd had been the largest employer in the practice area. Therefore, all the other local firms were approached in seeking control subjects. Seven firms, dealing in a variety of products and services, were each able to provide a minimum of 10 long-term employees who fulfilled criteria analogous to the employees at the Harris factory but they had not been subject to redundancy at any time during the study period.

Study period

The study period was taken to be 1 July 1976 to 30 June 1984. The eight years of the study period were denoted as years one to eight. The study period allowed observation of the study cohort during six years of continuous employment and during the two subsequent years after redundancy. Similarly it allowed observation of the control cohort for eight years, a period in which they remained continuously and fully employed.

Observations

Consultations, reported episodes of illness and referrals to specialists were recorded as defined in the instructions for the third national morbidity study (1981–2) (OPCS, 1981). However, attendances at antenatal clinics and other similar patient-contacts were not recorded. The number of attendances at hospital casualty and out-patient departments and the number of admissions to, and number of days in hospital were also recorded for each year. At no stage were any of the subjects approached personally – all the information was obtained from their medical records.

A search was also made in the medical file of each employee for any written record of their place or type of occupation. For the group employed by Harris Ltd, it was also ascertained whether or not there were any comments intimating unemployment.

A data card was constructed for each individual and these were filed in family groups.

Statistical testing

In this study the Mann–Whitney U test was applied to the data concerning consultations and episodes of illness while the Wilcoxon rank sum test was used for the data concerning referrals to, and attendances at hospital out-patient departments.

Results

The study group originally consisted of 133 Harris employees. Four of these employees left Calne in the two years after redundancy and they were omitted from the study. The remaining 129 employees consisted of 80 men (62 per cent) and 49 women (38 per cent). Seventy-four of their spouses were registered with the practice and 72 of their children. During the study period a further 16 children were born, five spouses died, seven employees married and one employee divorced.

There were 99 employees in the control group – 77 men and 22 women. Sixty-six of their spouses were registered with the practice as were 55 children. A further 16 children were born during the eight years of the study. No deaths were recorded, three employees married and one employee divorced.

Consultations

The preliminary results showed an obvious change in the number of consultations made per annum by the Harris group between years four and five (Table 16.1). The findings were therefore aggregated and examined during three time periods: years one to four (representing 'jobs secure'); years five and six (representing, for the Harris workers, 'jobs insecure') and years seven and eight (representing, for the Harris workers, 'jobs lost'). No significant differences were found when testing years five and six against years seven and eight. Therefore all subsequent analyses

Table 16.1   *Annual consultation and episode rates*

	Year	Mean number of consultations per patient per annum		Mean number of episodes per patient per annum	
		Harris families (275 patients)	*Control families (220 patients)*	*Harris families (275 patients)*	*Control families (220 patients)*
Jobs secure	1	2.66	2.78	1.54	1.68
	2	2.44	2.48	1.58	1.58
	3	2.44	2.66	1.46	1.71
	4	2.32	2.28	1.30	1.38
Jobs insecure	5	2.87	2.11	1.54	1.34
	6	3.06	2.40	1.68	1.54
Jobs lost	7	2.86	2.53	1.66	1.40
	8	3.05	2.51	1.68	1.49

were performed on data aggregated for years one to four inclusive and years five to eight inclusive.

Three sets of comparisons were made: (1) data for Harris employees in years one to four were compared with years five to eight, and the same for the control subjects. (2) data for Harris employees in years one to four were compared with data for control subjects in these years. (3) data for Harris employees in years five to eight were compared with data for control subjects in these years.

For the purpose of analysis, families were studied as units and then subdivided so that employees, spouses and children could each be examined as separate groups.

Table 16.2 shows those groupings for which significant increases in consultation rates were found between the years when jobs were secure (years one to four) and the years when jobs were insecure or had been lost (years five to eight) for the Harris employees. The second part of Table 16.2 shows significant differences between Harris employees and controls in the number of consultations over years five to eight. No significant differences in consultation rates were found between Harris employees and controls in years one to four.

Episodes of illness

The same statistical comparisons were applied to episodes of illness as for

Table 16.2 Significant differences in consulting behaviour

Group	Number of families	Number of individuals	Number of consultations over four years		Percentage increase	Significance level for years 1–4 versus years 5–8
			Years 1–4	Years 5–8		
All Harris families	129	275	2792	3353	20.1	$P<0.01$
All Harris employees	—	129	1202	1400	16.5	$P<0.05$
Families of female Harris employees	49	81	748	1000	33.7	$P<0.05$
Female Harris employees	—	49	528	605	14.6	$P<0.05$

Group	Number of individuals	Number of consultations over four years (years 5–8)	Mean number of consultations per individual	Significance levels for Harris versus control employees
Male Harris employees }	80	807	10.1	$P<0.05$
Male control employees }	77	603	7.8	
Spouses of Harris employees }	74	930	12.6	$P<0.05$
Spouses of control employees }	66	733	11.1	

Note: 1–4 = jobs secure; years 5–8 = jobs insecure or lost.

consultations. There was a 10.6 per cent increase in episodes of illness reported by the Harris families in the period when jobs were insecure or lost compared with a 9.3 per cent decrease for the control families over the same period. Although neither of these changes were significant, a decrease from 419 episodes (years one to four) to 330 episodes (years five to eight) reported by the control employees ($n = 99$) was found to be significant ($P = 0.05$).

The female Harris employees ($n = 49$) had significantly fewer ($P = 0.05$) episodes of illness than their control counterparts ($n = 22$) in the first four years and subsequently caught up.

Hospital referrals

The number of referrals to and attendances at hospital out-patient departments also showed obvious changes around 1980 and not, as had been expected, in 1982 (Figure 16.1). About one patient in seven only attends hospital in any one year in Britain and this severely reduces the data from the sample populations studied here. Therefore, the Wilcoxon rank sum test was the most appropriate statistical test and the results for the comparison of Harris employees in years one to four with years five to eight and the same comparison for control employees are presented in

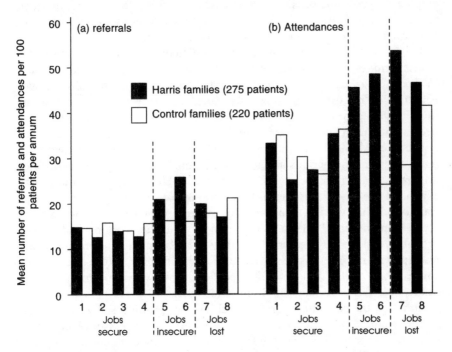

Figure 16.1   *(a) Referrals to and (b) attendances at hospital outpatient departments*

Table 16.3. No other comparison could be examined statistically since the Wilcoxon rank sum test requires paired samples.

No clear trends were apparent in the rates of admission to hospital in-patient departments. The mean hospital admission rate was 3.5 per cent of patients per annum and a much larger study would be necessary to detect consistent changes.

Notification of occupation and/or redundancy

The search of the records for details concerning the type or place of occupation of the patients revealed a written record for only 31 of the Harris employees (24 per cent) and 20 of the control employees (20 per cent). Details of redundancy had been recorded in the notes of only 18 Harris workers (14 per cent) by July 1984, that is, in the two years since they had been made redundant.

Discussion

This study demonstrates that unemployment results in a negative effect on health and not merely on welfare and morale. The results show a significant increase in the number of times that both men and women employees consult their doctors when subjected to compulsory redundancy. This increase is also shown by their spouses and when all the individuals studied are integrated into their family units.

The increase in stress exhibited was sufficient not only to provoke the Harris families into seeking the help of their doctors more often but also to give them symptoms which necessitate more frequent specialist advice. An equally important finding was quite unforeseen: the increase in morbidity began two years before redundancy – at the time when it became apparent to the Harris families that their economic futures were not secure. All other studies of factory closures have been performed over much shorter time periods and none were able to demonstrate the distinct importance of the threat of redundancy. However, one study has examined the psychiatric morbidity of the threat of unemployment and it was found that there was a decrease in symptoms when the threat was lifted (Jenkins *et al.*, 1982). The majority of the working population probably experience concern that they may be made redundant when unemployment rates rise and perhaps there is now more evidence to suggest that, during an economic recession, those with a job may also feel under stress, as postulated by Brenner (1979).

Although the consultation rates for the Harris group rose by 20 per cent in the second four-year period, the number of new episodes of illness increased by only 11 per cent. Therefore, the number of consultations per episode of illness increased during the period of job insecurity and unemployment. Similarly, the number of attendances as hospital out-

Table 16.3   Referrals to and attendances at hospital outpatient departments

Group	Number of individuals	Number of referrals per 100 patients		Significance levels for years 1–4 versus years 5–8	Number of attendances per 100 patients		Significance levels for years 1–4 versus years 5–8
		Years 1–4	Years 5–8		Years 1–4	Years 5–8	
All Harris employees	129	53	76	P < 0.05	84	145	P < 0.05
All control employees	99	65	82	NS	130	130	NS
Dependants of Harris employees	146	58	92	P < 0.01	147	230	P < 0.01
Dependants od control employees	121	58	69	NS	123	120	NS

Notes:
NS = not significant. Years 1–4 = jobs secure; years 5–8 = jobs insecure or lost.

patients departments per referral increased for the Harris group while the same ratio dropped for the control group. The Harris families either developed an increased doctor-dependency or the symptoms with which they presented proved more difficult to diagnose and treat. It is possible that their problems were less clear-cut, their distresses more psychosomatic in type or their disorders less responsive to simple measures. These hypotheses are being tested at present by classifying the illnesses which were presented.

If the consultations with the Harris families were proving ineffective, were they also frustrating? Higgs has stated 'We do not always know what really brings a patient to the doctor' (1984). Many consultations are unsatisfactory because the real reasons for the consultation do not emerge and there is an increased risk of chronicity. The results of this study lend credence to this for redundancy was only recorded in a minority of cases.

The reluctance of the unemployed to admit to their predicament is well-known – they see it as a stigma. Other major events such as marriage or divorce, changes of address and even foreign holidays more usually come to the notice of family doctors because of the necessary documentation. Fourteen per cent of the workforce in Britain are now suffering, together with their families, from what might correctly be called an epidemic, and for only a small minority is that fact recorded in their notes. Extrapolation of the observations made in this small study to the population at large is probably valid but several points could influence such projections. First, the rate of unemployment in the Calne area is lower than the national average. Secondly, the population of North Wiltshire is largely stable and closely-knit, has not been subject to any recent large migration and has no significant ethnic minorities. In addition, the employees themselves were a stable working group who were settled in their jobs (many for over 25 years) and worked in an unskilled or semiskilled capacity. However, it is interesting that the consultation and referral rates before 1980 for the Harris group and those for the controls throughout the study match closely the results of the second national morbidity study (OPCS, 1974).

At present it is not known how many of the ex-Harris workers have been successful in finding employment. It is hoped that a comparison of those remaining out of work for a long period with those who found a new job quickly will form the basis of a future study and that further analysis of the data might reveal other significant findings, such as the effect of the age of the employees. It had been expected that large numbers of the Harris families would have left the area in search of new work which would have complicated both the collection of data and the interpretation of the results. It is surprising that only four of the 133 Harris employees originally studied have moved away from the town in the two years since losing their jobs. This initial study shows that the information already stored in general practice records can provide useful facts about a population subjected to changes in its environment.

The organisation of the National Health Service was an advantage in this study. When there is no cost to the patient at the point of service, those subject to financial hardship, such as unemployment, are not inhibited from seeking help. This would not be so in other countries where the inability to pay could obscure a real increase in morbidity or even result in an apparent decrease. On the other hand a 20 per cent increase in consultations (65 per cent of which generally end with a prescription) and a 60 per cent increase in visits to hospital out-patient departments by the families of the 3.3 million unemployed in Britain is a projection of startling economic consequences to the National Health Service.

Acknowledgements

This study was supported by a grant from the Scientific Foundation Board of the Royal College of General Practitioners and we are grateful for their support. We thank our families for their patience. Dr Ian Russell for his advice, all the staff at Calne Health Centre: in particular Miss Barbara Farquhar, Mrs Maureen Comley, Miss Beverly Earl and Miss Eloise Self. Dr Andrew Thornton for his critique of the script and the whole partnership for their cooperation. Space does not permit us to thank, individually, all those who helped us in local industry but we must acknowledge the cooperation and hospitality of Mr Radford, Personnel Manager of Harris (Ipswich) Ltd . Finally we also acknowledge Miss Kate Clarke and her staff of the Medical Library, Postgraduate Centre at the Royal United Hospital, Bath.

References

Brenner, M. H. (1979). Mortality and the national economy, *Lancet*, 2, 568–573.

Dewi-Rees, W. and Lutkins, S. G. (1967). Mortality of bereavement, *British Medical Journal*, 4, 13–16.

Fisher, A. L. (1965). Psychiatirc follow-up of long term industrial employees subsequent to plant closure, *International Journal of Neuropsychiatry*, 11, 267–274.

Harrison, R. (1976). The demoralising experience of prolonged unemployment, *Department of Employment Gazette* (April issue), 339–348.

Higgs, R. (1984). Life changes, *British Medical Journal*, 288, 1556–1557.

Iverson, L. and Klausen, H. (1981). *Lukningen af Nordhavns (The closing of Nordhavns shipyard)*, 13. Vaerflet: Institute for Social Medicine, University of Copenhagen, 199–207.

Jacobsen, K. (1972). Afskedigelse og sygelighed (Dismissal and morbidity), *Ugeskr Laeger*, 134, 352–354.

Jahoda, M. (1979). The impact of unemployment in the 1930s and the 1970s, *Bulletin of the British Psychological Society*, 32, 309–314.

Jahoda, M., Lazarfield, P. I. and Zeisel, H. (1973). *Marienthal – the sociography of an unemployed community*. London: Tavistock Publications (first published in 1933).

Jenkins, R., MacDonald, A., Murray, J. and Strathdee, G. (1982). Minor psychiatric morbidity and the threat of redundancy in a professional group, *Psychological Medicine, 12,* 799–807.

Kasl, S. V. (1983). Strategies of research on economic instability and health. In John, J., Schwefel, D. and Zouner, H. (eds) (1983). *Influence of Economic Instability on Health.* Berlin: Springer-Verlag.

Kasl, S. V., Cobb, S. and Brooks, G. W. (1968). Changes in serum uric acid and cholesterol levels in men undergoing job-loss, *JAMA, 206,* 1500–1507.

Kasl, S. V., Gore, S. and Cobb, S. (1975). Reported changes in health, symptoms and illness behaviour, *Psychosomatic Medicine, 37,* 106–122.

Murray Parkes, C. (1971). Psycho-social transitions, *Social Science Medicine, 5,* 101–115.

Office of Population Censuses and Surveys, Royal College of General Practitioners and Department of Health and Social Security (1974). *Studies on medical and population subjects, 26. Morbidity statistics from general practice. Second national study, 1970–71.* London: HMSO.

Office of Population Census and Survey (OPCS), Royal College of General Practitioners and Department of Health and Social Security (1981). *Morbidity Statistics from General Practice: 3rd study (1981–82). Manual of definitions and procedures.* London: HMSO.

Watkins, S. J. (1984). Unemployment and health, *Lancet, 2,* 1464.

Westin, S. and Norum, D. (1977). *Nar sardinfabrikken nedlegees (When the sardine factory is shut down).* Bergen: Institute for Hygiene and Social Medicine, University of Bergen.

17 Health education and health promotion: planning for the 1990s*

Andrew Tannahill

Plans for health *promotion* invariably recognise the instrumental role of health *education*. Thus, in deciding how we should – and should not – plan for health promotion, it is logical to consider what makes for sound health education. More specifically, since health education may be seen essentially as the communication sphere of health promotion (Tannahill, 1985), it is important to devise programmes of health promotion which are consistent with principles of good communication. An important criterion is the capacity to establish *two-way* communication: between professionals, between agencies; and with the public. This is in keeping with central themes of the World Health Organisation strategy 'Health for All by the Year 2000' (HFA 2000) (WHO, 1985), namely multi-disciplinary and intersectoral collaboration, and community participation.

In the search for a solid health education foundation for health promotion planning, it is helpful to distinguish and assess three categories of health education: *disease-orientated, risk factor-orientated, and health-orientated.*

Disease-orientated health education

Scrutiny of this category (see Figure 17.1) takes us a long way towards appraising the hitherto dominant style in health promotion planning, since disease-orientated health education has been a cornerstone of most strategies for health promotion to date. In this type of orientation, priorities are defined in terms of specific diseases, and action is directed at the various risk factor sets associated with these diseases. The inherent assumption is that each major preventable disease category, such as CHD or cancers, is best tackled through a specific preventive programme directed at the relevant risk factors.

A number of fundamental organisational problems are inherent in this approach. Firstly, there are difficulties with inter-professional communication. Individual professionals or groups are apt to work on

* From *Health Education Journal*, 49, (1990), pp. 194–198.

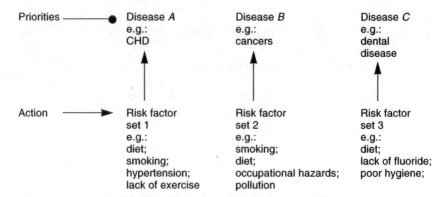

Figure 17.1   *Disease-orientated health education*

single topics in relative (or even absolute) isolation from one another. Given the overlap in risk factors between various diseases (Figure 17.1), duplication of effort is inevitable. As well as being wasteful of resources, this may lead to over-saturation and a 'switch-off' response amongst members of the public.

Moreover, there is a considerable propensity for inconsistency of 'messages'. For instance, 'CHD preventers' may throw up their hands in horror at dental colleagues who encourage children to avoid sweets in favour of crisps. Such inconsistency damages overall professional–community communication: it leads to public confusion and militates against behavioural change. Communication problems also arise in the relationships between health promoters and important gatekeepers to the community, including professionals both within and outside the health service. In a single community there may be, for example, a CHD prevention programme, one aimed at preventing cancers and another concerned with dental disease (Figure 17.1). Leaders of each separate initiative may approach the various gatekeepers individually. Thus headteachers, for instance, may feel besieged by requests for inclusion in already crowded timetables, and may reasonably feel aggrieved at having been excluded from earlier stages of programme development.

Returning to the question of professional–public communication, criticism can be levelled at the fact that this is an expert-dominated orientation, not one in which community participation is emphasised. Borrowing from the vocabulary of clinical practice, the approach involves professionals making a community 'diagnosis' and issuing a population 'prescription', without any public consultation', and expecting mass 'compliance'. This deficiency is compounded by the common tendency to focus on individuals' health related behaviour, rather than recognising the impact of social factors on lifestyle.

The disease-orientated model is also open to attack on the grounds that it entails an incomplete view of health: the positive dimension – embracing well-being and fitness is neglected. Related to this, it is commonly argued that a disease-orientated approach is less valid educationally than one which emphasises more immediate and positive health benefits. It has to be said that, as yet, the scientific evidence in favour of this premise is limited. Nevertheless, it is plausible that advocating behavioural change purely on negative grounds is less likely to be successful in motivational terms than an approach which emphasises positive benefits in addition to the preventive. Why should people give up valued practices, or adopt new behaviours which they may perceive to be unpleasant, on the strength of some speculative, intangible, preventive benefit? This line of argument is especially applicable to those who have the worst health problems, for whom the present is a grim struggle, whose pleasures are few (and often damaging), and who have little perception of a future worthy of investment or even amenable to personal control. It is also of particular relevance in considering health education with young people.

Risk factor-orientated health education

This second category of health education (see Figure 17.2) is aimed at eliminating particular risk factors in order to prevent the various diseases with which they are associated. It has some advantages over the disease-orientated approach, most notably in its recognition that a single risk factor may have an impact on more than one disease category. For example, an anti-smoking programme can highlight associations with cancers, CHD and chronic obstructive airways disease. Thus, although the model is still an incrementalist one, there are fewer problems with professional duplication and public confusion.

However, the approach is otherwise open to the same criticisms as disease-orientated health education: it is expert-dominated rather than properly participatory, and the positive dimension of health is neglected. Moreover, problems relating to co-ordination between programmes – duplication, and so on – arise from the fact that the two orientations are

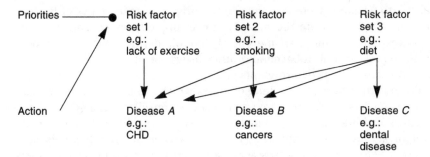

Figure 17.2   *Risk factor-orientated health education*

often combined (for instance, a single health board may have separate programmes for smoking and CHD). Indeed, the approach currently dominant in health promotion planning is, in essence, based on an amalgam of disease- and risk factor-orientated health education.

Health-orientated health education

This model avoids the pitfalls of the first two orientations. The major organisational and communication problems of disease- and risk factor-orientated health education are overcome by setting as priorities *people* and the *places* in which they may be reached (rather than the diseases and the risk factors). Effort is directed towards developing *comprehensive programmes* of health education in *key community settings* (for example, schools, primary care, the workplace, deprived localities) and with *key groups* (for instance, old people, unemployed people, and ethnic minority groups). These key settings and groups are determined locally, with sensitivity to public opinion.

Multi-disciplinary and intersectoral collaboration is facilitated. Relevant gatekeepers (school teachers, primary care teams, industrial and commercial managers, to name but a few) can be involved from the start, rather than having a hotch-potch of initiatives dropping on them from above. Programmes can thus be properly co-ordinated, cutting out inefficient and ineffective duplication. Moreover, content, timing and methodology can be tailored to the needs and characteristics of the particular setting or group.

Tailoring is also helped by the fact that there is scope for true public participation. A cardinal principle is that the people in the settings and groups should be involved in defining health issues of relevance to them, in identifying factors which affect their health and health-related behaviour, and in shaping and implementing action for better health.

The health factors referred to in Figure 17.3 do include 'medical' risk factors, but this is not all. Instead of dealing with individual aspects of lifestyle *in vacuo*, underlying circumstances, including social factors, are taken into account. Common links in the origins of many types of health-damaging behaviour are recognised – for example, peer and other social pressures (such as those arising out of multiple deprivation) – in relation to the use of alcohol, tobacco and other drugs. In other words, a holistic view of health and its determinants prevails.

The health factors also include qualities which are components of well-being as well as conferring protection against unhealthy behaviour. These 'positive health attributes' (Tannahill, 1988) (various lifeskills, and a high level of self-esteem) contribute to the *empowerment* of individuals and groups – helping them towards achieving a greater control over their own destinies. Such considerations, fundamental to health education theory,

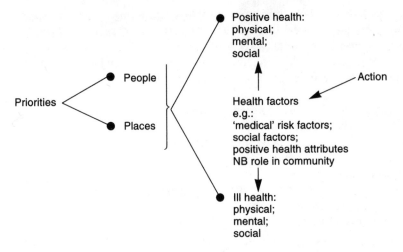

Figure 17.3   *Health-orientated health education*

have tended to be eclipsed in practice by the domination of disease- and risk factor-orientated programmes.

The broad view of health which characterises the health-orientated approach includes recognition of its positive dimension. The focus is dual: the aims are to enhance positive health while preventing ill-health. The positive (and not just preventive) benefits of a healthy lifestyle are stressed, and the myth that 'it has to be hell to be healthy' is actively dispelled. For example, a healthy diet is presented (accurately) as rich, varied and enjoyable, rather than as something Calvinistic and inevitably less palatable than 'chips with everything', to be tolerated for some speculative deferred benefit. Preventive advantages are not ignored, but are regarded as additional to more immediate (and more reliable) benefits in terms of well-being and fitness. Common sense – and insight into our own motivations in life – tell us that this approach should be more fruitful than gloomy catalogues of prohibitions.

The broader view of health also encompasses the physical, mental and social facets of both positive health and ill-health, and accommodates lay perspectives.

Health education planning

Clearly the health-orientated approach should be the preferred model for planning health education. Instead of relying exclusively on disease- or risk-factor orientated schemes, we should aim to set up, in key settings and with key groups, comprehensive, co-ordinated, and properly participatory programmes, which acknowledge the positive dimension of health . . .

It is necessary to look more closely at the situations in which single-topic initiatives – in health education and in other aspects of health promotion – may be advantageous, and to scrutinise how single-topic and comprehensive approaches relate to one other. Single-topic health education initiatives are appropriate in the following circumstances:

1. Agenda-setting – raising awareness of the significance of preventable diseases and risk factors. . .
2. Responding urgently to new threats to health, such as Aids.
3. Promotion of the uptake of specific preventive services, such as immunisation and screening.
4. Opportunistic education for instance, advising on smoking cessation during a medical consultation.
5. Meeting special needs, including those of patients who wish to avoid the recurrence or progression of a disease, and those of people at particular risk of developing a given disease. . .
6. Advocacy of policies aimed at promoting health (health protection measures), for instance, non-smoking or healthy eating policies.
7. Responding to specific needs identified by individuals or communities.

In addition, the comprehensive programmes of health education proposed in this paper will themselves involve specific work on lifestyle, diseases, and so on. The crucial point; however, is that such programmes will be developed in a *co-ordinated* manner, rather than growing haphazardly from a series of single-topic efforts. Furthermore . . . it must be ensured that single-topic initiatives in the circumstances outlined above are *complementary* to the more general population strategy.

This clarification of the respective roles of comprehensive and specific approaches, and of their interconnections, has helped break down false

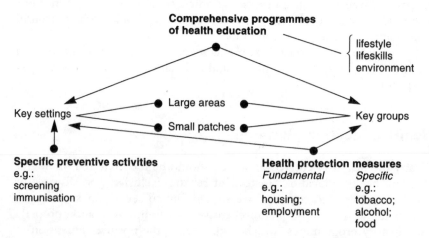

Figure 17.4   *A framework for integrated health promotion planning*

and damaging polarisations and barriers to collaboration between professional groups, notably between health service managers and public
health physicians on the one hand, and health education and promotion
officers on the other.

Finally, it should be acknowledged that the non-educational aspects of
health promotion–specific preventive services, and health protection
measures – will, by their very nature, be geared towards particular health
problems or factors influencing health.

Health promotion planning

An integrated approach to health promotion planning involves dove-
tailing comprehensive programmes of health education, in key settings
and with key groups, with specific preventive services and with health
protection measures, appropriate to the places and people concerned
(Figure 17.4).

This planning framework may be used either at the level of a relatively
large community (such as a health board area or health district), or on the
scale of smaller patches (in keeping with trends towards locality planning
of community services). Thus, services may be organised on an area or
district-wide basis in key settings and with key groups. Alternatively, and
arguably preferably, professionals and others, working in locally-sensitive
teams, may seek to gain access to key settings and groups within their
patches.

Whichever means of 'delivering' health promotion in the community is
chosen, larger-scale efforts (national and sub-national) will be required to
plan, co-ordinate and manage preventive services (such as breast
screening) and health protection measures.

Research challenges

The paucity of research evidence in support of a positive approach to
health education has been referred to above. Indeed, in general, the
advocacy of a health-orientated basis for health promotion planning arises
more from pragmatic or common-sense considerations than from rigorous
scientific appraisal. The lack of a supportive research base is attributable
to the lack, hitherto, of an adequate commitment to a health-orientated
approach, rather than to any demonstration that the approach is flawed.
Despite this, however, the approach has commonly been rejected on
scientific grounds, in favour of disease and risk factor-orientated
approaches – weaknesses of which *have* been demonstrated. Moreover,
research funding is often ear-marked for the more specific approaches.

This state of affairs should not be allowed to continue. Health boards and authorities, grant-awarding bodies, research institutions, and others concerned with health promotion, must channel resources into the development, implementation and evaluation of health promotion strategies built on comprehensive, health-orientated, programmes of health education. Public health physicians, in partnership with health education and promotion officers, have an important part to play in bringing this about.

References

East Anglian Regional Health Authority (1988). *Health promotion. A new strategy to 1994.* Cambridge: East Anglian Regional Health Authority.

Tannahill, A. (1985). What is health promotion? *Health Education Journal, 44,* 167–168.

Tannahill, A. (1988). Health promotion and public health: a model for action. *Community Medicine, 10,* 48–51.

World Health Organisation (1985). *Targets for health for all.* Copenhagen: WHO.

18 Randomised controlled trial assessing effectiveness of health education leaflets in reducing incidence of sunburn[*]

Paola Dey, Stuart Collins, Sheila Will and
Ciaran B. J. Woodman

Exposure to the sun and severe sunburn are associated with an increased risk of malignant melanoma (Østerlind, 1992). Health education leaflets are often part of primary prevention strategies which aim to modify high risk behaviour related to the sun[1]. This study aims to assess the effectiveness of a health education leaflet in reducing sunburn.

Subjects, methods, and results

The study population comprised holidaymakers travelling on Air UK Leisure flights from Manchester airport during August 1993. The unit of randomisation was the flight. Flights were stratified into long haul (North America and Jamaica) and short haul (Europe) and randomly allocated to the intervention or control arm. Before boarding, the health education authority leaflet *If You Worship The Sun, Don't Sacrifice Your Skin* was placed in seat pockets on flights in the intervention arm but not in the control arm. Cabin crew distributed questionnaires to passengers on Air UK Leisure return flights to Manchester. A history of sunburn was elicited by the question 'Did you suffer from any sunburn during your recent holiday?' and, if so, whether this was associated with one or more of: redness of the skin, blistering of the skin, pain for less than a day, pain for more than a day. Adults completed the questionnaire for children. The study endpoint, severe sunburn, was defined as any episode of sunburn which was either painful for more than a day or resulted in blistering. Randomisation by group was undertaken to reduce contamination between the study arms. A clustering parameter was calculated for the study endpoint. Brier's adjusted χ^2 was used for baseline comparisons

* From *British Medical Journal*, 311 (21 October 1995), pp. 1062–1063.

Table 18.1   *Baseline characteristics and incidence of severe sunburn in intervention and control groups. Values are numbers (percentages) of subjects unless stated otherwise*

	Intervention (n = 6276)	Control (n = 6109)
Age group (years):		
Median	32	33
Range	0–97	1–88
Sex:		
Male	2885 (46.0)	2777 (45.5)
Female	3273 (52.1)	3233 (52.9)
Not recorded	118 (1.9)	99 (1.6)
Duration of holiday:		
0–7 days	841 (13.4)	1058 (17.3)
8–21 days	5435 (86.6)	5051 (82.7)
Hair colour:		
Blonde	2152 (34.3)	2065 (33.8)
Red	230 (3.7)	271 (4.4)
Brown/black	3699 (58.9)	3566 (58.4)
Other	107 (1.7)	97 (1.6)
Not known	88 (1.4)	110 (1.8)
Skin colour:		
Fair, never tans	160 (2.5)	185 (3.0)
Fair, gets a pale tan	2161 (34.4)	2066 (33.8)
White skin, tans easily	3114 (49.6)	3057 (50.0)
Mediterranean	593 (9.5)	580 (9.5)
Brown	151 (2.4)	136 (2.2)
Black	37 (0.6)	17 (0.3)
Other	31 (0.5)	26 (0.6)
Not known	29 (0.5)	32 (0.5)
Incidence of severe sunburn[a, b]		
All flights	1013 (16.1)	1053 (17.2)
Short haul	717 (16.3)	793 (17.1)
Long haul	296 (15.7)	260 (17.7)

Notes:
a χ^2 (1 degree of freedom)
b 95% confidence interval for difference in proportion:
  All flights 0.731 ($P = 0.392$); –0.014 to 0.036
  Short haul 0.276 ($P = 0.6$); –0.022 to 0.038
  Long haul 1.288 ($P = 0.256$); –0.014 to 0.052.

(Brier, 1980), and 95 per cent confidence intervals were constructed for the difference in proportions using methods appropriate to group randomised trials (Donner and Klar, 1993).

Sixteen long haul and 62 short haul flights were randomised to the intervention arm and 15 long haul and 62 short haul flights to the control arm; 21,611 questionnaires were distributed and 14,956 (69 per cent) returned. A total of 2483 questionnaires completed by passengers who had not departed from Manchester airport during the study period and 88 inconsistent or illegible questionnaires were excluded from the analysis, leaving 12,385 evaluable questionnaires. The clustering parameter was 0.02. The study had a power of 90 per cent to show a 5 per cent difference between the two groups at the 5 per cent two sided significance level. There was no significant difference between the two groups in the distribution of baseline characteristics or the proportion reporting severe sunburn (see Table 18.1).

Comment

This leaflet did not seem to reduce the incidence of severe sunburn. Passengers were not asked if they had seen or read the leaflet as this might have influenced their response to the questionnaire. Therefore it is not possible to determine if the intervention failed because subjects had not read the leaflet, they had ignored its messages, or the messages were inappropriate. However, unsolicited distribution of leaflets is a common practice.

Randomised controlled trials provide the most compelling evidence of effectiveness. We have found no other randomised controlled trials of the effectiveness of health education leaflets in the prevention of sunburn and few trials of health education leaflets in other settings (McAvoy and Raza, 1991). Although leaflets are perceived as low cost and unlikely to cause harm, there are substantial opportunity costs associated with promoting strategies of unproved effectiveness. We commend the more extensive use of randomised controlled trials in the evaluation of primary prevention programmes.

Acknowledgements

We thank the management and staff of Air UK Leisure and Manchester airport for their invaluable help in administering the study and the Health Education Authority for supplying the leaflets.

Funding: North Western Regional Health Authority.

Conflict of interest: None.

Note

1 PLC/MO(93)6 Ultraviolet radiation and skin cancer.

References

Brier, S. S. (1980). Analysis of contingency tables under cluster sampling, *Biometrika*, 67, 591–596.

Donner, A. and Klar, N. (1993). Confidence interval construction for effect measures arising from cluster randomization trials, *Journal of Clinical Epidemiology*, *46* (2), 123–131.

McAvoy, B. R. and Raza, R. (1991). Can health education increase uptake of cervical smear testing among Asian women?, *British Medical Journal*, *302*, 833–836.

Østerlind, A. (1992). Epidemiology of malignant melanoma in Europe, *Reviews in Oncologica*, *5* (2), 903–908.

19 *Is prevention better than cure?*[*]

Christine Godfrey

Introduction

Most health-care systems have been focused on illness services. Preventive health interventions have been far less developed than those for acute care. Is prevention better than cure? Which prevention strategies are cost-effective? What incentives are needed within health services to ensure that the correct balance of preventive and curative services is achieved?

Purchasers require answers to these questions if they are to maximise the health of their populations, given finite resources. However, many treatments remain to be evaluated and economic studies of prevention, especially health promotion interventions, are even rarer (Drummond *et al.*, 1987). Decisions are made based on limited information. An economic approach can give some guidance to setting priorities. . .

Future mortality and morbidity – the potential for prevention

To examine future changes in mortality, morbidity and costs accruing from current prevention activities requires sophisticated epidemiological techniques.

PREVENT is a simple simulation model which predicts changing patterns of deaths likely to occur if risk factors such as smoking, drinking, high blood-cholesterol or hypertension are reduced (Gunning-Schepers, 1989; Godfrey *et al.*, 1993). Figure 19.1 shows some results from the model using English and Welsh data. The prevention simulation was based on the *Health of the Nation* (HON) smoking targets: that prevalence of smoking should be reduced to 20 per cent, by the year 2000 and overall consumption of cigarettes should be reduced by 40 per cent over the same period.

It can be seen from Figure 19.1 that, although the interventions to achieve these targets would take place between now and the year 2000, the peak reduction in the number of deaths is well after this period and

---

[*] From M. Drummond and A. Maynard (eds) (1993). *Purchasing and Providing Cost Effective Health Care*, Chapter 13, pp. 183–197 ©Edinburgh: Churchill Livingstone.

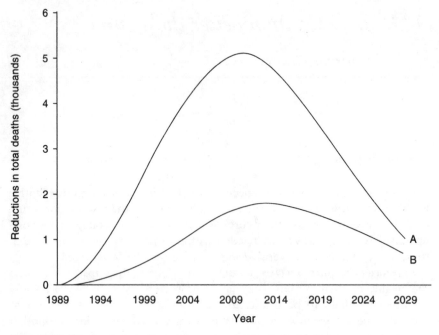

Figure 19.1   *Reductions in the total number of deaths in England and Wales associated with achieving HON smoking targets: A for men B for women*

reductions in mortality are predicted over the whole period. If the results are expressed in terms of life years gained, then the risk factor reduction is predicted to lead to the saving of more than 54,000 life years between now and the year 2000, and a cumulative total of nearly three million life years by the year 2029. These simulations are based on all age groups, not just the under-65s.

Results from epidemiological models such as PREVENT (Gunning-Schepers, 1989) indicate that there are large potential health gains from reducing risk factors such as smoking. However, in terms of life years, gains occur over a long time period.

Considerable analyses can be undertaken to examine the potential benefits from prevention in terms of gains in the quantity of life. Far less information is available, however, about other indicators of ill-health and the potential gain in positive health if risk factors are reduced. Consideration of these potential benefits are likely to change the ranking between conditions. It should also be noted that these health gains to the quality of life may be realised in a shorter time period than those extending the quantity of life.

Identifying the options for prevention

Given the information on the potential for health gain, what are the means available to reduce risk factors and prevent disease? Health-care treatments are generally concerned with the consequences of disease or infirmity and are intended to restore some of the lost health status. Prevention activities are concerned with both preventing ill-health and with enhancing positive health, i.e. increasing current health status.

Examining the full range of prevention options can be an important component of a purchasing strategy. Prevention can be directed at the population as a whole – for example, media campaigns – or patients in the early stages of disease. There are many different prevention activities ranging from education through to legislation which can be undertaken and targeted at different groups in the population.

Defining prevention activities

There are a number of different levels of prevention activity but few common definitions. In this chapter, these levels are defined following Downie *et al.* (1992). Primary level health promotion – exercised before the onset of any disease – includes activities such as health education on smoking for children and drug therapy for hypertension or high blood-cholesterol. Health promotion directed at halting the progression of disease or health deterioration would be considered secondary level prevention and would include screening for disease symptoms and any subsequent intervention. Tertiary level prevention consists of measures to help prevent the recurrence of an illness, and would include rehabilitation for heart attack patients.

The domains of health promotion

Most of the policy statements, in the United Kingdom and elsewhere, have concerned primary level health promotion and, in particular, the prevalence of certain risk factors, such as smoking, drinking, obesity, lack of exercise and poor diet. While secondary and tertiary level activities tend to be disease specific, some primary level activities overlap. Also behavioural change could be affected by many different interventions, not only from the health-care sector.

Tannahill (1985) developed a model in which health promotion activities are divided into three overlapping domains: health protection measures, comprising legal, fiscal or workplace controls, prevention activities (for example, immunisation) which reduce the risk of occurrence; and health education activities.

Further divisions can be made by disease (or condition) and lifestyle behaviours. Such divisions are not mutually exclusive. A heart programme could cover smoking, diet and exercise and a smoking programme cover cancer and heart disease. Health promotion, particularly health education, can also be given in a number of settings.

The range of options that could be considered by a purchaser wishing to reduce coronary heart disease through health education is illustrated in Table 19.1. The choices include programmes with several elements directed at a single risk factor, such as smoking or exercise, and multi-risk, multi-element programmes, such as the Look After Your Heart initiatives.

Targeting health promotion

The final set of options available is whether health promotion or prevention is targeted at the whole population or at certain sub-groups. The sub-groups considered could be selected by age, sex, ethnic group or socio-economic circumstance. The reasons for choosing different groups may be due to disease and illness patterns, or the prevalence of adverse lifestyles. Another form of targeting can take place if health promotion activities are concentrated on those at highest risk of disease.

The options for prevention for any disease or risk behaviour are considerable. Some activities will be controlled by purchasers or providers but many, such as tax levels or advertising restrictions, are not. Agenda setting activities may, however, help to influence policy.

Is prevention cost effective?

There are few economic evaluations of health promotion activities in which comparisons to treatments have been made and results are mixed. For example, opportunistic advice from general practitioners to stop

Table 19.1   *Options for coronary heart disease health promotion*

Main health promotion interventions	Intervention influences	
	Several risk factors	*One risk factor*
Workplace	Option A1	Option B1
School	Option A2	Option B2
Community based	Option A3	Option B3
Primary healthcare	Option A4	Option B4
Mass media/public education	Option A5	Option B5
	Programme A (e.g. HEA Look After Your Heart Programme)	Programme B (e.g HEA Smoking Programme)

smoking frequently heads QALY or well year league tables . . . Other activities, such as breast cancer screening, have been found to be less cost-effective. What determines the cost-effectiveness of different types of prevention activities?

The factors influencing both costs and benefits can be considered in two ways: in relation to whether prevention is more cost-effective than cure, and in relation to which mixture of prevention activities (for example, which of the options set out in Table 19.1) represents the best buy.

Treatment or prevention: numbers and time

Treatment only involves those who contract the disease or condition, whereas prevention can involve large numbers who may or may not develop the disease. Hence, the cost per individual for treatment can be much higher than the cost per individual for prevention, producing the same total cost for either option (Russell, 1986).

For some conditions, such as lung cancer, which are associated with adverse lifestyles, the survival rates may be poor and in other instances treatment may not restore the individuals to full quality of life.

A further issue is the time lapse before prevention results in health gains. In economic evaluations it is usual to discount future sums to a lower present value. However, if a discount rate is applied to future health benefits from prevention, the 'present' value of the health gains is reduced. Using the PREVENT simulation, a cumulative health gain of 2.8 million life years over the period 1989 to 2029 was predicted to result from achieving the *Health of the Nation* smoking targets. Discounting these health gains at 5 per cent to a present value for 1989, however, reduces the health gain to 720 000 life years.

Health economists continue to debate which discount rate should be used for health benefits. It has been suggested that all studies of health-care programmes should include the undiscounted figures, i.e. a zero discount rate (Parsonage and Neuburger, 1992). Purchasers face a considerable dilemma when, at the same time as current (and often identified) cases are waiting for treatment, they are being urged to commit resources to prevention where the health gains are anonymous and way in the future. It is likely that some discounting of future health benefits occurs in practice.

The timing of future health benefits also affects calculations about the potential for resource saving from prevention activities. This is an issue raised especially in areas where treatment is unlikely to prolong life. The avoidance of future treatment has been seen as a way of 'financing' prevention. However, such savings are often difficult to realise, due partly to the costs of prevention. Also, especially when considering behavioural changes, a decline in disease – and hence fewer patients requiring treatment often occurs with a time lag. Where the prevention activity involves screening for early signs of disease, which require some treatment, health-care costs may rise in the short term.

Treatment versus prevention – indirect costs

One of the indirect costs associated with prevention is the possibility of higher expenditure from increased longevity. These types of consequences can form part of a cost-effectiveness analysis where the value of the health benefits of a longer and healthier life and the indirect benefits from increased productivity would also be assessed. Such costs may also be less than predicted from the current pattern of health-care costs among the elderly. It has been argued that, for those who adopt healthy lifestyles in their older age, morbidity may be compressed and health-care expenditures reduced (Fries, 1989).

For many secondary prevention activities there may be some risk of side-effects. Although the risk is small per individual, the total cost of these adverse effects could be sizeable. There are also costs associated with screening procedures. The intangible costs through worry and anxiety can be extremely high for conditions such as HIV/AIDS (Godfrey *et al.*, 1992).

The balance between preventive measures and treatment, or non-treatment, is likely to change over time. For example, immunisation may become less cost-effective if previous activities have reduced the overall risk of disease.

Choices and costs and benefits of prevention activities

Other factors may influence the choice between different types of prevention activity. Secondary prevention will generally involve lower numbers than primary prevention. The costs of identifying a disease at an early stage, especially when it is asymptomatic, can be high. Also screening for disease precursors can only be worthwhile if early treatment is effective in enhancing quality and or quantity of life. A further problem in screening (and health promotion clinics) is the difficulty of getting some of the population at highest risk to attend (Holland and Stewart, 1990).

Some health education campaigns may have adverse effects in creating a 'worried' well group. Early campaigns directed at raising awareness of HIV and AIDS, for example, were thought to have caused anxiety among those at low risk. However, the receipt of health information may have benefits as well as costs (Cohen and Henderson, 1988).

Another factor affecting the costs of different prevention activities is the frequency with which they have to be administered. Screening may need to be repeated. One question which may be addressed using cost-effectiveness techniques is the optimum timing of repeat screening.

Repetition may also be a factor in achieving behavioural change. For example, many smokers try quitting several times before finally succeeding and interventions at each attempt may influence the outcome.

Cost-effectiveness of targeting health promotion activities

The economics of targeting health promotion activities depend on the cost consequences of targeting and the effectiveness of a population approach. For example, screening the population to identify those with elevated blood-cholesterol levels, to give them either dietary advice or drug therapy, will be expensive but the health gain per individual could be high. In contrast, population approaches such as mass media campaigns or work with food companies to produce healthier products are likely to give a lower gain per individual but because of their coverage could give a higher overall gain. Most research in this area has concerned the most cost-effective strategy for lowering risk factors such as high blood pressure and cholesterol levels through primary care. Calculations by the Standing Medical Advice Committee (1990) suggested that population screening for elevated blood-cholesterol levels would not be cost-effective and that drug therapy should be considered as a last resort for the older age group with high cholesterol levels.

There are only a limited number of studies which can be used to illustrate the different factors influencing policy choice. Many studies of primary prevention have been based on assumptions about costs and benefits, rather than actual policy evaluations, to make conclusions about cost effectiveness (Williams, 1987; Cummings *et al.*, 1989; Hall *et al.*, 1988). Extensions of this type of work may be a first step in determining health promotion priorities.

The economic evaluation of health promotion activities presents a number of challenges, especially in designing studies to give robust results as not all initiatives are suitable for randomised controlled trials. There is also great difficulty in measuring the health outcomes from health promotion activities (Tolley, 1993). Models such as PREVENT (Gunning-Schepers, 1989) are a useful tool in providing predictions of health gains occurring over a time period. Most available models are, however, limited to mortality measures and it is important to attempt to measure changes in morbidity, especially those changes which may occur in the short term from different prevention activities.

Rosen and Lindholm (1992) list the factors often ignored when considering the cost-effectiveness of lifestyle interventions. This list includes intangible costs and benefits from different prevention strategies, the morbidity as well as the mortality effects, and the effects of a lifestyle change on the full range of diseases. They also consider how changes in behaviour by one person may also influence others (social diffusion).

Conclusions

Whether prevention is better than cure or lifestyle change is better than other prevention activities remains to be fully investigated. All ineffective interventions are a waste of scarce resources. This raises problems for both purchasers and providers, especially when some prevention activities, such as those directed at HIV/AIDS, involve diseases with devastating consequences. Systematic reviews are suggesting some effective prevention strategies while others have little value (Holland and Stewart, 1990; Fisher, 1989). Russell (1990) illustrates that cost-effectiveness criteria may alter some of the recommendations arising from such reviews. An economic approach as outlined has the potential for giving some initial guidance for purchasers. There is, however, a need to improve the monitoring and evaluation of prevention activities to ensure resources are being used cost-effectively.

It is clear that cost-effectiveness criteria have not been a primary concern at the initial policy planning stage of many recent reforms designed to encourage more health promotion. Scott and Maynard (1991) suggest for example, that the services that general practitioners were required to provide after a new contract was negotiated in 1990 were not proven cost-effective. They conclude 'examining the contractual obligations for health checks, it can be seen that the evidence points to the fact that such activities provide little or no benefit to the patient in terms of reducing mortality and morbidity, and incur substantial costs'. New arrangements have been proposed for the reimbursement of general practitioners for health promotion work. These should allow the encouragement of more opportunistic screening and advice, but initially requirements for health checks are to remain for the present.

Similar problems could occur as the *Health of the Nation* initiative is implemented (Akehurst et al., 1991). The selection of areas to target and the level at which they were set were not driven by cost-effective criteria. Local circumstances may suggest different priorities than those given as national targets. There is, therefore, a danger that the pursuit of targets may neither maximise health gain nor use resources efficiently.

While there is widespread support for prevention, there are still many barriers to its implementation. A number of steps can be taken to identify activities which purchasers may consider have the best evidence for being good buys but change cannot be implemented without the right incentives. More attention is needed to provide both evidence of the cost-effectiveness of different prevention activities and the structures needed to ensure that where evidence is strong change takes place.

Acknowledgements

The author gratefully acknowledges the support of the Health Education

Authority for funding some of the research used in this chapter and the ESRC Data Archive and the OPCS for the provision of data used with the PREVENT model. The views expressed are those of the author alone.

References

Akehurst, R., Godfrey, C., Hutton, J. and Robertson, E. (1991). 'The Health of the Nation': an economic perspective on target setting, *Discussion Paper, 92*. York: Centre for Health Economics.

Cohen, D. B. and Henderson, J. B. (1988). *Health, Prevention and Economics*. Oxford: Oxford Medical Publications.

Cummings, S. R., Rubin, S. M. and Oster, G. (1989). The cost effectiveness of counselling smokers to quit, *Journal of the American Medical Association, 261*, 75–79.

Department of Health (1992). *The Health of the Nation*, Cm 1986. London: HMSO.

Downie, R. S., Fyfe, C. and Tannhill, A. (1992). *Health promotion models and values*. Oxford: Oxford Medical Publications.

Drummond, M. F., Ludbrook, A., Lowson, K. and Steele, A. (1987). *Studies in economic appraisal in health care*, vol 2. Oxford: Oxford University Press.

Fisher, M. (ed) (1989). *Guide to Clinical Preventive Services*. Baltimore: Williams & Wilkins.

Fries, J. F. (1989). Health promotion and the compression of morbidity, *British Medical Journal, 289*, 481–483.

Godfrey, C., Tolley, K. and Drummond, M. (1992). The economics of promoting sexual health. In Curtis, H. (ed). *Promoting sexual health*. London: British Medical Association.

Godfrey, C., Hardman, G. and Tolley K. (1993). Cost effectiveness of health promotion: application to coronary heart disease. London: Health Education Authority.

Gunning-Schepers, I. (1989). The health benefits of prevention – a simulation approach, *Health Policy, 12* (special issue).

Hall, J. P., Heller, R. F., Dobson, A. J. *et al.* (1988). A cost-effectiveness analysis of alternative strategies for the prevention of coronary heart disease, *Medical Journal of Australia, 148*, 272–277.

Holland, W. W. and Stewart, S. (1990). Screening in health care – benefit or bane? London: Nuffield Hospital Trust.

Parsonage, M. and Neuburger, H. (1992). Discounting and health benefits, *Health Economics, 1*, 71–76.

Rosen, M. and Lindholm, I. (1992). The neglected effects of lifestyle interventions in cost-effectiveness analysis, *Health Promotion International, 7*, 163–169.

Russell, L. B. (1986). *Is Prevention Better than Cure?* Washington, DC: The Brookings Institution.

Russell, L. B. (1990). The cost effectiveness of preventative services. In Goldbloom, R. B. and Lawrence, R. S. (eds). *Preventing Disease: Beyond the Rhetoric*. New York: Springer-Verlag, 433–437.

Scott, T. and Maynard, A. (1991). Will the new GP contract lead to cost effective medical practice?, *Discussion Paper, 82*. York: Centre for Health Economics.

Standing Medical Advisory Committee (1990). Blood Cholesterol testing: the cost-effectiveness of opportunistic cholesterol testing. London: Department of Health.

Tannahill, A. (1985). What is health promotion?, *Health Education Journal, 44*, 167–168.

Tolley, K. (1993). Evaluating the cost-effectiveness of health promotion. London: Health Education Authority.

Williams, K. (1985). Screening for syphilis in pregnancy: an assessment of the costs and the benefits, *Community Medicine, 7*, 37–42.

Williams, A. (1987). Screening for risk of CHD: is it a wise use of resources? In Oliver, M. (ed). *Screening for Risk of Coronary Heart Disease*. Chichester: John Wiley.

20 The efficacy of health promotion, health economics and late modernism

Roger Burrows, Robin Bunton, Steven Muncer and Kate Gillen

Introduction[1]

All contemporary health care systems are interested in the efficacy and cost-efficiency of different modes of intervention Although there are various philosophies of evaluation it has become apparent that the discourse of health economics is increasingly being turned to. More and more the organisation and delivery of health care is being framed and articulated in terms of 'value for money' rather than any alternative moral discourses. . .

In reviewing the literature on this topic it became apparent that a variety of economic analyses had recently been carried out. However, despite their level of technical sophistication the nature of the conclusions reached were, without exception, lacking in specificity, and thus practically were of little use to policy makers and/or purchasers of health care. In this paper we argue that the inability of health economics to deliver practical guidance highlights important epistemological issues concerning both the nature and evaluation of health promotion, that no amount of technical advance in health economics will solve. . .

[U]ntil the 1990s there had been very few major published studies on the cost effectiveness of either health promotion or health education activities (Drummond *et al.*, 1987; Cohen and Henderson, 1990). However, in the 1990s things changed in this respect, as the language of health economics entered ever more deeply into considerations of health care efficacy. Just as had happened in other organisational contexts (Burrows, 1991), the discourses of business, enterprise and efficiency have, despite resistances, increasingly become codified as *the* legitimating articulating principles of the British health service. This codification finds its most sophisticated expression in the frameworks and models of health economics.

* From *Health Education Research, Theory and Practice*, 10, (2) (1995), pp. 241–249. © Oxford University Press 1995.

There is an irony here, because although the language of organisational calculus is increasingly a rational one the 'reality' of contemporary organisational life is anything but. The process of socio-economic restructuring experienced by almost all (what used to be) public sector organisations (Burrows and Loader, 1994) over the last decade has resulted in a chaos and confusion within organisational life with which most of us are familiar. However, this has been accompanied by a language of legitimation based upon economic *prioritisation* and systematic *evaluation*. Our argument is that the emergence of this language in this context has little to do with modernist rationality and much to do with a desperate search for some form of [what the influential social theorist Anthony Giddens (1990) calls] *'ontological security'*. At just the point when, as Marx would have it, '[a]ll that is solid melts into air, all that is holy is profaned' the late modern subject searches for the apparent surety, rationality and solidity that the discourse of economics provides. The rise of health economics in the context of health care has then, in the end, more to do with the power of rhetoric than it has to do with rational decision-making (Ashmore *et al.*, 1987). In short, the indeterminant, complex and contradictory world of late modern health care has found in economics a touchstone with which to ease its aching head.

In summary our argument is that the procedures designed for the economic evaluation of modernist clinical and experimental work are often not appropriate for the evaluation of much non-clinical public health work, emblematic of late modern medicine, where data is more often than not based upon non- or, at best, quasi-experimental social survey research designs where there is no, or very little, possibility of using control groups. Further, unlike much biomedical research where statistical and causal relations are often more readily unravelled by experimental techniques, social survey-based research interested in environmental, sociological and psychological variables related to lifestyles and behavioural changes, are often more opaque, contingent and sometimes just simply impossible to relate to a causal view of the world.

The framework

The framework consists of seven elements (Tolly, 1993, pp. 53–5); defining the study problem; expressing the economic objectives; identifying the alternative options; choosing a study design; identifying and measuring costs; identifying and measuring outcomes; and calculating cost-effectiveness indicators.

Defining the study problem

This has two dimensions: the *level of analysis* and the *perspective* adopted.

There are four possible levels of analysis. First, the assessment of the cost-effectiveness of alternative, but analytically similar interventions, such as different health education programmes. Second, the assessment of the cost-effectiveness of one style of health promotion, such as health education, compared to alternative health promotion or prevention interventions. Third, the assessment of the cost-effectiveness of health promotion activities compared to treatment and curative interventions. For example, the economics of the new public health compared to more clinically-based medicine. Fourth, the assessment of the cost-effectiveness of health promotion compared to the allocation of additional resources to other areas of the public sector which, although beyond the domain of health policy as narrowly conceived, still have a considerable impact upon health outcomes: education, housing, transport, social security, environment and so on. These different levels of analysis can be viewed from three possible perspectives. First, that of a single agency such as a District Health Authority (DHA), a GP surgery, a Trust or even the Health Education Authority. Second, that of many agencies when health promotion strategies involve multi-agency collaborations such as community-based prevention programmes involving DHAs, Family Health Service Authorities, Social Services, Voluntary Organisations and so on. Third, that of society as a whole – the broadest perspective possible – where the costs and outcomes relevant to all agencies *and* members of the public are considered. Clearly, depending upon the perspective taken, one's economic conclusions can be dramatically different. Such a rational approach is, of course, in practice rarely possible. The messy world of health policy and resource allocation is only very infrequently articulated in terms of such alternatives.

Economic objectives

The stated objectives of *The Health of the Nation* (Department of Health, 1992) are the prevention of ill health and the promotion of good health and wellbeing. Thus, the economic objectives of health promotion can be viewed in terms of (1) the reduction of both mortality and morbidity levels, and (2) improvements in the quality of life at lowest cost. Thus, from the perspective of health economics health promotion strategies should be selected which produce the lowest cost per life year saved or, alternatively and perhaps more realistically, the greatest number of life years saved for a given cost. Thus, as has occurred in so many spheres of cultural, political and social life over the last decade, it is the calculus of cost, rather than any other basis of decision-making, which has come to predominate (Burrows, 1991). Under this regime the multiple and complex determinants of the 'irrationalities' of organisational life, i.e. tradition, morality, expert knowledge, culture, ecology, etc. are reduced to the supposed 'rationality' of economic calculation. Health economics promises an objective basis for the allocation of health care resources driven by a clear set of objectives (Ashmore *et al.*, 1987).

Health promotion options

There are a myriad of different health promotion strategies which can be followed. However, health economics demands a clear delineation of the different alternatives available if it is to be able to make rational comparisons of the costs and benefits of different approaches. Economics demands a systemic approach to health policy options. This involves the clarification of (1) the full range of different types of health promotion on offer, (2) a consideration of which 'risk factor strategy' to follow within each type of health promotion, (3) a consideration of the most appropriate location or setting for the strategy and (4) consideration of whether a 'high risk' or 'population' approach is to be followed. This systemic approach has led to some clear analytic distinctions being made in the conceptualisation of health promotion as a generic set of practices, which is to be welcomed. One of the clearest conceptualisations is that offered by Tannahill (1985) and Downie *et al.* (1991). This is based upon a typology, which in its most simple version (Tolley, 1993, p. 21), makes distinctions between the four broad health promotion options: *prevention* (e.g. immunisation/screening), *health education* (e.g. empowering individuals to be able to influence their own health), *health protection and support* (e.g. the provision of exercise facilities, no-smoking policies, etc.) and *progressive health education* (e.g. community development strategies). These four basic approaches can, of course, be combined in various different ways in order to construct more complex strategies.

These different strategies also have to be considered within the context of another set of possible options. First, what *risk factor strategy* is to be followed? A single risk factor strategy focuses on just one issue – smoking, high blood pressure, lack of exercise and so on, whilst a *multi-risk factor strategy* involves a programme which simultaneously attempts to modify a range of risk factors associated with a particular cause of morbidity and/or mortality such as heart disease. Next, consideration has to be given to what setting or site is most appropriate for the health promotion activity selected. Possible settings might include workplaces, schools, the 'community', primary health care sites, the mass media or public education channels, etc. Finally, decisions need to be made on whether *high risk* or *population-based* strategies are to be followed. For example, whether GP advice on smoking should only be given to those patients already identified as being 'at risk' or whether it should be aimed at all patients.

Study designs

The most rigorous study design is one based upon *experimental procedures* using random control trials. However, there are great problems in applying such research designs in the context of the real social settings of health promotion activities. Much more common in actual settings are *quasi-experimental designs*. This approach usually relies upon the statistical 'matching' of participants in health promotion programmes with individuals with similar social characteristics from a site not involved in the programme. Obviously, although more practicable, such designs possess a much lower level of reliability in controlling for the influence of variables outside of the health promotion programme. Finally, *non-experimental* designs, although perhaps the most common in health promotion research, are the least rigorous and reliable method for establishing the efficacy of health promoting activities. They, most commonly, rely upon 'before and after' study designs in which, for example, patterns of diet are measured prior to and then following a 'healthy eating' campaign in order to ascertain the extent to which the desired changes in the pattern of diet have occurred.

Social research is very different to clinical research not because it is any better or any worse, but because the object of its attention – the social – is a very different phenomena to the human body. It is an 'open system' subject to highly complex patterns of determination and, crucially, it is the product, at least in part, of the meaningful actions of intentional agents who reflexively monitor their performances in a way in which purely biological and physical entities do not. Experimental methods in such a context are, in large part, simply not possible (Stacey, 1987). Thus. evaluations of the 'measurable' efficacy, or otherwise, of health promotion is difficult, perhaps impossible, to determine. The usual response to this is to argue that radical methodological developments in the evaluation of health promotion interventions are required. However, little in the way of practical guidance as to what these methodologies might look like is available. As things stand the efficacy, and so it must follow, the cost-effectiveness of health promotion, is difficult to determine because the methods associated with measuring social interventions orientated to health are so blunt.

Costs

The costs included in any analysis of cost-effectiveness will obviously be a function of the perspective the study takes (see above). If a single agency approach is taken only direct costs to the agency might be included. If a multi-agency approach is taken the costs to all the agencies should be included. Finally, if a society perspective is adopted then the costs of all provider agencies *and* the costs to all individuals receiving the intervention (such as travel costs, the cost of other activities foregone, etc.) should be included. In addition future cost savings (such as GP time saved in the future due to health promotion activity now) should, in theory at least, be included in any evaluation. This process of costing is, in practice, extremely difficult if not impossible to carry out. Further, the cost of collecting the cost data can itself be very high. Thus, it might be that the cost effectiveness of a given intervention could be undermined by the very process of economic evaluation. Further, the nature of the assumptions made about costs at this stage can, and do, have a dramatic impact upon the conclusions of any study.

Outcomes

There are three interrelated measures of outcome. First, necessary but of least overall importance, are *process indicators* which provide an indication of both the supply and demand of health promotion artifacts. An example of a supply indicator would be the number of smoking cessation leaflets distributed, and an example of a demand indicator would be the extent of public awareness of a mass media campaign on the risks associated with smoking. Second, *intermediate outcomes* relate to the influence that health promotion has on behaviours and lifestyles. For example, the impact a smoking cessation campaign has upon rates of smoking. These then are the mediating factors between health promotion interventions and changes in health status. Finally, and crucially, final outcomes relate to such measurable changes in health, if any, associated with the mediating changes in behaviour and/or lifestyle. These might be measured in terms of reductions in prevalence of a given disease, life years saved or Quality Adjusted Life Years (QALYs) gained from changes in mortality and/or morbidity rates due to the original health promoting intervention.

However, the measurement of outcomes are, like costs, very difficult. First, as discussed above, research designs in health promotion tend, for good reason, to be non-experimental and thus efficacy is very difficult to quantify. Second, as is well known, the use of final outcome measures based upon QALYs and the various other scales available, originally designed for clinical settings, tend to be insensitive in the context of health promotion. Outcome measures of qualitative changes of subjective wellbeing amongst the population due to interventions are notoriously difficult to construct. Third, the health gains from health promotion tend to occur over the mid to long term and are thus difficult to quantify within short-term research designs.

The only 'solution' to some of these problems has been to use epidemiologically-based simulation models such as PREVENT (Gunner-Schepers, 1989; Godfrey, 1993) in order to provide crude estimates of the possible outcome measures associated with various health promotion interventions. Although problematic, such an approach may be the only really viable option available to agencies who have neither the time nor the resources to undertake large-scale, long-term research projects. PREVENT and similar simulations are statistical models which are able to estimate changing aggregate patterns of death given estimates of relevant risk factors such as smoking, drinking. high blood cholesterol, hypertension and so on. Such models are analogous to econometric simulations of the economy which attempt to estimate changes in variables such as growth, unemployment and inflation given changes in other variables such as taxation, interest rates, government expenditure and so on. Parameter estimates for the evaluations which constitute the model can be derived from the (few) long-term cohort studies which do exist and/or other sources of evidence.

The problems with such an approach to the estimation of outcomes are, however, numerous. Two problems in particular are important. First, there is only very limited evidence for the reliability of the strength of associations between both health promotion interventions and risk factor modification and between risk factor modification and disease outcomes. In short, evidence for the link between behavioural change and physiological impact is, to say the least, limited. Second, most models concentrate on mortality rather than morbidity and have great difficulties in dealing with changes in the rather opaque area of 'quality of life' which may be the only outcome of some styles of radical community based health promotion and education interventions Nevertheless despite these problems the development of such simulation models appear to be the only viable source of estimates of outcome data in most analyses short of the funding of large-scale cohort studies over two or more decades.

Cost-effectiveness indicators

The final stage of the framework is to bring together cost data and outcome data and, ideally, present it in such a manner as to inform rational decision making as to the most appropriate allocation of resources. This would normally be expressed in terms of a comparison between calculations of, for example, costs per life saved or costs per QALY. It will be clear from the discussion above that such calculations are rarely unproblematic. Even if reliable data is available on both costs and outcomes – and we have been unable to find any such studies (Bunton *et al.*, 1994) – a view still has to be taken on how best to deal with two other crucial issues.

First, consideration has to be given to what the most appropriate *discount rate* should be. This refers to the idea that people and/or organisations tend to prefer to delay costs but to obtain immediate benefits: hence, e.g.:

> consumers . . . prefer to pay for a washing machine using interest-free credit or will only deposit their money in a restricted access savings

account if a high rate of interest is paid on the sum. (Tolley, 1993, p. 53)

In relation to health, the Department of Health suggests that a 'zero' discount rate is appropriate, i.e. health benefits in the future are worth as much as they are in the present. However, this is unrealistic given the seemingly inherent 'short-termism' of much public sector funding. Whatever the rhetoric might be, at the moment at least, health service organisations are going to value measurable gains in health *now* more highly than any future gains. Given that the cycle of performance measures for individuals in such organisations tends to be annual as well, this also reinforces a favourable disposition towards policies aimed at short-term rather than long-term results. A discount rate of greater than 'zero' will clearly – if it can be measured – reduce cost-effectiveness. However, it is apparent from the literature that such discount rates are – and this despite the 'technical' character of much of the justifactory discourse which surround them – essentially subjective imputations, which tend to vary from between about 5 to 10 per cent.

Second, although not a priority for *The Health of The Nation*,[2] equity has been demonstrated to be an important correlate of national mortality rates (Wilkinson, 1992) and is, consequently, an important element of many local strategies for public health (e.g. NRHA, 1992). Considerations of cost-effectiveness should then perhaps include pre-defined equity objectives (McGuire *et al.*, 1988). This might result in the (possibly) higher costs of health promotion activities being justified in order to have an impact upon socially deprived localities if equity objectives are explicitly built into the calculus of considerations. Indeed, unless equity objectives are explicitly considered in cost-effectiveness considerations they will be implicitly excluded on cost grounds. In short, it may be that the most effective strategies are not the most cost-effective.

Conclusion

The framework is the most sophisticated one available to health economists. It can be used, for both retrospective reviews of existing studies – a kind of ideal typical template against which any particular study might be 'deciphered – or in a prospective manner, in any future research and/or evaluation designs. However, as we have already indicated few, if any, of the studies which exist on the economics of health promotion can live up to the demands of this ideal type. In short, although conceptually coherent in terms of the paradigm of health economics it is, and we argue will remain, empirically unoperationalisable because of the nature of the phenomena to which it is being directed. In short, the problem is not one of methodological refinement, it is a problem inherent to life under late modernism. . .

Notes

1. This paper derives from work carried out for Bunton *et al.* (1994), a report commissioned by the (then) Northern Regional Health Authority (NRHA). We gratefully acknowledge the support of the NRHA. The views expressed here are, however, only those of the authors and do not in any way represent the views of the NRHA.
2. However, it is interesting to note that in November 1993 the Department of Health commissioned a review and evaluation of interventions which attempt to address the issue of health inequalities.

References

Ashmore, M., Mulkay, M. and Pinch, T. (1987). *Health and Efficiency*. Buckingham: Open University Press.

Bunton, R., Burrows, R., Gillen, K. and Muncer, S. (1994) *Interventions to Promote Health in Economically Deprived Areas: A Critical Review of the Literature*. Northern Regional Health Authority.

Burrows, R. (ed) (1991) *Deciphering the Enterprise Culture*. London: Routledge.

Burrows, R. and Loader, B. (eds) (1994). *Towards a Post-Fordist Welfare State?* London: Routledge.

Cohen, D. and Henderson, J. (1990). *Health Prevention and Economics*. Oxford: Oxford Medical Publications.

Department of Health (1992). *The Health of the Nation: A Strategy for Health in England*. London: HMSO.

Downie, R., Fyfe, C. and Tannahill, A. (1991). *Health Promotion: Models and Values*. Oxford: Oxford University Press.

Drummond, M. F., Ludbrook, A., Lowson, K. and Steel, A. (1987). *Studies in Economic Appraisal in Health Care*, vol 2, Oxford: Oxford Medical Publications.

Fox, N. (1994). *Postmodernism, Sociology and Health*, Buckingham: Open University Press.

Giddens, A. (1990). *The Consequences of Modernity*. Cambridge: Polity Press.

Giddens, A. (1991). *Modernity and Self-Identity: Self and Society in the Late Modern Age*. Cambridge: Polity Press.

Godfrey, C. (1993). Is prevention better than cure? In Drummond, M. and Maynard, A. (eds), *Purchasing and Providing Cost-Effective Health Care*. Edinburgh: Churchill Livingstone.

Gunner-Schepers, L. (1989). The health benefits of prevention – a simulation approach, *Health Policy*, *12*, 12–55.

Hall, S., Held, D. and McGrew, T. (eds) (1992). *Modernity and its Futures*, Cambridge: Polity Press.

Kelly, M. and Charlton, B. (1995). The modern and the postmodern in health promotion. In Bunton, R., Nettleton, S. and Burrows, R. (eds), *The Sociology of Health Promotion*. London: Routledge.

McGuire, A., Henderson, J. and Mooney, G. (1988). *The Economics of Health Care*. London: Routledge.

Northern Regional Health Authority (NRHA) (1992). *How Do We Create a Healthy North?* Northern Regional Health Authority.

Stacey, M. (1987). The role of information in the development of social policy. *Community Medicine*, *9*, 216–225.

Tannahill, A. (1985). What is health promotion? *Health Promotion Journal*, *44*, 167–168.

Tolley, K. (1993). *Health Promotion: How to Measure Cost-Effectiveness*, London: Health Education Authority.

Wagner, P. (1994). *A Sociology of Modernity: Liberty and Discipline*, London: Routledge.

Wilkinson, R. (1992). National mortality rates: the impact of inequality? *American Journal of Public Health*, *82*, 1982–1084.

21 Towards a critical approach to evaluation *

Angela Everitt and Pauline Hardiker

. . . In the market economy of social welfare, a rational–technical approach to performance measurement, underpinned by the notion of causality relating input and output, is being applied to such an extent that a form of managerial evaluation is emerging. Evaluation thus is rapidly becoming part of the repertoire of those controlling policy and resource allocation mechanisms . . .

In this chapter, we now explore evaluation approaches located within alternative paradigms, acknowledging the significance of subjectivity, values and power in the shaping of understandings of programmes, projects and practice . . .

Interpretivist evaluations

The first responses to the criticisms of rational–technical evaluations came from evaluators approaching understandings of the world within an interpretivist, sometimes called naturalistic, paradigm . . .

[This] assume[s] that the social world is fundamentally different from the physical and natural one in that it is made up of people with subjectivities. Subjectivity cannot be eliminated by controlling it. To pretend to such an endeavour is to fail to capture the richness and variety of people's subjective understandings. And to assert that values can be eliminated through control is to negate the inevitable influence of values on data collected and on their analysis: thus leaving such values intact and implicit. This applies to the subjectivities and values of all involved in the evaluation process. So, rather than knowledge of practices and programmes being generated through supposedly neutral and objective data collection and analysis processes, these are treated as being given meaning by the range of actors involved in the practice. It is these meanings that are sought by the evaluator. This position is clearly articulated by Smith and Cantley, for example, in proposing:

* From A. Everitt and P. Hardiker (1996). *Evaluating for Good Practice*, Chapter 5, pp. 83–215. London: Macmillan, as part of BASW series Practical Social Work.

the need to develop a more pluralistic approach which could cope with diversity and conflict. A more subjectivist methodology would promote the collection of multiple perspectives on the programme (not necessarily in agreement with each other) and would incorporate them into the evaluation exercise. Ambiguity and lack of agreement in perception between parties of the policy-shaping community would then be a central feature of the research, rather than an embarrassment as is the case when the presumption of consensus fails. (Smith and Cantley, 1985, pp. 8-9)

These evaluations, then, reject the notion of value-free, neutral objectivity. Instead, evaluation:

- Seeks to capture people's understandings of what is going on and to what effect, recognising that these will not be the same for all people;
- Reflects on the subjectivity of the evaluator, recognised as important to the development of understanding;
- Focuses on processes through which meanings are attached to practices and programmes;
- Reveals understandings rather than causal explanations;
- Tends to generate qualitative data and analyses these as such;
- Focuses on meanings ascribed by people;
- Does not control or pretend to eliminate values but treats them as fundamental to the meanings people attach to their experiences.

Having regard to equality, this approach is clearly an advance on the managerial, rational–technical model in that it accords all involved, including users, the right to know and be heard. And the evaluators must make their own subjective values explicit. The approach holds evaluators accountable for their values . . .

Towards a critical evaluation

Critical theorists criticise interpretivists for their failure to take account of the structures and processes through which subjectivities are shaped and maintained. There are theories of power which help locate people's views of their experiences and their expectations of, and aspirations for, social welfare projects and programmes. These theories, too, help to decide who to include on the list of stakeholders and, furthermore, to actively draw into the process those who otherwise might be excluded. In informing and facilitating the evaluation process, theories of power help to understand whose interests may be actively articulated, by themselves and others, at the expense of whom. Structural and interpersonal expressions of power render some as powerful and others as powerless. It is these forms of power that can provoke both conflict and consensus in the project or organisation. If evaluation is to be effective in ensuring 'good' practice and revealing or inhibiting 'poor' and 'corrupt' practice, it needs to develop ways to puncture consensuses that produce taken-for-granted, uncontested ways of understanding and intervention that may not be in everyone's interests.

Critical social science can help in a number of ways in our search for such an evaluation model. It:

- Locates social welfare projects, programmes and practices, and people's understandings and evaluations of them, historically and in their social, political and economic contexts;
- Reveals how dimensions of oppression such as social class, gender, race, age, disability and sexuality generate and maintain certain practices and understandings;
- Deconstructs commonly accepted ways of doing things and understandings so that these are not taken-for-granted but are exposed for the extent to which they both influence and are influenced by prevailing ways of thinking; is informed by theories of democracy and social justice that help to guide both the processes of judgement making and the judgements to be made; is committed to provoking change in the direction of equality . . .

The evaluation process may be conceptualised in two phases although in practice these are interrelated. First is the phase of generating evidence about the practice, the programme or project. Critical social science theorises the ways in which people's views, experiences, aspirations and expectations are shaped through dimensions such as age, class, gender, race, sexuality and disability. Through their understanding of the ideological shaping of subjectivities, critical social scientists claim that they are able to generate a more true version of reality than interpretivists who accept subjectivity at face value. Rather than generate ideologically constructed versions of reality, through their methods of data collection and analysis, critical social scientists claim that they can take account of ideology in their search for truth.

The second interrelated phase of evaluation is that of making judgements about whether the practice is 'good', 'good enough' or 'poor' or 'corrupt'. Critical social science provides us with standards against which to make such judgements: standards of justice and equality.

Case example

The evaluation of the young women's project based in an area of social and economic disadvantage did not only involve stakeholders who could readily be identified as being associated with the project. Certainly, there were such people who were involved in the evaluation from the beginning: the workers in the project; the local authority personnel who were responsible for recommending to the authority that it continue to grant-aid the project; members of the voluntary management committee, there as professionals, feminists and/or former and current users; volunteers; and workers in other agencies such as a nearby family centre and the area office of the social services department which refer young women to the project. The project's aims included a commitment to making the project accessible to all young women, Black and white. The evaluation adopted this commitment as a statement of equality and justice by which the work of the project could be evaluated.

Generating evidence about the project revealed that the meaning of this commitment was becoming increasingly contested as the project employed Black workers with different views about the needs of young Black women. Some workers, Black and white, felt that it was alright that Black young women did not use the project. They argued that the project was not appropriate for young Black women who would be better served by developing their own activities like sewing groups. The project currently offered discussion groups and activities that would facilitate discussion around issues such as single parenting, child abuse, and domestic violence. Other workers, Black and white, argued strongly that the project and all of its activities should be more accessible to Black young women. Additionally there should be some Black-only groups to provide space for Black women to share accounts of their experiences and develop understandings of racism.

Taking a critical social science perspective, the evaluation did not accept all the workers' views at face value, a process which would have resulted in a plurality of perspectives being documented. It theorised race and racism as influencing the views of white and Black workers. It engaged in a process of data generation and debate in the project to address more critically the processes that resulted both in the de-politicising of the lives of young Black women and in leaving invisible to the project young Black women living in the locality. The evaluation team was expanded to include a Black woman and data were collected to identify potential stakeholders, potential users. The picture that emerged was of a predominantly white locality with issues of racism being experienced directly by women of mixed ethnicities who sometimes identified themselves as white, sometimes as Black. There were also issues of racism for young white mothers with Black children.

The Black member of the evaluation team conducted a study day with the project to facilitate informed debate about race and ethnicity in the project. For debate, or critical dialogue, the project had before it the data that had been generated in such a way as to take account of race and racism. The study day also was concerned to develop some agreed priorities for the future work of the project. (Everitt and Johnson, 1992).

This analysis of evaluation approaches and their development across positivist, interpretivist and critical paradigms shows a continuing struggle on the part of evaluators to refine their methodologies and methods to generate the truths of the practice, programme or project. What is going on? What is being achieved? Is it 'good', 'good enough', 'poor' or 'corrupt'? Who thinks so and who doesn't? Who decides?

These are the difficult questions that have troubled evaluators. However, for us, those evaluators who take account of subjectivity and have an understanding of relationships between subjectivity and power are more likely to generate sensitive and political understandings of practice and its value. A critical approach to evaluation that recognises dimensions of power and treats evaluation, practice and the policy arena as political processes would seem to meet our conditions for effective evaluation.

At this stage it is useful to reflect . . . on those conditions to test the relevance of critical social science approaches:

- The importance of moral debate and everybody, irrespective of power, status and position, having the right to legitimate opinions.

Critical social science puts faith in what is called the process of emancipatory reasoning. Through reasoning and debate, the truth of practice and the extent to which it is moving in the direction of the 'good' would become evident.

- Scepticism of rational–technical modes of practice.

Critical evaluators understand the rational–technical mode for the ways in which, through supposed control of values, it fails to take them into account, leaving them unchallenged. It thus maintains the status quo and serves powerful interests.

- The recognition of power, powerlessness and empowerment.

Critical evaluators have an understanding of structural and interpersonal processes of power and engage in evaluation as a tool for empowerment, or, in other words, to achieve practice and policy change for equality.

- The development of genuine dialogue between users and those within the organisation, and within the organisation itself.

Critical evaluation engages with users in dialogical processes to provide opportunities for them to develop greater understandings, and through these, enhanced control of their lives. Consciousness-raising is valued as a process through which people lift the mantles of ideology to reveal their true experiences, feelings and views. Users of services within social welfare would be regarded as people likely to be discriminated against through dimensions of race, gender, disability, age and sexuality.

- Attention to be paid to the fundamental purpose of the organisation and caution about becoming diverted into demonstrating productivity.

The critical evaluator would pay attention to the purpose of the organisation regarding this as a statement not only of goals and objectives but of values. This would be used by the critical evaluator to facilitate judgement-making about the programme, project or practice.

- The encouragement of openness, questioning, complaints and criticisms from outside and within the organisation.

Critical evaluation is about opening up the influence of ideology. It questions what appears to be, scrutinising the taken-for-granted, ensuring that people are not saying about a service, policy, organisation what they think they are supposed to say. Evaluation within this paradigm would provide space so that people may feel free to be critical without fear of being penalised.

- The removal of 'otherness' that may be attributed to those lower in the hierarchy, to users and to those relatively powerless in the community.

Critical evaluators, having an awareness of power and powerful processes, would be alert to those who usually are excluded from meaningful decision-making about services, policies and their development. Critical evaluation would ensure that such people, particularly workers and users, have a say in judging the effectiveness of projects. It would ensure that people are not marginalised through racism and/or sexism or because of their social class, age, disabilities or sexual orientations.

We are still not sure however about claims that critical social scientists make to the effect that they are able to lift the mantle of ideology to discover the real views and experiences of people. This reliance on reasoning as a way of seeking out the truth does not fit with our experience of the ways in which such judgements are made in organisations. In our view, the social world of practice is such as to suggest that there are potentially many truths. There is no one answer. Processes of generating and debating evidence of practice in evaluation do not produce the truth of practice. They may produce an agreed version that will do for the moment. The processes of generating and scrutinising evidence do not obviate the need, in the end, to make moral judgements about whether practice is 'good', 'good enough', 'poor' or 'corrupt'. . .

References

Everitt, A. and Johnson, C. (1992). *A Young Women's Project: An evaluation.* Social Welfare Research Unit, University of Northumbria at Newcastle.

Smith, G. and Cantley, C. (1985). *Assessing Health Care: A study in organisational evaluation.* Milton Keynes: Open University Press.

Promoting health
in a wider context

Health promotion is a multi-layered activity and many of the contributions in Sections One and Two have argued that people's health is
more than a matter of individual responsibility. The influence of physical,
social, cultural and economic environments on the health chances of the
individual have been emphasised many times. The focus of health
promotion over the last decade has been to take action within the domains
identified in the Ottawa Charter of 1986: building healthy public policy;
creating supportive environments; strengthening community action;
developing personal skills; re-orienting health services. The contributions
in Section Three are concerned with the wider agenda that arises from
these priority areas.

Yolande Coombes sets the scene in 'An International Perspective on
Primary Health Care' (Chapter 22). She argues that primary health care
lies at the heart of the health promotion vision set out in the Alma Ata
declaration but that in global terms primary health care embraces the
whole community and is not confined to the rather narrower view held in
the United Kingdom, where it is synonymous with General Practice. The
late Wendy Farrant, Chapter 23 in 'Addressing the Contradictions:
Health Promotion and Community Health Action in the United
Kingdom' explored the community development approach based on
participation and community involvement. She argued that in spite of the
WHO global strategy this was largely located outside the NHS. It was not
until the late 1980s that the NHS began to embrace the principles of user
involvement in health with initiatives such as 'Listening to Local Voices'
and moves to make General Practice more community oriented. Wendy
Farrant exposed some of the contradictions in the increased NHS
support for community development approaches and warned of the
dangers of 'colonisation'. This issue is given a further airing in extracts
from the writings of Paulo Freire (Chapter 24) whose work inspired much
of the community development movement in the 1960s and 1970s.
Although written from the perspective of developing countries these

extracts from his influential book *Pedagogy of the Oppressed* remind us today of the dangers of 'cultural invasion', where

> the ultimate seat of decision regarding the action of those who are invaded lies not with them but with the invaders. And when the power of decision is located outside rather than within the one who should decide.

The empowerment of communities is a major part of the agenda of community action for health and in Chapter 25 Alan Beattie asks how effective community action is, and poses the dilemma of evaluating such a diverse activity.

In Chapter 26, Stephen Jan takes up the issues of community participation and asks 'how community preferences can more effectively shape equity policy'. Equity, Stephen Jan points out, is about fairness and social justice and is incompatible with the existence of wide social inequalities in health. Jenny Douglas explores this theme in relation to Black and minority ethnic groups. In Chapter 27 she analyses work at the local level which has identified key issues and concerns involved in trying to improve the health of people from Black and minority ethnic groups. She concludes that whilst work at the community level is vital there is a need for health promotion to operate at the policy level on issues such as employment and immigration policy which are germane to the health of Black and minority ethnic groups.

Building healthy public policy involves putting health on other agendas especially those which have hitherto not focused on health. Chapters 28–30 discuss health in relation to environmental and transport policies as well as an innovative project which uses sport as a vehicle for health promotion. Ronald Labonté (Chapter 28) sets out principles for building a healthy environment. He suggests that health and environmental issues have converged and that health promoters cannot afford to ignore issues such as pollution, global warming, species decline or excessive industrial development. Think globally – act locally is becoming a new watchword for health promoters as well as environmentalists.

Billie Corti and her colleagues offer us in Chapter 29 a glimpse of an innovatory and potentially transformatory approach to health promotion. The notion of sponsorship raises important questions about effectiveness and the marketing of health messages.

In the final contribution in this part Adrian Davis (Chapter 30) examines the politics and policy issues in relation to sport, physical activity, transport and health policy. We explore some of the complexities, of interagency and intersectoral working which are central if health is to be put on wider agendas.

22 An international perspective on primary health care*

Yolande Coombes

Introduction

Primary health care (PHC) is a term that is used in many different ways. PHC is used synonymously in the United Kingdom with primary medical care or community-based care, and is often referred to as 'primary care'. But PHC in the international context involves much more than simply the provision of primary care services. It is an approach to health which embraces the WHO definition of 'complete mental, social and physical well-being' and it has a distinct emphasis on health promotion and disease prevention. PHC involves the participation of the community as well as the organisation of health professionals and other sectors, and it is also (but not just) concerned with the organisation and delivery of health services.

Background

It has been argued (Macdonald, 1993) that PHC offers a fundamental challenge to the dominance of the philosophy of 'western medicine' with its emphasis on curative services and the absence of disease as the definition of health. During the 1970s within the international health arena it became apparent that the inequalities between (and within) countries in terms of health status were continuing to widen. In addition it was recognised that improvements in health status could not happen in isolation and needed to be accompanied by improvements in social and economic conditions. Thus at the thirtieth World Health Assembly in 1997 what has become known as the Health For All by the year 2000 declaration (HFA 2000) was set down. The declaration was that the main *social* goal for governments and WHO should be 'the attainment by all the people of the world by the year 2000 of a level of health that would permit them to lead a socially and economically productive life'. (WHO, 1988). At the same time it was acknowledged that there was a need to re-

---

* Commissioned for this volume.

orientate health services and that there was an over-reliance on technical curative medical interventions which were expensive and limited to a small proportion of the population, in both developed and developing countries.

Primary health care as an approach

In 1977 a conference jointly organised by WHO and UNICEF (United Nation's Children's Fund) in Alma-Ata in the then USSR unanimously endorsed the aim that an acceptable level of health for the world's population could be achieved through a better use of the world's resources. At this conference the key to achieving 'an acceptable level of health throughout the world in the foreseeable future as part of social development and in the spirit of social justice' (Dhillon and Philip, 1994) would be through primary health care (PHC), which offered a way forward for both developed and developing countries alike.

Eight key factors were selected on which PHC would place emphasis:

- Education concerning prevailing health problems and the methods of preventing and controlling them;
- Promotion of food supply and proper nutrition;
- Adequate supply of safe water and basic sanitation;
- Maternal and child health care, including family planning;
- Immunisation against major infectious diseases;
- Prevention and control of locally endemic diseases;
- Appropriate treatment of common diseases and injuries;
- Provision of essential drugs.

WHO identified four key elements or 'pillars' on which action for health should be based:

- Political and social commitment and determination to move towards health for all as the main social target for the coming decades;
- Community participation, the active involvement of people and the mobilisation of societal forces for health development;
- Intersectoral co-operation between the health sector and other key development sectors such as agriculture, education, communications, industry, energy, transportation, public works and housing;
- Systems support to ensure that essential health care and scientifically sound, affordable health technology are available to all people.

These four pillars translate to the concepts of equity, community participation, intersectoral working, and reorientation of health services, which are commonly used concepts within health promotion, and underpinned the Ottawa Charter on health promotion developed in 1986. It could be argued that the differences between PHC as outlined at Alma-

Ata and health promotion are merely semantic. This point is supported by the emphasis on community participation, which was further developed within PHC and the declaration of Alma-Ata, to take an explicit 'people-orientated' approach (in both developing and developed countries) aiming:

- To enable people to seek better health at home, in schools, in fields and in factories;
- To enable people to prevent disease and injury, instead of relying on doctors to repair damage that could have been avoided;
- To enable people to exercise their right and responsibility in shaping the environment and bringing about conditions that make it possible and easier to live a healthy life;
- To enable people to participate and exercise control in managing health and related systems and to ensure that the basic prerequisites for health and access to health care are available to all people. (Dhillon and Philip, 1994)

The idea was that each country would take these principles and approaches towards primary health care and translate them into practical programmes of action that would be specific to the context of that country. The early 1980s saw many countries (mainly within Africa, Asia and Latin America) embracing the PHC approach. Macdonald (1993) points out that this concept of PHC as outlined by the Alma-Ata declaration is far more common in developing than developed countries. Research by Walton (1985) showed that in Europe public health and medical trainees were not aware of the PHC approach, and saw primary care as the provision of 'medical' services within the community.

Although the PHC approach gained widespread support during the early 1980s as the key model for the restructuring of health service provision and health development within developing countries, there were also problems associated with trying to put into place some of the core principles of PHC within these countries. Many countries were politically unstable and were experiencing huge difficulties associated with their economic and social development. For example Farrant (1991) discusses how the importance of equity, participation and intersectoral working implicit to the PHC approach were assumed to be able to be attained without any radical restructuring of society. She cites the WHO publication 'Health by the People' which acknowledged that countries such as China, Tanzania and Cuba which initiated the changes to their health systems through a political process had clear advantages over those countries which had separated health interventions from politics.

Fry and Hasler (1986) acknowledge that there are often remarkable differences between the commitment given to a PHC approach that is down on paper in the form of national policies and the practical implementation of those policies. They discuss a number of case studies which demonstrate that many interventions are haphazard and/or poorly planned. They are often under-resourced and are not controlled. In their conclusion these authors point to the main problems of implementation of the PHC approach being due to the low morale and low enthusiasm of staff due to the practical difficulties associated with translating the principles of equity, participation and multi-sectoral working within the constraints as listed above. Within more developed countries they point to the tensions between GP-led primary care and other PHC health provision as hampering the more comprehensive approach to PHC as outlined at Alma-Ata.

Baum and Sanders (1995) point out that the Alma-Ata declaration was reflective of its time when there was a belief that things would get better. The third world debt crisis of the early 1980s had not appeared, and the market forces which dominated industrialised countries were only just beginning. Although PHC was picked up in the early 1980s by many developing country governments, it was not in the comprehensive form outlined by Alma-Ata but in a more selective and targeted approach 'Considerations of equity, intersectorality and community involvement were dismissed in favour of technical feasibility and cost-effectiveness of programmes' (Baum and Sanders, 1995, p. 150).

Comprehensive versus selective primary health care

Briefly, the distinction between comprehensive and selective PHC can be delineated as the former relating to a philosophy or developmental process towards health and health care and the latter to selective vertical programmes or interventions such as immunisation or screening. These are often designed to increase the health status of the highest possible number of individuals that is cost-effective to cover. Rifkin and Walt (1986) suggest that the main differences between these two views lie in who controls the inputs and outcomes of health improvements, and the time frame in which the outcomes are expected – comprehensive PHC focuses on process and selective PHC on programmes. Selective PHC is seen as a pragmatic approach to the 'idealism' of PHC as outlined at Alma-Ata.

Rifkin and Walt (1986) suggest that comprehensive and selective PHC approaches the concepts of health, equity, inter-sectoral working, and community participation in fundamentally different ways. Selective PHC views health as the absence of disease, does not take account of poverty in the determination of targets for interventions, focuses solely on mobilising health services, and sees community participation in terms of compliance. It could therefore be argued that although pragmatic in its approach, selective PHC is a retrograde step in terms of health promotion.

Although the descriptions of comprehensive and selective PHC seem to be placed at opposite ends of the spectrum, in practice most countries are implementing some form of PHC inclusive of the basic elements (as outlined at Alma-Ata), and with a focus on preventive and clinical aspects. However very few countries have acknowledged PHC as a strategy for organisation of their health systems. Malcom (1994) argues that this has re-emphasised the importance of high-cost curative medical interventions and to hospitals being 'empowered' to dominate the strategic role. PHC is often seen purely as complementing hospital-based services.

Funding PHC

Within developing countries, PHC has mainly been supported by outside donors. Development aid has mainly come from North America and Europe, and PHC has been a high priority for funding since the 1970s. However as Engelkes (1993) points out over the past decade the initial optimism has been replaced by scepticism, and criticism. He suggests that this is mainly due to the decision by some many governments to opt for selective PHC, introducing vertical medical interventions. A number of evaluations have been carried out on PHC programmes and some donors have subsequently given up on funding PHC on the basis of them. Although there are difficulties associated with the way PHC has been put into practice, Engelkes questions the reliability, validity and relevance of many of these evaluations and thus whether important policy decisions should be based on them. It has been argued that people are expecting positive outcomes within too limited a time scale and that this has also contributed to the movement towards selective PHC.

There have been suggestions that the failure of comprehensive PHC has been due to the influence of donors. De Winter (1993) examined the ways that donors have externally funded developing countries. He found that there was a tendency to provide money in terms of PHC 'projects', which has led to a lack of innovative comprehensive PHC programmes. This is partly because people are under the pressure of the daily running of an institution or other facilities/services, and partly because the funding does not permit more creative or innovative ideas. De Winter advocates an institution solely devoted to the development of innovative PHC programmes, and suggests that this should be a priority for donor funding which might lead to the long-term sustainability of PHC within developing countries.

Maclure (1995), in a case study of two PHC programmes in Burkino Faso, suggests that donor aid has induced dependency on the money. The author suggests that donor dependency is directly opposed to the idea of self-reliance and empowerment which are central to the PHC approach. LaFond (1994) suggests that donors need to introduce a staged withdrawal of funds which encourage initial mobilisation and participation within programmes but then move to the promotion of self-reliance and longer-term sustainability.

PHC: Success or Failure?

In an editorial, Malcom (1994) suggests that PHC has not been successful because the inequality between rich and poor countries has continued to grow. WHO (1988) in reporting the progress half way towards the year 2000 at the Riga meeting in 1988, point to both the successes and failures of PHC. They acknowledge that the gaps between developed and developing countries in terms of health status are still apparent, but they claim that the situation is dynamic. They point to indicators of achievement such as that in 1960 there were 72 countries with under-five mortality rates of 178 or more and by 1985 that number had halved to 34 countries (p. 21).

Baum and Sanders (1995) contend that since Alma-Ata progress towards HFA 2000 has been limited, and in part this is due to the global economic recession which in turn has been aggravated by IMF imposed structural adjustment policies, and this has subsequently led to a deterioration of health status in many countries. They note that in some sub-saharan countries mortality rates have increased. Some diseases like malaria and TB have spread back into areas where they had been controlled and HIV/AIDS has appeared.

Baum and Sanders outline the link between poverty and health, and go on to demonstrate how global inequalities contribute to this. They outline four global trends that are detracting from achieving HFC 2000:

1. Goals and targets approach to health promotion – they suggest that this is not practical at the local level, it is a reductionist approach to health and tends to put the focus or responsibility on the individual, and thus ignores the structural causes of ill health.
2. Dominance of market ideology – i.e. minimising the role of the state, and contributing to the increase in private medical care and thus the widening of inequalities.
3. Individualism – a philosophy antithetical to public health, but part of the new right ideology. They advocate a need to restructure the global economy in order to alleviate poverty.
4. Environmental degradation – they argue that this is a qualitatively different public health problem that transcends national boundaries and generations.

These daunting problems may contribute to the move towards selective PHC as those involved feel powerless to overcome these larger global issues, which are nevertheless having an affect at the national and local level.

Other more specific problems associated with PHC stem from the inadequate resources devoted to training. Walker (1995) and Stock-Iwamoto and Korte (1993) both highlight the fact that many PHC programmes in developing countries rely on minimally trained staff. In some cases this was a pragmatic approach to the problems experienced in rural populations, but this has been perpetuated even in urban areas.

Collins and Green (1994) feel that one of the strengths of the PHC approach has been the decentralisation of services and this has aided the responsiveness of services to local needs, has facilitated community participation, improved access to services and resources and is more flexible. However, they also suggest that decentralisation can be a negative part of PHC and indicate examples of where it has strengthened political domination.

Monekasso (1992) argues that the perceived failure of PHC as advocated at Alma-Ata stems from the numerous short-cut attempts and introduction of selective PHC. He argues that when the concept of PHC was re-visited at Riga, 10 years after Alma-Ata it was still apparent that there was consensus for the PHC approach. He argues that what is needed is a better framework to facilitate implementation towards achieving HFA 2000.

The future of PHC

Baum and Sanders (1995) argue that in order for PHC and health promotion to succeed a fundamental restructuring which addresses global inequities in health and the distribution of resources is needed. They suggest a broader vision of health as outlined in the Alma-Ata declaration which concentrates on the processes of change and not static goals. They reassert the need for multi-sectoral approaches, and policy decisions rather than an emphasis on the individual.

Just as the conference in Riga, 10 years after Alma-Ata reaffirmed the goals of PHC it appears that those original ideas still offer the way forward. What is apparent is that the time scale for implementation may take longer than originally envisaged, and that they may not be achieved by the year 2000. The short-cuts in the form of selective PHC have not been successful, as they have proved to be unsustainable. If PHC is truly going to promote the health of the world's population then there needs to be a return to the original ideas of Alma-Ata.

References

Akin, J., Griffin, C., Guilkey, D. and Popkin, B. (1985). *The Demand for Primary Health Service in the Third World*. New Jersey: Rowman & Allanheld.

Baum, F. and Sanders, D. (1995). 'Can health promotion and primary health care achieve Health for All without a return to their more radical agenda?', *Health Promotion International, 10* (2); 149–160.

Collins, C. and Green, A. (1994). 'Decentralisation and Primary Health Care: Some negative implications in developing countries', *International Journal of Health Services, 24* (3); 459–475.

De Winter, E.R. (1993). 'Which way to sustainability? External support to health projects in developing countries', *Health Policy and Planning, 8* (2); 150–156.

Dhillon, H. S. and Philip, L. (1994). *Health Promotion and Community Action for Health in Developing Countries*. Geneva: WHO.

Engelkes, E. (1993). 'What are the lessons from evaluating PHC projects? A personal view', *Health Policy and Planning, 8* (1); 72–77.

Essomba, R. O., Bryant, M. and Bodart, C. (1993). 'The re-orientation of primary health care in Cameroon: rationale, obstacles and constraints', *Health Policy and Planning, 8* (3); 232–239.

Farrant, W. (1991). 'Addressing the contradictions: Health Promotion and Community Health Action in the United Kingdom', *International Journal of Health Services, 21* (3): 423–439.

Ferrinho. P., Robb, D., Cornielje, H. and Rex, G. (1993). 'Primary health care in support of community development', *World Health Forum, 14*; 158–162.

Fry, J. and Hasler, J. (1986). *Primary Health Care 2000*. Edinburgh: Churchill Livingstone.

LaFond, A. (1994). *Sustaining Primary Health Care*. London: Earthscan Publications.

MacDonald, J. (1993). *Primary Health Care: Medicine in its place*. London: Earthscan Publications.

Maclure, R. (1995). 'Primary Health Care and donor dependency: A case study of non government assistance in Burkino Faso', *International Journal of Health Services, 25* (3); 539–558.

Malcom, L. (1994). 'Primary Health Care and the hospital: Incompatible organisational concepts?', *Social Science and Medicine, 39* (4); 455–458

Modeste, N. (1996). *Dictionary of public health promotion and education: terms and concepts*. Thousand Oaks: Sage Publications

Monekosso, G.L. (1992). 'Achieving health for all: a proposal from the African Region of WHO', *Health Policy and Planning, 7* (4); 364–374

Rifkin, S. B. and Walt, G. (1986). 'Why health improves: Defining the issues concerning comprehensive primary health care and selective primary health care', *Social Science and Medicine, 23* (6); 559–566.

Stock-Iwamoto, C. and Korte, R. (1993). 'Primary health workers in North East Brazil', *Social Science and Medicine, 36* (6); 775–782.

Walker, L. (1995). 'The practice of primary health care: A case study', *Social Science and Medicine, 40* (6); 815–824.

Walton, H. J. (1985). 'Primary health care in European Medical Education: A survey', *Medical Education, 19;* 167–188.

World Health Organisation (1978). *Primary Health Care. Report of the international conference on primary health care.* (Alma-Ata, USSR, 6–12 September 1978), 'Health for All' series, *1.* Geneva: WHO/UNICEF.

World Health Organisation (WHO) (1988). *From Alma-Ata to the Year 2000: Reflections at the midpoint.* Geneva: WHO.

23 Addressing the contradictions: health promotion and community health action on the United Kingdom*

Wendy Farrant

Introduction

In the United Kingdom as elsewhere, the last decade has seen a rapid growth and development of the community health movement (Community Projects Foundation, 1988; Blennerhassett *et al.*, 1989). The emergence of the UK community health movement in the late 1970s can be linked to a number of influences, including the women's movement, health action by black and minority ethnic groups; increasing public dissatisfaction with conventional approaches to health care; community workers becoming involved with local health issues; and health workers seeking more democratic ways of working that address the social, economic and political determinants of health. The movement encompasses a diverse and increasing number of groups, projects and initiatives that are applying a community development approach to health. Central to these initiatives is a concern with redressing inequalities in health, by facilitating collective responses to community-defined health needs and enabling powerless and disadvantaged groups to have an effective voice in policy decisions that affect their lives and health. During the 1980s the movement gained added strength and cohesion through the setting up of the National Community Health Resource (NCHR), a national voluntary organisation with responsibility for supporting, developing and promoting the community health movement. Accounts of the development, composition and activities of the UK community health movement and descriptions of individual community development health initiatives, are contained in various publications produced by the NCHR [which changed its name to Community Health UK in 1993], for example see Kenner (1986).

Up until the mid-1980s, there was little meeting point between the community health movement and the National Health Service (NHS). The initial wave of local community development health projects in the

* From *Critical Public Health*, (1994), 5, pp. 5–19. © Baywood Publishing Co. Inc. 1991.

late 1970s and early 1980s were largely initiated, funded and located outside the NHS, mainly in the voluntary sector (Rosenthal, 1983). Although some NHS workers, particularly health education officers, were pioneering community development approaches, health and prevention policy and practice within the NHS continued to be dominated by an individualistic perspective. A study carried out during the first half of the 1980s highlighted the marginalisation of community development approaches to health education at both central and local levels within the NHS, and the perceived political constraints that militated against the national Health Education Council and local Health Education Departments taking this approach on board (Farrant and Russell, 1986).

The latter half of the 1980s, in contrast, was marked by increasing lip service within the NHS to community development in health, stimulated in part by the World Health Organizations' 'Health for All by the Year 2000' (HFA 2000) and Health Promotion initiatives. A development project in an inner city health district during this period highlighted the possibilities, as well as the constraints and dilemmas, of utilising HFA 2000 principles as a framework for promoting a community development approach to health promotion policy (Farrant and Taft, 1989). It also underlined the profound contradictions of 'community participation for health for all' coming into vogue at a time of major national policy shifts toward inequality and non-accountability.

This article focuses on the contradictory implications for the community health movement of recent developments in health promotion policy within the United Kingdom, and aims to illuminate the contradictions by locating them within a historical and international context. The NHS interest in community development in health is examined in relation to broader health and welfare policy of the 1980s, the history of community development in health in former British colonial territories, and the background to the WHO health promotion initiative. The possibilities and limitations of utilising the rhetoric, to support community health action, are explored with reference to moves by the UK community health movement to 'reclaim' Health for All . . .

Community participation or community manipulation?

For those involved in community health action outside the NHS, the later 1980s saw the opening up of opportunities, contradictions and dilemmas. Within mainstream health promotion, there were signs of community development moving from the periphery to centre stage and being seen as less of a threat than a panacea. Terms such as 'community participation' and 'community empowerment' became commonplace in the literature.

The principles of community development received endorsement from

WHO in its HFA 2000 strategy. As noted by the WHO Regional Office for Europe: 'It is a basic tenet of the health for all philosophy . . . health developments in communities are made not only for but with and by the people' (WHO, 1985). References to HFA 2000 became increasingly prominent in UK policy statements. There was little evidence, however, of this official endorsement being translated into increased support for community development health initiatives and devolution of power in decision-making. Health promotion and 'the new public health' were becoming arenas for intersectoral competition as much as collaboration, and in the power struggles between different professional groups and statutory sectors for resources and control the community health movement was hardly getting a look-in (NCHR, 1988). Health promotion priorities were adopting the language of community development without taking on board the fundamental principal of community control over the definition of health needs and solutions.

Meanwhile, as government policies served to intensify inequalities in health, the burden of caring was being thrown ever more on the shoulders of unpaid women in the family and the voluntary sector. Under such circumstances, the notion of health by the people begins to look like a convenient cover-up for the erosion of health *for* the people.

Community development and ideology

Beattie (1986), in arguing for the crucial importance of a critical analysis of the relationships of power and control embedded in different approaches to community development, observed: 'Too often in the health promotion field, the community development approach has been seized upon uncritically and simplistically, as offering radical promise in and of itself . . . It is essential to see that community work is bound up with the whole historical development of the social welfare sector in the modern state.'

Accounts of the historical emergence of community development suggest that far from being inherently radical, it has often been employed to safeguard and further the interests of the ruling class (Cockburn, 1977). The label 'community development' has been applied to many different, often coexisting activities and approaches, ranging from the programme initiated by the British Colonial Office in response to demands for self government for the colonies and by the UK and US governments in response to urban unrest in the 1960s, to oppositional forms of community-based action, and comprehensive development strategies introduced by countries such as China in pursuit of major social transformation. If the potential of community development for challenging rather than reinforcing power relations is to be realised, then it is essential to identify where the impetus for community development is coming from and to differentiate between the ideologies underlying various approaches.

Community development health work in the UK largely originated outside the NHS, in response to the rapid growth of public interest in health from the late 1970s onward. The belated interest of the NHS in community development needs to be seen in relation to the crisis of the welfare state, and broader debates around such issues as community care, volunteerism, decentralisation and consumerism. It is also illuminating to examine the much longer history of state interest in community development in health in the third world, and the background to the WHO health for all initiative.

The NHS policy content

The increasing reference to concepts of community development/participation/involvement/empowerment in the health promotion literature in the late 1980s was backed up by the rhetoric about responsiveness to community needs in Department of Health policy documents such as *Care in Action* (DHSS, 1981), the Griffiths Report on NHS management (1983) and the Cumberledge report on community nursing (DHSS, 1986).

Davies analysed a series of policy interventions within the NHS introduced during the first two administrations of the Thatcher government, which can be seen as amounting to successful establishment of the conditions for a new mix of services, public and private, statutory, voluntary and commercial, in the arena of heath care delivery. She argues that 'self-help, new forms of volunteering, and community empowerment are some of the terms in which a more limited statutory involvement is being cast' (Davies, 1987). This trend toward welfare pluralism has been subjected to more critical scrutiny in the field of social services than in the health sector. Although the opening of the door for expansion of the commercial sector might be regarded as perhaps the most serious implication of the ideology of welfare pluralism, a major focus of the debate has been the relationship between the state and the voluntary sector. While the potential of voluntary and community initiatives for challenging the non-accountability of state bureaucracies and official definitions of need is recognised by both the advocates and critics of welfare pluralism, Beresford and Croft (1984) point out that it is essential to distinguish between allocation of resourccs to the voluntary sector versus promotion of unpaid voluntary and informal care, and between voluntary initiatives that seek to change statutory provision versus those that provide a substitute for it. It is the notion of unpaid voluntary and informal care as a substitute for statutory provision that is so strongly supported by Tory government policy: the negative implications for women as the main providers of unpaid care in the family and the community have been well documented (Finch and Groves, 1983).

Debates around policies of decentralisation highlighted the ways in which concepts such as 'decentralisation', 'patch planning', 'accountability', 'community participation', 'public involvement', 'partnership with the voluntary sector' and so on, can have very different meanings and very different implications in practice, depending on where they are coming from and the political ideology of their advocates (Hambleton and Hoggett, 1984). The model of decentralisation that can be seen as dominating the growing popularity of 'pack' and locality planning within health authorities is a managerialist–consumerist approach that has little to do with notions of democratisation and shifting of the balance of power between providers and users of service (Dun, 1987) . . .

Health for who by the year 2000?

The limitations of conventional approaches to health development were documented in WHO-commissioned studies published in the mid-1970s. The search for alternative solutions (Djukanovic and Mach, 1975), drew heavily on the socialist development strategies of China, Cuba and Tanzania. The major conditions for success identified by WHO analysts were: a commitment to reallocation of resources toward meeting the basic health needs of the impoverished majority; integration of the health sector within a comprehensive programme of social and economic development; and community participation in health planning and implementation. These principles formed the basis of the 1978 Alma-Ata declaration on Primary Health Care (PHC) and the subsequent global HFA 2000 strategy . . .

Health promotion: a new panacea?

Whereas the initial impetus for HFA 2000 came from demands for new approaches to health development in the third world, the WHO health promotion initiative can be linked to the health crisis and social movements in advanced capitalist societies. To quote from the introduction to the report of the First International Conference on Health Promotion (1987):

> This first conference was intended primarily to bring together people from industrialised countries . . . In the industrialised countries inequalities in health are increasing between social groups while health costs continue to rise. The gap between the potential for health of people in industrialised countries and their current health status has indicated a need for new strategies and programmes . . . Moreover, the public interest in health, self-care and mutual aid has led to the questioning of professional approaches and definitions in

health problems . . . Health promotion is an effort to crystallise a wide range of activities that have contributed towards a changing model of public health.

Some insight was provided by Stacey (1988) at a workshop in which she shared her experiences as a social scientist on the WHO European Committee for Research for Health for All (RFHFA). She described the background of the RFHFA strategy as a continual struggle between individualistically oriented biomedical approaches and more socially oriented perspectives.

Such tensions are reflected in the products of WHO consultations on health promotion. The WHO concept of health promotion is explicitly informed by a sociological perspective that sees health and lifestyle as inextricably linked to the social and economic environment, and acknowledges the social nature of the movement for health (Kickbusch, 1986). In many places, however, the publications of the WHO Regional Office for Europe continue to reflect the influence of the biomedical model. A clear example is the 'Targets for HFA' documents, in which the socially oriented perspective of the 'lifestyle' section is juxtaposed with the biomedical perspective of the section on disease prevention.

Although the underlying principles of the WHO concept of health promotion can be seen as profoundly radical in their implications, the model of social change that is implicit in policy statements is inevitably constrained by the political and ideological position of WHO discussed above (Ineson, 1986). Whereas the central HFA focus on redressing inequalities would imply an emphasis on empowering oppressed and disadvantaged groups, 'the community' and 'the public' are frequently referred to as a homogeneous whole, with little encouragement to systematically analyse power relations within and between communities. Insofar as mention is made of the need to secure the participation of the disenfranchised, it is rarely acknowledged that participation involves conflict and confrontation as well as consensus and co-operation and, to be effective, would require a fundamental shift in the distribution of power. While support of spontaneous community action around health is encouraged, community activists tend to be treated as just one set of actors in an equal partnership between the powerful and powerless. The profound significance of the community health movement in challenging social relations that are antithetical to health is at best underplayed.

As with the implementation of HFA in the third world, the contradictions inherent in the strategy documents of the WHO Regional Office for Europe leave them open to misappropriation by professional and other vested interests. There are clear parallels, for example, between the promotion of selective PHC in the third world and the selective interpretation of HFA targets by some health authorities within the UK to support a conventional medical model (Farrant, 1987).

Reclaiming Health for All

In contrast to the gap between the rhetoric and reality of official health promotion, the HFA principles of redressing inequalities, community participation and intersectorial collaboration are central to the aims, values and ways of working of community development health projects and initiatives.

The growth of the UK community health movement has been paralleled by similar developments in other industrialised countries. As indicated above, the WHO health promotion initiative can be seen as, in part at least, a response to this movement. As noted in the report of the workshop on 'Strengthening Communities' at the First International Conference on Health Promotion (1987):

> Though this has been an international conference of local, national and international delegates, the deliberations were primarily a response to the rising and changing expectations of populations around the world, who are demanding assistance in achieving their self-set goals . . . People are seeking a broader social response to improving their personal, social and health environments.

If the potential of this social movement is not be be stultified, then a priority for all concerned about Health for All must be to safeguard against its appropriation.

The Ottawa Charter for Health Promotion (1986) emphasises that 'Health promotion works through concrete and effective *commtunity action* in setting priorities, making decisions, planning strategies, and implementing them to achieve better health. At the heart of this process is the *empowerment of communities,* their *ownership* and *control* of their own destinies'. Endorsement of this principle implies at the very least:

- *Acknowledging* inequalities in power, ownership and control, and vested interests in maintaining inequalities;
- *Challenging* professional control of health promotion; and
- *Validating* and *supporting* community health initiatives that are seeking to transform the distribution of power, ownership and control.

As the implications of professional misappropriation of HFA 2000 have become more apparent, the response of the UK community health movement to 'Health for All' has shifted from detached cynicism to active attempts to 'reclaim' it. An important trigger was the First UK Healthy Cities Conference in Liverpool in 1988, at which community activists produced a statement commenting on the contradiction between the rhetoric of community participation and the planning and structure of the conference, which precluded the participation of local community groups and particularly women and the black community (Thornley, 1988). A week later, at the other end of the world, community activists representing the Central Australian Aboriginal Congress similarly seized possession of the podium at the Second International Conference on Health Promotion, to challenge the Australian Health Minister's expressed commitment to reducing the health gap between white and aboriginal peoples and to seek support for a community health initiative by and for aboriginal women (Farrant and Taft, 1988).

The implications of HFA 2000 for the UK community health movement were the subject of the Summer 1988 issue of *Community Health Action*, the newsletter of the (then) NCHR. A leading article noted that:

> an important point – which seems to have been misused by some who are keen to leap on to the Health for All bandwagon – is that the fundamental principles of Health for All are also principles of community development. More importantly, there is already a wealth of experience and expertise in this area, which needs to be recognised and acknowledged. Health for All might currently be 'flavour of the month', but those who have been battling for years to get community development work adequately resourced might take a more cynical view of what really lies behind the enthusiasm. (National Community Health Resource (1988).

Conclusion

This article has focused on the contradictory implications for the community health movement of developments in health promotion policy during the late 1980s, whilst the scarcity of resources to back up the rhetoric about strengthening community action remained a major contradiction, the trend toward increased NHS support for community development health projects inevitably gave rise to a new set of dilemmas.

At the national level, some of the contradictions were played out in the relationship between the community health movement, the Health Education Authority and government. As HFA 2000 began to capture the imagination of the community health movement and progressive local government and health authorities, and staff within the Health Education Authority began to utilise it as a framework for a systematic strategy of support for community development, there were signs of the government's response to HFA 2000 shifting from apathy to opposition. An indication was a widely publicised ministerial review of the Health Education Authority's 1989/90 operational strategy, when pressure was placed on the Authority to channel its activities even more narrowly into high-profile government-initiated mass media campaigns, and questions were asked about 'the proposed concentration on a community development approach' (West and Jones, 1989). This reaction was not new, but was an endemic feature of the relationship between government and the central body for health education.

The research community did not escape the backlash. A study of dampness and health, carried out by the Edinburgh Research Unit for Health and Behavioural Research at the initiation of, and in collaboration with, a local tenants' group, came under critical scrutiny at the Unit's review by its main funding body, the Scottish Office (West and Jones 1989). The Scottish Office made clear that it would not welcome a continuation of such research. In terms of both the content and process of the research, the study in question was an exemplary model of 'Research for Health for All'.

Despite the contradictions, the HFA 2000 principles of redressing inequalities, community participation and intersectoral collaboration provide a useful framework for:

- Monitoring the gap between the rhetoric and reality of official health promotion policy and practice;
- Stimulating debate about the structural barriers to translating HFA principles into practice;
- Challenging the monopolisation of health promotion by health professionals;
- Legitimising and promoting approaches that are rooted in community health action.

The indications are that the last decade before the year 2000 will be marked by further retrenchment of material support for community health action, accompanied by the continued propagation of consumerist notions of community participation that undermine the fundamental principles of community development. The challenge for the community health movement will be to utilise the rhetoric, at the same time as exposing the contradictions and safeguarding against its own colonisation. For activists both within and outside the statutory sector, there is a need to critically re-examine the meaning of *In and Against the State* (London Edinburgh Weekend Return Group, 1979) in the current cold political climate.

References

Beattie, A. (1986). Community development for health: from practice to theory? *Radical Health Promotion 4*, 13.

Beresford, P. and Croft, S. (1984). Welfare pluralism: the new face of fabianism, *Critical Social Policy*, *9*, 19–39.

Cockburn, C. (1977). *The Local State*. London: Pluto Press.

Community Projects Foundation (1988). *Action for Health: Initiatives in Local Communities*. London: Health Education Authority and Blennerhassett, S., Farrant, W. and Jones, J. (1989). Support for community health projects in the UK: a role for the National Health Service, *Health Promotion*, *4(3)*, 199–206.

Davies, C. (1987). Viewpoint: things to come: the NHS in the next decade, *Sociology of Health and Illness*, 9 (*3*), 302–17.

Department of Health and Social Security (DHSS) (1981). *Care in Action*. London: HMSO.

Department of Health and Social Security (1986). *Neighbourhood Nursing – A focus for care*. London: HMSO.

Dun, R. (1987). *Going Local? A Study of West Lambeth District Health Authority*. London: West Lambeth Health Authority.

Djukanovic, V. and Mach, E. P. (1975) *Alternative Approaches to Meeting Basic Needs in Developing Countries*. Geneva: World Health Organization.

Farrant, W. (1987) Health for WHO by the year 2000? – choices for district health promotion strategies. *Radical Community Medicine* 28, 19–26.

Farrant, W. and Taft, A. (1988). WHO Healthy Public Policy conference, *Community Health Action*, 9, 16–7.

Farrant, W. and Taft, A. (1989). Building healthy public policy in an unhealthy political climate – a case study from Paddington and North Kensington. In Evers, A., Farrant, W. and Trojan, A., (eds), *Healthy Public Policy at Local Level*. Boulder, Col.: Westview Press, 135–143.

Farrent, W. and Russell, J. (1986). *The Politics of Health Information: 'Beating heart disease' as a case study in the production of Health Education Council Publications, Bedford Way Papers, 28*. London: Kogan Page.

Finch, J. and Groves, D. (1983). *A Labour of Love: work and caring*. London: Routledge & Kegan Paul.

Griffiths, E. R. (1983). *NHS Management Inquiry*. London: HMSO.

Hambleton, R. and Hoggett, P. (eds) (1984). *The Politics of Decentralisation: Theory and practice of a radical local government initiative*. Bristol: School of Advanced Urban Studies.

Ineson, A. (1986). O Is for obscurantism – a review of Health Promotion Glossary 1, *Radical Health Promotion*, 3, 49–51.

Kenner, C. (1986). *Whose Needs Count? Community action for health*. London: Bedford Way Press.

Kickbusch, I. (1986). Lifestyles and health, *Social Science Medicine 22*, 117-24.

London Edinburgh Weekend Return Group (1979) *In and Against the State*. London: Publications Distributions Co-op.

National Community Health Resource (1988) Health for All by year 2000? *Community Health Action* 9, 4–6.

Report of the First International Conference on Health Promotion (1987). *Health Promotion*, 1 (*4*), 407.

Rosenthal, H. (1983). Neighbourhood health projects – some new approaches to health and community work in parts of the United Kingdom, *Community Development Journal*, *18*(2), 120–30.

Stacey, M. (1988). Background to the Research for Health for All initiative, unpublished paper presented at Workshop and Information Exchange on Research for HFA, convened by the British Sociological Association Medical Sociology Group, Aston University, Birmingham (March).

Thornley, P. (1988). Community participation – rhetoric or reality?, *Community Health Action*, 9, 7–10.

West, J. and Jones, L. (1989). Bound, gagged and blindfolded, *Health Matters*, 2, 12–3.

World Health Organisation Regional Office for Europe (1985). *Targets for Health for All*. Copenhagen: WHO.

World Health Organization (1986). *Ottawa Charter for Health Promotion*. Copenhagen: WHO.

24 Pedagogy of the oppressed: an extract

Paulo Freire (trans Myra Bergman Ramos) *

Cultural invasion

In this phenomenon, the invaders penetrate the cultural context of another group, in disrespect of the latter's potentialities; they impose their own view of the world upon those they invade and inhibit the creativity of the invaded by curbing their expression.

Whether urbane or harsh, cultural invasion is thus always an act of violence against the persons of the invaded culture, who lose their originality or face the threat of losing it. In cultural invasion (as in all the modalities of antidialogical action) the invaders are the authors of, and actors in, the process; those they invade are the objects. The invaders mold; those they invade are molded. The invaders choose; those they invade follow that choice – or are expected to follow it. The invaders act; those they invade have only the illusion of acting, through the action of the invaders.

All domination involves invasion – at times physical and overt, at times camouflaged, with the invader assuming the role of a helping friend. In the last analysis, invasion is a form of economic and cultural domination. Invasion may be practiced by a metropolitan society upon a dependent society, or it may be implicit in the domination of one class over another within the same society.

Cultural conquest leads to the cultural inauthenticity of those who are invaded; they begin to respond to the values, the standards, and the goals of the invaders. In their passion to dominate, to mold others to their patterns and their way of life, the invaders desire to know how those they have invaded apprehend reality – but only so they can dominate the latter more effectively.[1] In cultural invasion it is essential that those who are invaded come to see their reality with the outlook of the invaders rather than their own; for the more they mimic the invaders, the more stable the position of the latter becomes.

For cultural invasion to succeed, it is essential that those invaded become convinced of their intrinsic inferiority. Since everything has its opposite, if those who are invaded consider themselves inferior, they must necessarily recognize the superiority of the invaders. The values of the

---

* From Paulo Freire (1972). *Pedagogy of the Oppressed*, Chapter 4, pp. 150–186. London: Sheed & Ward.

latter thereby become the pattern for the former. The more invasion is accentuated and those invaded are alienated from the spirit of their own culture and from themselves, the more the latter want to be like the invaders: to walk like them, dress like them, talk like them.

The social *I* of the invaded person, like every social *I*, is formed in the socio-cultural relations of the social structure, and therefore reflects the duality of the invaded culture. This duality (which was described earlier) explains why invaded and dominated individuals, at a certain moment of their existential experience, almost 'adhere' to the oppressor *Thou*. The oppressed *I* must break with this near adhesion to the oppressor *Thou*, drawing away from the latter in order to see him more objectively, at which point he critically recognizes himself to be in contradiction with the oppressor. In so doing, he 'considers' as a dehumanizing reality the structure in which he is being oppressed. This qualitative change in the perception of the world can only be achieved in the praxis.

Cultural invasion is on the one hand an *instrument* of domination, and on the other, the *result* of domination. Thus, cultural action of a dominating character (like other forms of antidialogical action), in addition to being deliberate and planned, is in another sense simply a product of oppressive reality.

For example, a rigid and oppressive social structure necessarily influences the institutions of child rearing and education within that structure. These institutions pattern their action after the style of the structure, and transmit the myths of the latter. Homes and schools (from nurseries to universities) exist not in the abstract, but in time and space. Within the structures of domination they function largely as agencies which prepare the invaders of the future.

The parent–child relationship in the home usually reflects the objective cultural conditions of the surrounding social structure. If the conditions which penetrate the home are authoritarian, rigid, and dominating, the home will increase the climate of oppression.[2] As these authoritarian relations between parents and children intensify, children in their infancy increasingly internalize the paternal authority.

Presenting (with his customary clarity) the problem of necrophilia and biophilia, Fromm analyzes the objective conditions which generate each condition, whether in the home (parent–child relations in a climate of indifference and oppression or of love and freedom), or in a socio-cultural context. If children reared in an atmosphere of lovelessness and oppression, children whose potency has been frustrated, do not manage during their youth to take the path of authentic rebellion, they will either drift into total indifference, alienated from reality by the authorities and the myths the latter have used to 'shape' them; or they may engage in forms of destructive action.

The atmosphere of the home is prolonged in the school, where the students soon discover that (as in the home) in order to achieve some satisfaction they must adapt to the precepts which have been set from above. One of these precepts is not to think.

Internalizing paternal authority through the rigid relationship structure emphasized by the school, these young people tend when they become professionals (because of the very fear of freedom instilled by these relationships) to repeat the rigid patterns in which they were miseducated. This phenomenon, in addition to their class position, perhaps explains why so many professionals adhere to antidialogical action.[3] Whatever the specialty that brings them into contact with the people, they are almost unshakably convinced that it is their mission to 'give' the latter their knowledge and techniques. They see themselves as 'promotors' of the people. Their programs of action (which might have been prescribed by any good theorist of oppressive action) include their own objectives, their own convictions, and their own preoccupations. They do not listen to the people, but instead plan to teach them how to 'cast off the laziness which creates underdevelopment'. To these professionals, it seems absurd to consider the necessity of respecting the 'view of the world' held by the people. The professionals are the ones with a 'world view.' They regard as equally absurd the affirmation that one must necessarily consult the people when organizing the program content of educational action. They feel that the ignorance of the people is so complete that they are unfit for anything except to receive the teachings of the professionals.

When, however, at a certain point of their existential experience, those who have been invaded begin in one way or another to reject this invasion (to which they might earlier have adapted), the professionals, in order to justify their failure, say that the members of the invaded group are 'inferior' because they are 'ingrates' 'shiftless', 'diseased', or of 'mixed blood'.

Well-intentioned professionals (those who use 'invasion' not as deliberate ideology but as the expression of their own upbringing) eventually discover that certain of their educational failures must be ascribed, not to the intrinsic inferiority of the 'simple men of the people', but to the violence of their own act of invasion. Those who make this discovery face a difficult alternative: they feel the need to renounce invasion, but patterns of domination are so entrenched within them that this renunciation would become a threat to their own identities. To renounce invasion would mean ending their dual status as dominated and dominators. It would mean abandoning all the myths which nourish invasion, and starting to incarnate dialogical action. For this very reason, it would mean to cease being *over* or *inside* (as foreigners) in order to be *with* (as comrades). And so the fear of freedom takes hold of these men. During this traumatic process, they naturally tend to rationalize their fear with a series of evasions.

The fear of freedom is greater still in professionals who have not yet discovered for themselves the invasive nature of their action, and who are told that their action is dehumanizing. Not infrequently, especially at the point of decoding concrete situations, training course participants ask the coordinator in an irritated manner: 'Where do you think you're steering us, anyway?' The coordinator isn't trying to 'steer' them anywhere; it is just that in facing a concrete situation as a problem, the participants begin to realize that if their analysis of the situation goes any deeper they will either have to divest themselves of their myths, or reaffirm them. Divesting themselves of and renouncing their myths represents, at that moment, an act of self-violence. On the other hand, to reaffirm those myths is to reveal themselves. The only way out (which functions as a defense mechanism) is to project onto the coordinator their own usual practices: *steering, conquering,* and *invading*.[4] . . .

Cultural invasion, which serves the ends of conquest and the preservation of oppression, always involves a parochial view of reality, a static perception of the world, and the imposition of one world view upon another. It implies the 'superiority' of the invader and the 'inferiority' of those who are invaded, as well as the imposition of values by the former, who possess the latter and are afraid of losing them.

Cultural invasion further signifies that the ultimate seat of decision regarding the action of those who are invaded lies not with them but with the invaders. And when the power of decision is located outside rather than within the one who should decide, the latter has only the illusion of deciding. This is why there can be no socio-economic development in a dual, 'reflex', invaded society. For development to occur it is necessary: (a) that there be a movement of search and creativity having its seat of decision in the searcher; (b) that this movement occur not only in space, but in the existential time of the conscious searcher. . .

Cultural synthesis

Cultural action is always a systematic and deliberate form of action which operates upon the social structure, either with the objective of preserving that structure or of transforming it. As a form of deliberate and systematic action, all cultural action has its theory which determines its ends and thereby defines its methods. Cultural action either serves domination (consciously or unconsciously) or it serves the liberation of men. As these dialectically opposed types of cultural action operate in and upon the social structure, they create dialectical relations of *permanence* and *change*.

The social structure, in order to *be*, must *become*; in other words, *becoming* is the way the social structure expresses '*duration*', in the Bergsonian sense of the term.[5]

Dialogical cultural action does not have as its aim the disappearance of the permanence–change dialectic (an impossible aim, since disappearance of the dialectic would require the disappearance of the social structure itself and thus of men); it aims, rather, at surmounting the antagonistic contradictions of the social structure, thereby achieving the liberation of men.

Antidialogical cultural action, on the other hand, aims at mythicising such contradictions, thereby hoping to avoid (or hinder insofar as possible) the radical transformation of reality. Antidialogical action explicitly or implicitly aims to preserve, within the social structure, situations which favor its own agents. While the latter would never accept a transformation of the structure sufficiently radical to over come its antagonistic contradictions, they may accept reforms which do not affect their power of decision over the oppressed. Hence, this modality of action involves the *conquest* of the people, their *division*, their *manipulation*, and *cultural invasion*. It is necessarily and fundamentally an *induced* action. Dialogical action, however, is characterized by the supersedence of any induced aspect. The incapacity of antidialogical cultural action to supersede its induced character results from its objective: domination; the capacity of dialogical cultural action to do this lies in its objective: liberation.

In cultural invasion, the actors draw the thematic content of their action from their own values and ideology, their starting point is their own world, from which they enter the world of those they invade. In cultural synthesis, the actors who come from 'another world' to the world of the people do so not as invaders. They do not come to *teach* or to *transmit* or to *give* anything, but rather to learn, with the people, about the people's world.

In cultural invasion the actors (who need not even go personally to the invaded culture; increasingly, their action is carried out by technological instruments) superimpose themselves on the people, who are assigned the role of spectators, of objects. In cultural synthesis, the actors become integrated with the people, who are co-authors of the action that both perform upon the world.

In cultural invasion, both the spectators and the reality to be preserved are objects of the actors' action. In cultural synthesis, there are no spectators; the object of the actors' action is the reality to be transformed for the liberation of men.

Cultural synthesis is thus a mode of action for confronting culture itself, as the preserver of the very structures by which it was formed. Cultural action, as historical action, is an instrument for superseding the dominant alienated and alienating culture. In this sense, every authentic revolution is a cultural revolution.

The investigation of the people's generative themes or meaningful thematics constitutes the starting point for the process of action as cultural synthesis. Indeed, it is not really possible to divide this process into two separate steps: first, *thematic investigation*, and then *action as cultural synthesis*. Such a dichotomy would imply an initial phase in which the people, as passive objects, would be studied, analyzed, and investigated by the investigators – a procedure congruent with antidialogical action. Such division would lead to the naive conclusion that action as synthesis follows from action as invasion.

In dialogical theory, this division cannot occur. The Subjects of thematic investigation are not only the professional investigators but also the men of the people whose thematic universe is being sought. Investigation – the first moment of action as cultural synthesis – establishes a climate of creativity which will tend to develop in the subsequent stages of action. Such a climate does not exist in cultural invasion, which through alienation kills the creative enthusiasm of those who are invaded, leaving them hopeless and fearful of risking experimentation, without which there is no true creativity.

Those who are invaded, whatever their level, rarely go beyond the models which the invaders prescribe for them. In cultural synthesis there are no invaders; hence, there are no imposed models. In their stead, there are actors who critically analyze reality (never separating this analysis from action) and intervene as Subjects in the historical process.

Instead of following predetermined plans, leaders and people, mutually identified, together create the guidelines of their action. In this synthesis, leaders and people are somehow reborn in new knowledge and new action. Knowledge of the alienated culture leads to transforming action resulting in a culture which is being freed from alienation. The more sophisticated knowledge of the leaders is remade in the empirical knowledge of the people, while the latter is refined by the former.

In cultural synthesis – and only in cultural synthesis – it is possible to resolve the contradiction between the world view of the leaders and that of the people, to the enrichment of both. Cultural synthesis does not deny the differences between the two views; indeed, it is based on these differences. It does deny the invasion of one by the other, but affirms the undeniable support each gives to the other. . .

Notes

1. To this end, the invaders are making increasing use of the social sciences and technology, and to some extent the physical sciences as well, to improve and refine their action. It is indispensable for the invaders to know the past and present of those invaded in order to discern the alternatives of the latter's future and thereby attempt to guide the evolution of that future along lines that will favor their own interests.

2. Young people increasingly view parent and teacher authoritarianism as inimical to their own freedom. For this very reason they increasingly oppose forms of action which minimize their expressiveness and hinder their self-affirmation This very positive phenomenon is not accidental. It is actually a symptom of the historical climate which . . . characterizes our epoch as an anthropological one. For this reason one cannot (unless he has a personal interest in doing so) see the youth rebellion as a mere example of the traditional differences between generations. Something deeper is involved here. Young people in their rebellion are denouncing and condemning the unjust model of a society of

domination. This rebellion with its special dimension, however, is very recent; society continues to be authoritarian in character.

3. It perhaps also explains the antidialogical behavior of persons who, although convinced of their revolutionary commitment, continue to mistrust the people and fear communion with them. Unconsciously, such persons retain the oppressor within themselves; and because they 'house' the master, they fear freedom.

4. See my 'Extansão ou Comunicação?', in *Introducción a la Acción Cultural* (Santiago, 1969).

5. What makes a structure a *social* structure (and thus historical–cultural) is neither permanence nor change, taken absolutely, but the dialectical relations between the two. In the last analysis, what endures in the social structure is neither permanence nor change; it is the permanence–change dialectic itself.

25 Evaluation in community development for health: an opportunity for dialogue*

Alan Beattie

For many of those active in community health and health promotion, stumbling across the recent debates about the relative merits of different approaches to evaluation may be somewhat discomfiting. In some places the battle is still raging just to raise awareness of the importance of evaluation as an aspect of health work, or to find ways of creating time and space for such evaluative activities to be undertaken at all. It might be thought something of a distraction or a disfavour to make life even more difficult by focusing on current disputes about how evaluation should be done. Nevertheless in this chapter I want to argue that the issues surrounding what counts as evaluation are of crucial importance to the future of the public health movement, and I hope to show that the widening debate about these issues is likely to be one of the most significant growth points for the future.

The shift towards pluralistic evaluation

For much of the past fifteen years, different approaches to evaluation have been polarised into two warring camps. On the one hand there have been the various traditions of quantitative evaluation – drawing either on scientific research in experimental or quasi-experimental modes, or on managerial audits using statistical or other numerical ways of 'figuring out performance' in terms of economy, efficiency and effectiveness. On the other hand there emerged – largely outside the worlds of medical research and management sciences and unknown to them – a range of alternative 'qualitative' strategies of evaluation which focused on the portrayal of people, places and processes through ethnographic and other kinds of description.

Slowly but surely, these other methods and strategies have been adapted from their sources in the evaluation of schooling, of community

* From *Health Education Journal*, 54 (1995), pp. 465–472. London: Health Education Authority.

work and the like, and have been applied in the field of community development for health (CDH). Their appeal was particularly strong in this field because they offered promise of a way of conducting evaluation which reflected many of the features of CDH itself as a way of working: emphasising process, working with people in a non-judgmental manner that is sensitive to local cultures, collecting and negotiating an agenda of concerns from the participants, and keeping firmly in view such issues as who owns the evaluation data and what action should flow from the data. In a national survey of evaluation reports from CDH projects in the United Kingdom covering the period 1979 to 1990, it was clear that at local level a wide variety of evaluation styles were being tried out, involving many different types of data and data-handling procedures drawing on the full range of tools and techniques known to social researchers. Box 25.1 summarises the approaches found to be most commonly used.

It was also clear from this review of evaluation reports in the CDH field (Box 25.1) that they sprang from a wide variety of accountability arrangements, and that the purposes for which they were prepared and the audiences to whom they were directed were likewise diverse – encompassing variously: managers, funders, purchasers, and other official decision-makers; the users of CDH project services in the local community; wider national networks, forums and interest groups (e.g. women's health); and a general audience of interested professional practitioners, academics and scientists.

Several of the reports in this series were also beginning to put together the multiple-portfolio approach (Beattie, 1984), which seeks to compile a range of different kinds of information in order to be able to respond to the questions posed by the diverse interest groups that may have a stake in a CDH project. It is therefore CDH projects that have begun most vigorously to develop and explore the kind of 'pluralistic evaluation' (Smith and Cantley, 1984, 1985) or 'fourth generation evaluation' (Guba and Lincoln, 1989) that is increasingly seen as the appropriate strategy for addressing questions of worth in situations that are marked by deep-seated disputes about what counts as success or a 'good outcome'. In so doing, such projects are also showing a way forward in listening to local voices (DoH, 1992; NHSME, 1992; Sykes, *et al.*, 1992) and in moving towards the corporate assessment of health needs (DoH, 1993; NHSME, 1991) that can help to extend public health beyond an exclusively biomedical model. But these new departures raise new issues and pose new challenges for evaluative research.

The challenges of partnership

One consistent feature runs through most of the energetic efforts that have

Box 25.1   *Evaluation styles prominent in CDH projects in the UK (Beattie, 1991)*

1. The historical approach typically assembles a chronological narrative of project activities, affording an overview of the main events, signiflcant turning points and key features. Arguments in favour of this approach in the community work field were offered by the London Voluntary Service Council (1978)

2. Participatory evaluation gives priority to the involvement of 'consumers', of lay people, in the process of project evaluation. The fullest statement of the case for this approach is that by Feuerstein (1978, 1998).

3. Action research evaluation is where the evaluator has a 'hands-on' role and seeks to make a direct ('formative') contribution to the processes of project management and steering. A classic and influential general description of this is provided by Powley and Evans (1979).

4. The practitioner-as-researcher is where project workers themselves carry out the evaluation of the project, as a kind of intemal evaluation or self-evaluation. Influential sources are the accounts of the 'teacher as researcher' by Stenhouse (1975), and of the 'reflective practitioner' by Schon (1983).

5. The independent external evaluator is where evaluation is conducted by an outside person who is not otherwise contributing to the project work. Descriptions of the processes and difficulties of this role have been offered by Room (1983) and Hunt (1987).

6. Objectives-based evaluation places the emphasis on checking systematically the progress made in achieving each of the specfic aims and objectives specified at the outset of the project. This approach has been described by Key and colleagues (1976) and in LVSC (1978).

7. Decision-led evaluation takes the explicit form of 'briefing for decision-makers', and focuses on informing a specific managerial decision on a particular occasion. It is a version of performance review or performance assessment described in management literature.g. Pollitt (1984).

8. Goal-free evaluation focuses on the process of the project and seeks to characterise this, taking into account, but giving no special emphasis to, original goals or eventual decisions. This was described in the context of educational evaluation by House (1976) and by Stake (1976), and is particularly recommended for CDH projects by Graessle and Kingsley (1986).

9. Critical review is where evaluation relies upon the professional judgement of an expert or panel of experts. In educational evaluation this approach has been described by Willis (1978) as akin to 'art criticism', 'book reviews', adjudication, etc, and in community work, it has been described by LVSC (1978) as the 'blue riband testimonial' method.

10. Negotiated or democratic evaluation puts close emphasis on checking accounts with the key informants whose work or experience is under scrutiny. The merits of this have been discussed by Pring (1984), and Simons (1987).

been made to define and apply pluralistic approaches to evaluation. This is that it involves the researcher in new and closer negotiating stances with informants – both as individuals and as groups or communities, and with practitioners, with managers, indeed with all who have a stake in local health planning and practice. These relationships are new because they were certainly not required by the experimental–statistical research tradition: nor were they (for the most part) typically called for by ethnographic research, in which the researcher has often (but not always) remained as aloof and removed from the key players in the scene as their counterpart undertaking positivist research. But central to the new styles of mixed portfolio evaluation (see Box 25.1) are such methods as action research, practitioner research, participatory research, all of which deliberately cross the boundaries between the researcher and the researched. The experience of those involved in evaluating CDH initiatives is therefore opening up to scrutiny the process of research itself, and is exposing to view and to critical debate some of the taken-for-granted features of the research process. In doing so, evaluators in CDH projects are helping to shape an agenda for debate about method that is becoming urgent in the wider academic world of applied social research. The list below sets out a number of features of research process that have emerged with particular prominence in connection with the evaluation of CDH projects. Many of these features have been much commented on in recent social research, and some have become highly prized among some of the most sophisticated academic commentators on research methodology.

Dialogical features of pluralistic evaluation

1. Research as collecting stories. One of the most powerful tools of the new evaluation (in common with much recent social research) is the eliciting of lifestories, vignettes and similar kinds of personal testimony around the focus of enquiry. This crucially registers a power shift: subjects are no longer asked to make their answers fit the researchers' questions (Graham, 1983, 1984), but rather are invited to unfold their own stories on their own terms (Plummer, 1983).
2. Moving from public to private accounts. Related to the first point is that if sufficient time and trouble are taken to put informants at their ease, they offer a much fuller, richer, more complex picture of the ways in which they think about health and related matters than they do in more brief encounters (Cornwell, 1984; Blaxter, 1990; Stainton-Rogers, 1991).
3. Reciprocity. When the researcher/evaluator exchanges with the informant some experience from her/his own life that echoes what the informant is disclosing, an important kind of mutuality is created

which often appears to be crucial to the trust and goodwill of the informant (Finch, 1984; Oakley, 1981).

4. Mutual aid. Instead of maintaining a strict 'objective' distance from the informant (one of the most obvious sources of discomfort and incomprehension for informants), it may on occasions be essential for the researcher/evaluator to be ready to switch into the role of helper, or adviser, or advocate (e.g. in response to urgent questions from the informant). This is a crucial way of helping to make the research/evaluation less of an imposition, more a shared exploration of issues and a search for action.

5. Transparency of process. Here the researcher/evaluator accepts every opportunity available to explain the process of research – how data is being collected, where it will go, who will see it, how it will be used, etc. This is another way of helping the informant to become a partner in the process.

6. Reflexivity. This is a feature that is achieved when researcher and informant each comment on their experience of the research process - what it feels like to undergo, what is most or least rewarding about it, what aspects of the process they might wish to change (Smith, 1989).

7. Consciousness-raising. The processes of education and community work pioneered by Freire have had a major influence on CDH work; and this way of working is in itself a kind of shared research, with the facilitator (teacher) and student/client working as 'co-investigators'. Crucial to the research is the stage of 'consciousness-raising' a key marker of which is a shift of self-understanding on the part of the informant Padila, 1992; Nichter, 1984).

8. The action research orientation. Also important as a strengthening of the commitment to a process of change and improvement – flowing out of points 4 and 7 above – is the explicit deployment of the action research mode. Here the researcher/evaluator would from the outset be a fully participating member of an action team, perhaps a practitioner in her/his own right, and on the lookout for a chance to use findings immediately and formatively as a basis for new development work (Carr and Kemmis, 1986; Oja and Smulyan, 1989; Rapoport, 1970; Susman and Evered, 1978).

This series of features all arise from a view that pluralistic evaluation is essentially a dialogical process of enquiry. They add up to a formidable challenge to many taken-for-granted assumptions about research and evaluation: and it is to be noted that many of these features are precisely those that are most central to the distinctive style of CDH work itself. They show the considerable overlap and common ground between the dialogical approach in health promotion practice and the dialogical approach in research and evaluation.

Health and the dialogical imagination

The fact that evaluation attempts in CDH projects have opened up dialogue on several fronts has a crucial consequence which I suspect has not yet been fully appreciated by those concerned, and certainly not yet fully exploited. This arises as follows. Once the channels of debate and discussion are opened, it becomes increasingly possible for some basic questions to get a hearing: 'what is health?', 'what are health services for?', 'what is the purpose of prevention?', 'who has a say in all these things?', 'who decides?'. Given the contested nature of health and the multiplicity of 'stories about health' that are in circulation in society, such opening up of dialogues about health can lead to an appreciation – sooner or later – of the narrative construction of all of our knowledge about health and illness, about care and prevention. We will thereby all be helped to see that the evidence on which we can base our health action is all in the form of 'stories', some told by scientists, some told by practitioners, some told by lay clients or patients, but all of them representing competing accounts of the same topic or issue. This can prompt (as it already has among many participants in community health projects) further questions along the lines of 'so what story are we in here?', and 'whose story are we in?'.

The literary theorist Bakhtin describes 'the dialogical imagination' - listening to a polyphony of multiple voice – as essentially 'transgressive' (Bakhtin, 1981). It constantly challenges our beliefs and what we think of as knowledge: it takes them apart and puts them back together again in new ways, it refuses to allow anything to remain for long 'taken-for-granted': it refreshes and recharges our ways of seeing and our ways of doing. For a future in a mixed economy of welfare, with a proliferating range of choices in community health and with widening circuits of local voices to be consulted, I suggest that investment in the kinds of research and evaluation that can inform and feed the dialogical imagination will be our best hope for 'making sense together' (O'Neill, 1974).

References

Bakhtin, M. (1981). In Holquist, M. (ed), *The Dialogic Imagination: Four Essays*. Austin: University of Texas Press.

Beattie, A. (1984) Evaluating community health initiatives: an overview. In Somerville, G. (ed). *Community Development in Health: Addressing the Confusions*. London: Kings Fund/NCHR.

Beattie A. (1991). The evaluation of community development initiatives in health promotion: a review of current strategies. In *Community Development and Health Education: Occasional Papers of the Health Education Unit 1991*. Buckingham: Open University, volume 1, 61–86.

Blaxter, M. (1990). *Health and Lifestyles*. London: Tavistock/Routledge.

Carr, W. and Kemmis, S. (1986). *Becoming Critical: Education, Knowledge and Action Research*. London: Falmer.

Cornwell, J. (1984). *Hard-earned Lives: Accounts of Health and Illness from East London.* London: Tavistock.

DoH. (1992). *The Health of the Nation: First Steps for the NHS.* London: DoH (NHSME).

NHSME (1992). *Local Voices: The Views of Local People in Purchasing for Health,* London: NHS Management Executive.

DoH. (1993). *The Health of the Nation: Local Target Setting.* London: DoH (NHSME).

Feuerstein M. T. (1978). Evaluation by the people, *International Nursing Review,* 25, (5),146–153.

Feuerstein, M.T. (1988). *Partners in Evaluation.* St Albans: TALC.

Finch, J. (1984). It's great to have someone to talk to: the ethics and politics of interviewing. In Bell, C. and Roberts, H. (eds), *Social Researching: Politics, Problems, Practice.* London: Routledge.

Graessle, L. and Kingsley, S. (1986) *Measuring Change, Making Changes.* London: NCHR.

Graham, H. (1983). Do her answers fit his questions? Women and the survey method. In Gamaikow, E., Morgan, D., Purvis, J. and Taylorson, D. (eds). *The Public and the Private.* London: Heinemann.

Graham, H. (1984). Surveying through stories. In Bell, C. and Roberts, H. (eds), *Social Researching: Politics, Problems. Practice.* London: Routledge.

Guba, E. G. and Lincoln Y. S. (1989). *Fourth Generation Evaluation.* London: Sage.

Hunt, S. M. (1987). Evaluating a community development project: issues of acceptability, *British Journal of Social Work,* 661–7.

Key, M., Hudson, P. and Armstrong, J. (1976). *Evaluation Theory and Community Work.* London: CPF.

LVSC (1978). *Evaluation of Community Work.* London: Voluntary Service Council. National Consumer Council (1986). *Measuring Up.* London: NCC.

Nichter, M., (1984). Project community diagnosis: participatory research as a first step towards community involvement in primary health care, *Social Science in Medicine,* 19 (3), 237–252.

NHSME (1991). *Assessing Health Care Needs.* London: NHS Management Executive.

Oakley, A. (1981). Interviewing women: a contradiction in terms. In Roberts, H. (ed), *Doing Feminist Research.* London: Routledge.

Oja, S. N. and Smulyan, L. (1989). *Collaborative Action Research: a Developmental Approach.* Brighton: Falmer.

O'Neill, J. (1974). *Making Sense Together.* New York: Harper & Row.

Padilia, R. (1992). Using dialogical research methods to study chicano college students. *The Urban Review,* 24 (3), 175–183.

Plummer, K. (1983). *Documents of Life: an Introduction to the Problems and Literature of a Humanistic Method.* London: Allen & Unwin.

Pollitt, C. (1984). Blunt tools: performance measurement in policies for health care OMEGA, *International Journal of Management Science,* 12, 131–140.

Powley T. Evans, D. (1979). Towards a methodology of action research, *Journal of Social Policy,* 8, 27–46.

Pring, R. C. (1984). Confidentiality and the right to know. In Adelman, C. (ed), *The Politics and Ethics of Evaluation.* London: Croom Helm.

Rapoport, R. N. (1970). Three dilemmas of action research, *Human Relations,* 23, 499–513.

Room, G. (1983). The politics of evaluation, *Journal of Social Policy,* 2 (12).

Schon, D. A. (1983). *The Reflective Practitioner.* New York: Basic Books.

Simons, H. (1987). *Getting To Know Schools in a Democracy: The Politics and Process of Evaluation.* Brighton: Falmer.

Smith, G. and Cantley, C. (1984). Pluralistic evaluation. In Lishman, J. (ed), Evaluation: Aberdeen University Research Highlights, 8.

Smith, G. and Cantley, C. (1985). Directions in evaluative research. Chapter 1 (pp. 1–13) in *Assessing Health Care.* Milton Keynes: Open University Press.

Smith, D. (1989). Sociological theory: methods of writing patriarchy. In Wallace, R. (ed), *Feminism and Sociological Theory*. London: Sage.

Stainton-Rogers, W. (1991). *Explaining Health and Illness: An Exploration of Diversity*. London: Harvester/Wheatsheaf.

Stake, R. (1976). Making school evaluations relevant, *North Central Association Quarterly*, 50, 347–352.

Stenhouse, L. (1975). The teacher as researcher, Chapter 10 in Stenhouse, L. *An introduction to Curriculum Research and Development*. London: Heinemann.

Susman, G. I. and Evered, R. D. (1978). An assessment of the scientific merits of action research, *Administrative Science Quarterly*, 234, 582–603.

Sykes, W., Collins, M., Hunter, D. J., Popay, J. and William, G. (1992). *Listening to Local Voices: a Guide to Research Methods*. Leeds: Nuffield Institute for Health Services Studies.

Willis, C. W. (ed) (1978) *Qualitative Evaluation*. New York: McCutcheon.

Further reading

Beattie, A. (1989) From quantity to quality: the 4 E's of evaluation, *Community Health Action*, 12 (Spring), 7–9.

Beattie, A. (1990) 'Knowledge and control in health promotion: a test case for social policy and social theory' in Calnan, M. and Gabe, J. (eds), *Sociology of the Health Service*. London: Routledge.

Beattie, A., (1991) Evaluation by portfolio: a way forward for community health projects? In Allen, S. (ed). *New Directions in Evaluation*. Edinburgh: Lothian Mental Health Forum, *Discussion Paper*.

Wales, K. (1988). Back to the future: Bakhtin, stylistics and discourse. In Van Peer, W. (ed), *The Taming of the Text*. London: Routledge.

Walker, R. (1978). The conduct of educational case studies: ethics, theory, and procedures. In Dockrell, B. and Hamilton, D. (eds), *Rethinking Educational Research*. London: Hodder & Stoughton.

Walker, R. (1982). The use of case studies in applied research and evaluation. In Hartnett, A. (ed), *The Social Sciences in Educational Studies*, London: Heinemann.

26 *How community preferences can more effectively shape equity policy*[*]

Stephen Jan

Introduction: what is equity?

There is no uniquely correct way of defining what is equitable. Equity is about fairness and can mean one thing to one person and something completely different to another. Therefore equity is essentially determined by values, both community values and/or individual values. At present, there does not appear to have been much attempt to ascertain either community or individual values within population-based resource allocation formulae. Most equity policy of this type has, to date, revolved around the equal distribution of resources or service use across population groups. However, within the framework of trying to define fairness, equality is but one candidate. The appropriateness of equality as a criterion for equity is potentially mitigated by the fact that not all individuals or groups in society are equal to start with.

This chapter aims to explore some of the issues surrounding equity as it is applied in health care policy making, particularly in population based resource allocation formulae. The next section attempts to define equity or fairness as a community concern rather than an individual one. In doing so questions are raised about the adequacy of conventional economic instruments to cope with these issues. Following this, there is a discussion of how equity is considered in resource allocation formulae as they currently operate in Australia. The scope for incorporating community values for equity into such formulae is examined with particular reference to recent work in Australia. Specifically, this is done by examining the needs of the Australian Aboriginal population where there are major health disadvantages. Finally, some general lessons for equity are considered.

How can we frame any notion of fairness?

Considerations of equity are essentially underpinned by some notion of

[*] From *Critical Public Health*, 6 (3), (1995), pp. 12–18.

fairness. As mentioned above, however, 'equality' will not always be deemed fair. For instance, in defining what is fair in health care, a range of possibilities is available beginning at one extreme with the idea of 'user pays' where services are provided only to those willing and able to pay and at the other extreme where fairness involves equal health for all. It is argued later in this section that discussion on equity in health care has to date been limited to the extent that it has generally focused on the notion of 'equality' and in particular the principle of 'the equal treatment of equals', i.e. horizontal equity. The way forward it seems is to introduce the possibility that fairness in some circumstances requires the unequal treatment of unequals (vertical equity) (Mooney, forthcoming). Given that equity involves a question of values, and as argued here, community values, then incorporating this dimension of vertical equity into policy will require some form of community input.

Conventional economics, as applied to health care, generally proposes that the ultimate aim of health services is to maximise the total 'welfare' to society of these services. This framework is rooted in utilitarian principles where the objective is to maximise social welfare and where social welfare is an increasing function of individual welfare or 'utility'. It is implied also that utility is some increasing function of health (but not necessarily that they are the same or that there is a uniform relationship between the two). Utilitarianism of this form is characterised by certain axioms, such as:

- With respect to social welfare, more is preferred to less;
- Increasing one person's utility, all else being equal, social welfare will increase;
- Increasing person A's utility but at the same time reducing person B's, social welfare will increase only if A can potentially compensate B and remain ahead (this is the Pareto principle underlying cost-benefit analysis).

In essence, it is implied that the maximum welfare for society is achieved by maximising the utility from health care to individuals. At its most basic level, it is also implied that the welfare of individuals is independent. It is well known and acknowledged, however, that this is often not the case in health care and that the welfare of individuals can be affected by the health of others. This interdependence is commonly referred to as 'externalities'. Equity generally fits into the conventional welfare economics view of health care as an externality. A concern for equity arises in this framework because individual A derives benefit from both the good health of individual B as well as the consumption of health care by individual B (and this is independent of the threat to individual A of infection). The interrelationship between the utility functions of separate individuals can therefore be put down to the idea that altruism somehow fits into each individual's utility function.

There is an apparent unease with which equity in health care fits into the conventional economics framework. This view of equity for instance suggests that one individual's concern for another's health only extends as far as it affects the first individual's welfare. In aggregate, equity policy in this context is shaped by this interrelationship between individual utility functions. It is built collectively on the welfare to individuals of the utility from consumption of health care to themselves and the utility their consumption provides to others. There appears to be something wrong with this concept of equity insofar as it is based essentially on a concern for individual welfare and where concern for others arises only incidentally. No recognition is given to the possibility that concern for the health and indeed the consumption of health care by others can be shaped by community values because there is in fact no recognition that 'community' values need to be considered at all. The upshot is that equity is deemed, to a large extent, to be able to take care of itself. Individuals with altruism in their utility functions will ensure some sort of equity in the distribution of health care, through their willingness to pay for the satisfaction of these altruistic concerns much in the same way as there is a willingness to pay for the consumer goods which also belong in the utility function.

An alternative method of examining these equity concerns is to recognise that equity is a reflection of community-wide values rather than simply a reflection of aggregate individual preferences. It takes equity outside the utilitarian framework and opens up the possibility for action at a collective level motivated by community concerns. Such concerns may be expressed in a number of ways such as through community surveys or citizen panels. One possible advantage of citizen panels is that they could overcome the fears that the community might come up with 'equity weights' which were 'unfair' and indeed bring out the worst prejudices in society. On the other hand, one potential problem with citizen panels is establishing their legitimacy in representing community concerns. Clearly there is a degree of legitimacy in the form of 'democracy' expressed through community surveys which otherwise needs to be established through citizen panels. Eyles examines in greater detail the issues associated with the process of incorporating community values through the latter approach (Eyles, 1993). The aim of this chapter is more about whether community values should be used in equity policy and at this stage the question of how is left open.

The distinction between such community concerns and individual preferences will become clearer in the next section where it is illustrated how such ideas can be applied in practice. Although the example will be based on community values derived through a survey, it is recognised that this is not necessarily the best way of getting at these values.

Drawing on community values in practice

In certain states of Australia as in Britain (under the Resource Allocation Working Party), New Zealand, Finland, Italy, Norway, and Sweden some forms of population-based resource allocation formulae have been in place to govern the equitable geographical distribution of resources (OECD, 1994). In relation to those formulae used in Australia, the distribution of resources has been determined by the principle of 'equal resources for equal need'. Need in these formulae represents health need and is measured by variables such as socio-economic status, standardised mortality rates and a rural index (NSW Department of Health, 1993; Queensland Health, 1994). Therefore, the aim of these formulae is to distribute more resources per head of population to those in higher 'need' and fewer to those in lower need.

There is an important characteristic which is implicit in this notion of need. Need is defined by the extent to which health falls short of the average rather than being defined by the capacity to benefit from the next dollar allocated. Although these two concepts are likely to be related, it is also probable that allocating resources on the basis of the latter will do more good than the former simply because the latter implies that the next dollar is directed towards where it will derive the most benefit. There is a superior logic in this principle of allocating to areas where resources will do the most good rather than based simply on the size of a problem.

Under these current formulae, more resources will, all else being equal, go to those populations in poorer health. Any greater weighting attached to those in poorer health is based solely on 'health need' as defined in these respective formulae. At present, there is no provision for including community values in the allocation of resources across groups such that various characteristics of these groups – age, sex, existing health status – might be weighted differentially according to community values.

The use of community values to assist in determining the equitable allocation of health care resources could require as a first step, some form of community survey. The vertical equity issues highlighted above may be addressed directly by specifically asking respondents to weight health gains to different groups. For instance one such question might be: 'how much will a health gain going to population group A be worth in comparison to the same health gain if it were to go to population group B?' The two populations groups could differ by characteristics such as age, sex, current health status, ethnicity, socio-economic status, etc.

In a pilot study, it was found from a convenience sample of health care decision makers that there was a distinct willingness to weight health gains differently on the basis of the characteristics of the groups that were to receive them (Mooney and Wiseman, 1995). Although the results from the study are very much preliminary, they nevertheless provided signs that this type of survey is feasible and that there were definite concerns for vertical equity in this particular survey population.

It would be possible to conduct a similar survey but directly of the community and use this to produce certain weights for health gains to different groups. For instance, a health gain to group A might be three times the value of a health gain to group B. It is important to note that these are *social* weights rather than weights which an individual might put on his/her own health. Individuals may weight their own health differently from other individuals, but this is an issue of individual preference and not directly related to the equity issues outlined in this paper. Social weights of the type proposed here are specifically based on the relative value the community puts on health gains to different groups independent of how much either the groups, or the individual within those groups, value health to themselves.

Having weighted health gains to various groups differently, it is possible to incorporate the interests or values of the community in a framework where resources are allocated to those areas where most good can be done. In this context, what is defined as 'good' is a function of what the community defines as 'good' (and this is what comes out of the social weights resulting from the survey). Incorporating these values into current resource allocation formulae would involve placing these social weights on population groups and doing so in addition to any weights currently being applied to need. Therefore, those in lower socio-economic groups might achieve a greater entitlement to resources due to the established association between poor health and socio-economic status (as they currently do) but also obtain, over and above this, an additional entitlement based on the fact that society places a higher value on this group attaining some given increase in health status than on some other group attaining a similar increase in health status.

An example of where social weightings can be incorporated – Aboriginality

The Australian Aboriginal population lags well behind the Australian non-Aboriginal population on every conceivable health indicator (Bhatia and Anderson, 1995). These disparities in health are well documented and are greater than the gap in health between indigenous and non-indigenous populations in other developed countries (Ring, 1995).

At present, the allocation of resources through population-based resource allocation formulae in place in certain states of Australia takes little direct account of Aboriginality. Aboriginality is indirectly accounted for because there are clearly established associations between Aboriginality and the need variables used. However, in relation specifically to Aboriginality, the allocation of resources through these formulae has strictly been based on a horizontal equity principle of 'equal resources for equal need' (except in the state of Queensland where there is an additional weighting of three, seemingly based on differences in mortality rates). No attempt has been made to incorporate explicitly some form of social valuation of health gains to an Aboriginal population vis-à-vis a non-Aboriginal population. The opportunity now exists for these factors to be included in such resource allocation formulae.

Conclusion

The use of some form of community input into the construction of equity policy is crucial if, as argued in this chapter, equity is seen as a social rather than an individualistic concern. One way suggested (but there are others) is to develop social weights attached to health gains going to different population groups based on some form of community survey. The problem with much of how equity has been considered in health care until now has been its focus on 'equality', for instance equality of service use, equality of resources, etc. There is no necessary reason why any particular notion of equality as such can, intrinsically, be considered fair. Equity is about fairness and fairness does not necessarily imply equal treatment particularly when individuals are unequal to start with. Therefore there has to be some form of social valuation to determine how different individuals are most equitably treated in different circumstances. An area in which there is the potential for such valuation to come into play is in respect of the Australian Aboriginal population.

Acknowledgements

The author would like to thank Gavin Mooney, Virginia Wiseman and Danny Ruta for their helpful comments.

References

Bhatia, K. and Anderson, I. (1995). *An Overview of Aboriginal and Torres Strait Islander Health: Present status and future trends.* Canberra: Australia Institute of Health and Welfare.

Eyles, J.(1993). The role of the citizen in health-care decision-making. *Centre for Health Economics and Policy Analysis Health Policy Community Services*, C93-1, Hamilton, Ontario: MacMaster University.

Mooney, G. And now for vertical equity? Some concerns arising from Aboriginal health in Australia, *Health Economics*, forthcoming.

Mooney, G., Jan, S. and Wiseman, V. (1995). Examining preferences for allocating health care gains, *Health Care Analysis*, 3, 138, 1–5.

NSW Department of Health (1993). *A Resource Allocation Formula for NSW Health System. 1993 Revision.* Service Development and Policy Branch, New South Wales Department of Health.

OECD (1994) *The Reform of Health Care Systems. A Review of Seventeen OECD Countries.* Paris: OECD.

Queensland Health (1994). *Queensland Health Resource Allocation Formula.* Policy and Planning Branch, Queensland Health.

Ring, I. (1995). An open letter to the President of the Public Health Association, *Australian Journal of Public Health, 19 (3)*, 228–230

27 *Developing health promotion strategies with Black and minority ethnic communities which address social inequalities* *

Jenny Douglas

Introduction

This chapter aims to explore the role of health promotion in opposing the impact of racism and racial discrimination on the health of Black and minority ethnic communities in the United Kingdom. First, it examines some of the constraints and dilemmas health promotion faces at present, particularly in relation to addressing inequality in these communities. Second, it considers information currently available on the health of Black communities, concentrating on differential health experience and health status in relation to mortality and morbidity and the way in which work on health issues has tended to be conceptualised within minority ethnic communities.

The chapter then discusses lessons emerging from health promotion strategies which do aim to tackle inequality in Black and minority ethnic communities, drawing upon work that has been developed in Sandwell and focusing on the Smethwick Heart Action Research Project. This project has set out to document the health experience of those communities, opening up the links between poverty, racism and health and highlighting gaps in service provision. The project has also encouraged the participation of voluntary organisations and community groups in determining appropriate methods for health promotion. However, its initiatives too emerge as subject to current constraints on health promotion.

The role of health promotion . . .

Current theories and concepts of health promotion do not tend to focus

* From P. Bywaters and E. McLeod (eds) (1996) *Working for Equality in Health*, Chapter 12, pp. 179–196. London: Routledge.

on the contemporary realities of racial oppression. Where anti-oppressive practice has been developed this has not arisen out of prevailing health promotion theories, but has tended to represent the attempt of individual practitioners to develop health promotion programmes and strategies that seek to address oppression (Douglas, 1995a). The predominant approach adopted within health promotion campaigns and strategies is a multi-cultural one which concentrates on the particular cultures of Black and minority ethnic communities. It attempts to develop health promotion programmes and resources targeted at specific Black and minority ethnic communities; but without acknowledging the association between material inequality and ill health in the communities concerned. It also fails to move beyond a focus on the biological cause of ill health and their treatment by medical intervention (Douglas, 1995b). In these respects it echoes some of the dominant assumptions informing medical research and health initiatives more generally within Black and minority ethnic communities. These are discussed next.

The health of Black and minority ethnic communities

An emphasis on the relative incidence of ill health

There is now a diverse and growing literature on the health of Black and minority ethnic communities. This has been reviewed by Smaje (1995) who demonstrates its continued emphasis on a biomedical model, with a focus on illness and disease affecting the afore-mentioned communities. He argues that epidemiological work on mortality and morbidity has tended to concentrate on two approaches in examining the health of particular ethnic groups. The first approach is to outline the frequency of disease within each ethnic group by looking at prevalence or incidence of particular diseases or conditions, whilst the second approach is concerned with differences between ethnic groups. This is measured by relative risk or standardised mortality ratios which indicate the degree of difference between such groups. Bhopal (1988) has argued that the medical literature on the health of Black and minority ethnic communities has been inappropriately dominated by studies of relative risk. There has been an over-emphasis on diseases with high relative risk among Black and minority ethnic populations as compared to the White population, considered as the norm. Such an approach reinforces an emphasis on diseases such as tuberculosis and thalassaemia, where the diseases in question are ones where occurrence may reflect geographical or genetic aetiology. This is rather than concentrating on illness and conditions which affect larger populations of Black and minority ethnic people, such as coronary heart disease, where there may be explanations that relate to racially disadvantaged economic and social conditions.

In relation to morbidity, there is also little literature on the subjective experiences Black and minority ethnic communities have in relation to illness or disability. Where there is information this is usually not available at a national level, but is based upon small local studies of chronic illness or self-reported morbidity (Pilgrim *et al.*, 1993; Thompson *et al.*, 1994a, 1994b). Moreover, most health and lifestyle surveys have also been based on predominantly White populations (Blaxter, 1990), and there is little national data available on the health and lifestyles of Black and minority ethnic communities. To counteract this tendency the Health Education Authority . . . commissioned MORI's Health Research Unit to carry out a programme of health and lifestyle research on its behalf (Rudat, 1994). This survey demonstrated that there were significant differences between White and other ethnic groups in relation to health status and perceptions of health. At least twice as many African Caribbean, Indian, Pakistani and Bangladeshi respondents defined their health status as poor when compared with White respondents.

The health agenda within Black and minority ethnic communities

The health agenda coming from Black communities has also tended to focus on the incidence of freedom from disease and on securing appropriate medical intervention. These have been important issues in their own right. For Black communities, community initiatives of campaigns around health issues have arisen out of the link between racial discrimination and the lack of appropriate service provision as in the case of sickle cell anaemia, thalassaemia, coronary heart disease, diabetes, hypertension and circumcision (Douglas, 1991) or misdiagnosis based upon racial and cultural stereotypes, as in the case of mental illness (Wilson, 1993). However, there has been little attention to the association between poverty, racism and ill health. Moreover, the women's health movement, has not focused on the needs of Black and ethnic minorities and on the possible association between sexism, relative poverty, racism and ill health (Douglas, 1992). Little attention has also been focused on learning why some minority ethnic groups experience lower levels of certain diagnoses than the White majority population (Blakemore and Boneham, 1993).

The association between socio-economic conditions and the health of Black and minority ethnic communities

A number of studies indicate that Black and minority ethnic communities experience relative disadvantage in relation to poverty and discrimination. With the exception of Chinese communities and East African Indians, unemployment rates for minority ethnic communities are much higher than for the White population (Amin and Oppenheim, 1992; Brown,

1984; Jones, 1993). Rates of long-term unemployment are greater for most minority ethnic groups and differential between minority ethnic groups and White communities has widened during the 1980s and is wider amongst young people (Amin and Oppenheim, 1992; Jones, 1993). Black people are also employed disproportionately in low paid occupations and in poor working conditions such as night work and shift work (Brown, 1984). A greater proportion of Black people are employed as home workers as compared to White people. Housing tenure shows ethnic patterns (Jones, 1993). Caribbean and Bangladeshi people are more likely to be living in rented council accommodation compared to the White population. Although people from Indian and Pakistani communities tend to be owner occupiers, there is evidence that such ownership may still reflect occupancy of less expensive housing stock (Rudat, 1994).

An association between low socio-economic status and poor health in the White population has been demonstrated, as referred to earlier; where poor health is shown to be associated with poverty, unemployment, poor housing and poor working conditions. We have also discussed an association between minority ethnic status and disadvantage. Therefore material disadvantage associated with racism is a plausible explanation for poor health amongst Black and minority ethnic groups. However, there has been little research on the direct impact of the material disadvantage associated with racism, upon the health experience of these groups. Some research has also suggested that poor health and ethnic differences in disease prevalence can be explained by other factors such as the geographical distribution of Black and minority ethnic populations who reside primarily in inner-cities (McIntyre, 1986; Williams *et. al.*, 1994).

At most, the evidence on the effect of material disadvantage on Black and minority ethnic communities' health in the United Kingdom is therefore circumstantial. But what follows from this is that at the least, this issue should be a focus for further research and should be taken into account as a possibly significant factor in health promotion projects . . .

Introduction to Smethwick Heart Action Research Project (SHARP)

The Smethwick Heart Action Research Project was located within the framework of Healthy Sandwell 2000 and was a collaborative project between a number of agencies – the health authority, family health services authority, Health Education Authority – but located within Sandwell Health Promotion Unit. SHARP grew from the community-based approach of Sandwell Health Promotion Unit, supported by and building upon networks and resources which had already been established. As a piece of action research in line with Torkington's discussion of similar work in Liverpool (1991), the project was designed to provide data which could reflect issues of relevance for local communities and hence influence local policies which aimed to improve the health of the population in general and Black and minority ethnic communities in particular.

The project was funded by the Health Education Council for three years from April 1991, its aims were to identify risk factors for Black and minority ethnic communities in Smethwick in relation to coronary heart disease and stroke. Although the focus was predetermined as being on the incidence of disease, we sought to examine social, economic and political factors which might affect the health of these communities in Smethwick and to identify the priorities that members of Black communities worked to in terms of improving health . . .

Key findings

Detailed discussion of further findings is provided elsewhere (Thompson *et al.*, 1994a, 1994b). Overall, on the basis of self-report evidence in this study, Bangladeshi communities and Pakistani communities appear to experience greater relative poverty, with higher rates of unemployment and more worries about money. However, the data outlines a complex picture of the differences between ethnic groups in terms of perception of health, social disadvantage, experiences of racial discrimination, money worries and debt, and communication. Focusing . . . on the first three issues:

- *Perception of health*
  The findings demonstrated clear differences between Black and minority ethnic groups and White groups in relation to perceptions of health status. When asked, 'How healthy do you feel?' at least 17/60 in each of the Black and minority ethnic groups, compared with only 5/60 in the White group, answered 'not healthy' or 'not healthy at all'. The numbers were greatest for Pakistani (23/60) and Bangladeshi (22/60) respondents (Thompson *et al.*, 1994a)

- *Social disadvantage*
  With the exception of Indian respondents, respondents from other minority groups were, for example, consistently less likely to be car owners than White respondents. When asked about housing problems, for example, damp, condensation or mould, major repairs outstanding or problems maintaining adequate heating – 63 per cent of people from the Bangladeshi group compared to 40 per cent of people from the Pakistani group, 28 per cent of African Caribbeans and Whites and 15 per cent of Indians stated they had housing problems.

• *Racial discrimination*
9 per cent of the Black and minority ethnic sample reported racial discrimination and attacks, as being a problem in the locality. This result can be compared to Pilgrim *et al.*'s Bristol survey (1993) where 11 per cent of people had experienced racial insults in the streets. Fifteen per cent of the Black and minority ethnic sample also felt that racism had affected their access to health services.

These findings illustrate the difficulty, but also the importance of beginning to disentangle such issues and their possible bearing on health, by obtaining information from different minority ethnic groups and not simply contrasting the position of members of one minority ethnic group and the White population.

The survey also sought to explore possible gender differences in health experience. The data relating to this is still being analysed. However, for example, in relation to experience of signs of stress; indications of women being at some disadvantage here have emerged, although such differences require some qualification and there is evidence of the interaction of gender and ethnic identity. Respondents were interviewed about feeling angry or irritable; feeling tired and finding it hard to relax. 43 per cent of women in the survey as compared to 25 per cent of men said that they often felt angry or irritable with those around them. However, this was more frequently experienced by African Caribbean and White women than other groups. In the African Caribbean and White group, just over half the women interviewed said that they often felt angry or irritable. At least one third of women in each group agreed that they felt very tired with little energy. Overall 47 per cent of women compared with 33 per cent of men experienced this. 41 per cent of women overall and 31 per cent of men found it very hard to relax and unwind.

Following on from such responses the people interviewed highlighted a range of initiatives which they felt would improve their health. Across both White and minority ethnic groups, these related not only to initiatives they could take as private individuals such as to take more exercise, eat more healthily and to take steps to be happier in close relationships. They also concerned initiatives which drew on social policy measures such as provision of employment, good working conditions, a good standard of housing, a good education, to be reunited with family members abroad who were separated by immigration legislation and to live in a safe, clean, environment. Thus the survey uncovered the way in which initiatives identified by Black and minority ethnic communities as having the potential to improve their health moved away from a 'medical model' focus. The respondents identified environmental, economic, political and cultural factors as affecting their health and their comments were much more aligned to the Health For All model of health (World Health Organization, 1978).

In the context of one-to-one interviews the SHARP project therefore picked up a much broader definition of health than that which earlier research or community consultations had featured (Douglas, 1991). The reason for this may be that previously, community consultations had often focused upon Black health issues which had already become politicised – sickle cell disease and thalassaemia, mental health and circumcision (Douglas, 1991). In responding to health concerns, health promotion workers must, however, be able to address both this narrower health agenda, and the wider health agenda revealed by our survey. As without addressing the lack of health service provision, community support and trust will not be harnessed in order to tackle the much bigger issues of poverty, poor housing, material and racial disadvantage.

Further outcomes of the project

The project therefore broke new ground in establishing that health promotion workers and respondents from Black and ethnic minority communities shared concerns about the impact of unequal social conditions on health, and about the importance of addressing these issues. This has also provided a focus for subsequent practice. A series of health promotion initiatives has arisen out of the needs identified by Black and minority ethnic communities during the survey. These have involved Black and minority ethnic communities in their planning, implementation and evaluation and have endeavoured to tackle aspects of disadvantage and discrimination injurious to health. Four are presented in detail here:

Interpreting services

In relation to communication the survey showed that a third of the Bangladeshi group was literate only in Bengali, approximately one quarter of the Pakistani group was literate only in Urdu and almost a quarter of the Indian group were literate only in Punjabi. Thus the research demonstrated that in Smethwick almost a quarter to a third of Asian communities were literate only in their first language, hence also demonstrating the need for appropriate translation and interpreting services. These research findings on language and experiences of discrimination were then fed directly into the health services commissioning machinery. This led to a further investigation of interpreting services and a review of the overall provision of multi-lingual information.

SHARP training project

This project aimed to develop skills and confidence among Black and minority ethnic people/community workers in organising health promotion activities. One of the reasons for this initiative was that during community consultations Black and minority ethnic people described how they felt that health promotion activities did not target Black and minority ethnic communities and that there should be more health promotion activities organised within temples, Gurdwaras, and community centres used by Black and ethnic minority groups.

A training course was developed on 'Organising groups and activities in the Community'. This course was acredited by the Black Country Access Federation. Eight people attended the course which provided:

- Personal development in a supportive environment:
- Demystification of 'health promotion' – enabling local people/community workers to develop skills in health promotion;
- Networking between local community workers;
- Development of health provision and awareness of health issues in organisations/community groups.

Promoting Asian foods as healthy

When asked about their health, one of the reasons people from Black and minority ethnic communities cited for feeling less healthy than the indigenous White population was their diet. Asian respondents described themselves as 'not eating right foods', and Asian foods as 'rich in fat', i.e., they appeared to view their food as unhealthy. Among respondents and workers, there was also the impression that White health professionals lacked awareness of Asian and African Caribbean foods and therefore perpetuated racist stereotypes about unhealthy Asian and Caribbean food customs/practices.

The Community Action Steering Group for this project therefore felt that it was important to:

- Challenge myths about Asian foods with local Asian women and health professionals;
- Promote healthy eating with Asian foods.

The health promotion project therefore organised one day seminars on Food and Diet in a multi-racial society, aimed at health visitors, community workers and local authority workers: to look at broader aspects of healthy eating in a multi-racial society and also at the difficulties of affording food in low-income families. This second focal point was a crucial matter of concern as in the SHARP survey, 24 per cent of respondents overall had said affording food was sometimes, often, or very difficult. Bangladeshi (41 per cent) and White groups (31 per cent) stressed that affording food was difficult. (25 per cent) of African Caribbean and 10 per cent of Indian and Pakistani groups said affording food was difficult.

Cookery demonstrations were also organised at a local community centre run by Asian Community liaison officers from the FHSA (Family Health Services Authority), who had been involved with the SHARP project. The aim of the workshops was to raise awareness of healthy eating with Asian foods, and to demonstrate methods of reducing the fat content of meals. The demonstrations also included the use of cheaper, English vegetables, for example, leeks and potatoes in place of more expensive traditional Asian vegetables but using Asian methods.

Sustaining health promotion initiatives
One of the shortcomings of SHARP was that it was a short term funded project and hence it was important to try to ensure that its activities and initiatives were sustainable, by building upon networks that had been created. In achieving sustainability it is important to work with existing structures and representatives and workers within existing localities. It is important to involve established organisations including youth and community services, voluntary agencies, places of worship, community centres, local shops and health centres in any health promotion initiatives. So, for example, the SHARP survey had indicated low rates of physical/leisure activity among the Muslim population and 'Asian' women. Bangladeshi and Pakistani groups participated least in leisure exercise, as there were few facilities which catered for the needs and wishes of these communities. Facilities clearly needed to become more generally user-friendly: providing privacy for women, women instructors and information available in Asian languages. Two key issues that emerged as the availability of appropriate facilities was explored were: the lack of local authority leisure services' provision of sessions for women only, in Smethwick; and stereotypical views among White professionals and organisations about Asian women, such as: religious beliefs prohibited them from participation in physical activity.

Consequently, two options were explored and developed in conjunction with the leisure department: providing Bhangra aerobics sessions at a community centre; and providing swimming sessions for Asian women in Smethwick. The local authority Leisure Services Department employed an Asian woman Sports Development Officer who worked with the SHARP team to develop the initiatives described above – which were then continued by the Leisure Services Department after initial piloting and evaluation through the SHARP project.

Democratic, participatory forms of evaluation also need to be built into all health promotion programmes and initiatives, which involve local people and communities not only in identifying their own ideal objectives but in reviewing the outcomes. Each health promotion initiative developed as part of the Smethwick Heart Action Research Project, had a community action steering group with members drawn from local Community groups and voluntary organisations, which consulted with local people and organisations not only before the development of health promotion programmes – identifying the possible options and in implementing the health promotion programmes – but also in evaluating their success (Malik *et al.*, 1994).

Conclusion

The Smethwick Heart Action Research Project has demonstrated that health promotion can start to identify key issues and concerns for local people trying to maintain and improve health against a backcloth of social disadvantage, notably for Black and minority ethnic communities: against racism and racial discrimination. The findings from SHARP show that Black and minority ethnic communities are in fact aware of the social, economic and environmental factors influencing their health. What is more difficult is to develop health promotion programmes which address such concerns, once having identified them. This project within the limitations of its funding, tried to achieve small changes in policies within health and local authorities and to empower local communities to develop health promotion programmes which focused not only on lifestyle approaches to heart health but which acknowledged the impact of material factors.

SHARP also demonstrates that it is possible to make progress on the self-direction of health promotion initiatives by members of the local community, which address these issues.

However, in other respects, the experience of SHARP makes sobering reading. More sophisticated methods need to be developed to assess the health needs of black and minority communities, which reflect diversity in terms of ethnicity, 'race', culture, class, gender and disadvantage. Nationally, the remit of current health promotion practice is constrained by the Health of the Nation strategy which does not offer an incentive to move beyond a narrow focus on individual behaviour change as affecting the incidence of disease.

It is important for health promotion to develop methodologies and practices which recognise the social, economic and environmental factors affecting health. In doing so as SHARP's experience demonstrates, there is a need for health promotion to develop strategies to work with other organisations which are better placed to effect changes in policy to improve health. Local respondents to SHARP's survey clarified, for example, that substantial improvements in employment conditions and immigration policy are germane to their health: matters which are beyond the remit of short-term health promotion projects.

Acknowledgements

The author was project manager for SHARP; Helen Thompson was research coordinator; Ameen Malik project officer; Dawn Henry and Minara Khatun were research assistants and Lorna McKee was the research consultant. The project was funded as a demonstration project by the Health Education Authority, Look After Your Heart programme,as part of the community grant scheme. The views expressed in this article are those of the author and do not represent the views of any other person or the views of the authorities concerned.

References

Amin, K. and Oppenheim, C. (1992). *Poverty in Black and White*. London: Child Poverty Action Group/Runnymede Trust.

Bhopal, R. (1988). *Setting Priorities for Health Care for Ethnic Minority Groups*. Newcastle upon Tyne: Department of Epidemiology and Public Health. University of Newcastle upon Tyne.

Blakemore, K. and Boneham, M. (1993). *Age Race and Ethnicity – A Comparative Approach*. Buckingham: Open University Press.

Blaxter, M. (1990). *Health and Lifestyles*. London: Routledge.

Brown, C. (1984). *Black and White Britain: The Third PSI Survey*. Aldershot: Gower.

Douglas, J. (1991). 'Influences on the community development and health movement – A Personal view'. In Health Education Unit Open University (ed), *Roots and Branches: Papers from the Open University Health Education Council Winter School on Community Development and Health*. Milton Keynes: Health Education Unit, The Open University.

Douglas, J. (1992). 'Black women's health matters: putting Black women on the research agenda'. In Roberts, H. (ed), *Women's Health Matters*. London: Routledge.

Douglas, J. (1955a). Developing anti-racist health promotion strategies. In Bunton, R., Nettleton, S. and Burrows, R. (eds), *The Sociology of Health Promotion*. London: Routledge.

Douglas, J. (1995b). Developing appropriate research methodologies for health and social care research with black and minority ethnic communities. Conference Report, West Bromwich: SHARP/Sandwell Health Promotion Unit.

McIntyre, S. (1986). The patterning of health by social position in contemporary Britain: directions for sociological research, *Social Science and Medicine, 23*, (*4*), 393–415.

Malik, A., Thompson, H., Douglas, J. and McKee, L. (1994). *Smethwick Heart Action Research Project – Developing Heart Health Initiatives with black and minority ethnic communities*. West Bromwich: SHARP/Sandwell Health Promotion Unit.

Pilgrim, S., Fenton, S., Hugest, T., Hine, C. and Tibbs, N. (1993). *The Bristol Black and Ethnic Minorities Health Survey*. Bristol: University of Bristol.

Rudat, K. (1994). *Health and Lifestyles. Black and Minority Ethnic Groups in England*. London: Health Education Authority.

Smaje, C. (1995) *Health, Race and Ethnicity – Making Sense of the Evidence*. London: Kings Fund Institute/SHARE.

Thompson, H. (1994a). *Smethwick Heart Action Research Project, Results of a Health Survey with the African–Caribbean, Bangladeshi, Indian, Pakistani and White communities in Smethwick*. West Bromwich: SHARP/Sandwell Health Promotion Unit.

Thompson, H., Malik, A., Douglas, J. and McKee, L. (1994b). *Smethwick Heart Action Research Project, Final Report*. West Bromwich: SHARP/Sandwell Health Promotion Unit.

Torkington, P. (1991). *Black Health – A political issue*. London: Catholic Association for Racial Justice.

Williams, D., Larizzo-Mourney, R. and Warren, R. (1994). The Concept of race and health status in America. *Public Health Reports, 109* (*1*), 26–41.

Wilson, M. (1993). *Mental Health and Britain's Black Communities*. London: Kings Fund Centre/NHSME Mental Health Task Force/Prince of Wales Advisory Group on Disability.

World Health Organization (1978). *Alma-Ata 1978. Primary Health Care*. Copenhagen: WHO.

28 *Econology: integrating health and sustainable development. Guiding principles for decision-making**

Ronald Labonté

Introduction

The concept of sustainable development ('development that meets the needs of the present without compromising the ability of future generations to meet their own needs', World Commission on Environment and Development, 1987) is becoming central to political and economic discourse in most countries, and in international fora. . .

Health has been embedded in the concept of sustainable development since its inception. Until recently, however, the health sector, and more specifically the public health sector, has not been actively engaged in decision-making or policy setting discussions on sustainable development. Three unique patterns of relationships emerge when health is placed alongside the two major dimensions of sustainable development, the environment and economy.

The health–environment relationship is described by research on the human health impact of environmental hazards. Traditional public health has focused on protecting individuals from environmental hazards; this comprises one set of health–environment relations. The obvious shift herein is from toxins (biological hazards) to toxics (chemical hazards). However, data on the human health effects of toxics is rarely unequivocal and largely absent. Environmental protection policy must begin to use biological markers (health effects in other species and experimental animal research) as proxy human measures where human data are equivocal or absent, and must begin to study subtle effects (e.g. immunotoxic, developmental) as well as gross effects (e.g. cancer, reproductive failures). At a paradigmatic-shift level, public health must also shift its emphasis from protecting humans from environmental hazards, to protecting the environment from human hazards. The most threatening, and least quantifiable or certain, threats to human health are those

* From *Health Promotion International*, 6 (2) (1991), pp. 147–156. Oxford: © Oxford University Press 1991.

relating to global ecosystem change, notably the enhanced greenhouse effect.

The health–economy relationship pertains to the well documented relationship between poverty and disease. Less well known is research linking improved health status to social support systems, psychosocial emotional states and relatively flat income or power hierarchies. When human health in its broadest sense becomes the endpoint for sustainable development decision-making, 'trickle-down' theories of wealth creation and continuous economic growth become far less important than the equitable distribution of wealth related resources within a community or nation. Indeed, the most powerful amendment public health can make to the concept of sustainable development is the fundamental relationship between social justice, environmental protection and economic development.

The final relationship, that of economy–environment, represents both a value shift from what Daly and Cobb (1989) describe as 'chrematistics' ('the manipulation of property and wealth so as to maximise short-term exchange value to the owner') to 'oikonomia' ('the management of the household so as to increase its value to all members of the household over the long run'); and a correction in market economics so that 'externalities' such as the costs of pollution control and resource renewal are internalised in commodity prices, thus sending consumers a true price of consumption while generating the revenues necessary to invest in environmental protection.

Respectively, these three relationships can be captured by the imperatives to consume less, share more equitably and account more accurately.

It is possible now to articulate a set of principles for sustainable development that give full expression to human health and its social and environmental underpinnings. . .

The principles offered below are intended to provide ethical and health-biased guidelines for addressing the most fundamental question: When conflicts arise within the environment–health–economy triad, what values will guide the process of conflict resolution? These principles are not given in any order of importance, nor are they separate from each other. One might increase intranational equity while worsening transnational inequities and increasing pollution, or vice versa. Neither situation is sustainable, nor healthy. The principles are a packaged set.

Principle 1: the necessity of principle-based decision-making

Principles are fundamental to the process of sustainable development decision-making. Scientific data can only inform, but neither predict nor dictate, sustainable development decision-making.

Comment

Greater support for scientific research into the health implications of sustainable development is required. Nevertheless, decisions on global-scale environmental effects (greenhouse gas emissions, stratospheric ozone depletion, loss of carbon sink capacity and increased appropriation of net primary product) cannot await scientific certainty . . . To anticipate is to make best guesses about what might happen, and to act upon those guesses.

Principle 2: inclusiveness of information

Scientifically generated data should encompass as broad a pattern of complex relations as possible: environment–health (risk assessments); economy–health (equity assessments); environment–economy (full-cost accounting). It should not be restricted to only one set of relationships.

Comment

With respect to environment–economy relationships, an ecosystems approach is required, and not one that separately assesses environmental impacts on air, water, flora, fauna, etc . . . [Very] small toxic emissions or system-wide perturbations may be sufficient to create profound and health damaging changes, and the need to integrate 'total carrying capacity' for ecosystems and humans into risk assessments. Whenever disputes over data interpretation arise, particularly concerning environment–health effects, the most health-conservative findings or models should be used, that is, any benefit of scientific doubt should be given to human health.

Principle 3: shrinking global inequities

Sustainable development, globally, requires that a proposed activity increase global equity, that is, it lessen the wealth (income) gap between nations.

Comment

The Third World debt is the global economy's current greatest threat to sustainable development. It was largely incurred for the benefit of few. It must be forgiven or postponed, and not simply through debt–equity swaps such as rainforest preservation which, by themselves, are inadequate to meet the population growth and resource depletion crises faced by most poor nations. This is a radical suggestion, though not without precedent. (It also begs an interesting question: what is more important, the health of the species and sustainability of the planetary ecosystem, or colourful pieces of paper with the faces of dead politicians and rulers?) At the very least, the implications of monetary policy on environmental sustainability must be made explicit.

There are several ways in which this principle can be implemented. In the case of transnational projects, international agreements could require the retention and reinvestment within the poor country of more earned income than is repatriated. In the case of strictly national projects within a rich country, this might be achieved through a combination of national taxation policies and untied foreign aid, or specific trading and sharing policies for poor countries related to the project's goods or production technology . . . One suggestion would have each nation pay a carbon tax based on consumption, with revenues collected by an international body and used, in part, to fund clean technology transfer to poorer countries . . .

The environmental and occupational conditions under which the products are manufactured should equal those required for First World production. Increased foreign aid to Second and Third World countries could be dedicated to supporting these countries in achieving this equity in sustainable development . . .

Emphasis should be placed not on international trade, but on intranational, bioregional market development. This approach would foster, rather than remove, trade barriers. Daly and Cobb argue that free trade, by allowing capital to move wherever labour is cheapest, lowers living standards for most of the world's workers, creating a global 'rush towards poverty'. This stimulates unsustainable economic activities in rich countries in order to compete with the cheap labour productivity of poor countries . . .

Principle 4: shrinking national inequities

Sustainable development, nationally, requires that a proposed activity increase national equity, that is, it lessen the wealth (income) gap between have and have-not citizens.

Comment
This principle might be achieved through taxation policies (e.g. negative income tax), and equity oriented development permits . . . [It] might also be also be achieved through various forms of employment equity policies (regarding the hiring of women, ethnic minorities, disabled workers, and so on) and legislation supporting more equitable forms of remuneration. Taxation and other fiscal policy instruments will need to be used to offset the income inequities that will arise as full-cost accounting of environmental resource use is achieved.

Principle 5: empowering equally

Sustainable development, both globally and nationally, requires that a proposed activity increase equity in power.

Comment

Power is not quite the same as wealth, although the two are certainly related. Empowerment requires an increase in access to decision-making by less powerful individuals, groups and communities. This might be achieved through provision of resources (economic, technical, organisational) to such groups to assist them in participating in the decision-making on the proposed activity. It takes as fundamental the participation by all interested parties and requires regular environmental audits and reporting by the private and public sectors, including reports of international activities.

Principle 6: producing fairly, healthily

Sustainable development requires that each proposed activity increase worker control and workplace democracy relative to past practices.

Comment

Increasing workplace democracy may include, but is not restricted to, unionisation of the labour force; specific agreements regarding health and safety measures that comply with, or exceed, legislated minimums; worker–ownership agreements; voting worker representation on management boards and committees; and the existence of workplace policies reflecting Emery's six basic criteria for healthful work (cited in Levi, 1983).

- The job should be reasonably demanding in terms other than sheer endurance, and should provide variety.
- The worker should be able to learn on the job, and to go on learning.
- The job should include some area of decision-making that the worker can call his or her own.
- There should be some degree of social support and recognition in the workplace.
- The worker should be able to relate what he or she does or produces to social life (that is, feel that his or her labour contributes to improved social welfare).
- The worker should feel that the job leads to some sort of desirable future, at a personal and collective level.

Principle 7: sustaining communities

Sustainable development requires that each proposed activity create, sustain or re-create 'community'. This means that the activity, at a minimum, must address how it will:

- Increase opportunities for social interaction and development of social networks;

- Diversify the community's economic base;
- Increase proximity between production, consumption and disposal;
- Support a more active, democratic participation of community citizens in political and economic decision-making, including that pertaining to the proposed project.

Comment

This principle together with principles 3 through 6, comprise a social contract between capital (business, economy) and community. This principle also requires novel methodologies to capture community perceptions and future scenarios that draw heavily on participatory learning theories, ethnographic research and sociology.

The notion of increasing proximity between what is produced, consumed and disposed is sometimes dismissed as urging a return to pre-industrial, agrarian forms of economic and social organization. This is not so. Rather, the need to increase proximity recognises the absolute necessity of decreasing fossil fuel use and greenhouse gas emissions. This requires a dramatic decline in the scale of transport, and in the energy inputs for food production . . . Relatively self-sufficient communities form the base of relatively self-sufficient nation-states.

Principle 8: replenishing and replacing

Sustainable development locates a proposed activity along a hierarchy that asks if the product the activity produces, or the process by which it is fashioned:

- Replenishes the planet, putting in more resources (i.e. 'carbon sink') than it extracts?
- Replaces what is taken, achieving a steady-state economy-environment systems relation?
- Reduces energy and renewable/non-renewable resource consumption, and reduces the production/consumption of toxics?
- Reuses (or allows for the reuse of) constituent materials ('resources')?
- Recycles (or allows for the recycling of) constituent materials?

This is a hierarchy of sustainable development. Human sustainability is commensurate with any given activity's ability to address higher tiered concerns. Any proposed activity that does not, at a minimum, replace what it takes (the notion of 'living off the interest') is not, by definition, environmentally sustainable.

Comment

Implementation of this principle includes a 'best available' precept, in which the best available technologies, legislation, regulations and standards, conditions, enforcement practices and policies internationally are incorporated into proposed activity decision-making.

Principle 9: Internalising all the costs

Sustainable development requires that each proposed activity employ full-cost accounting, and internalise all of its externalities to the fullest extent that these externalities can be estimated.

Comment

Externalities are effects that create costs outside of the market-mediated relationship between producer and consumer, e.g. replacement of natural resources, clean-up of pollution. The costs of these externalities are to be borne by the proposer(s) of the activity. Since full-cost accounting is a novel activity and subject to debate over value estimates, preference should be given to those estimates most conservative in terms of human health and environmental integrity. Full-cost accounting must take place in public, and be accompanied by an 'open-book' policy by government and industry.

Principle 10: sustaining diversities

Sustainable development requires that each proposed activity respects, by not actively or passively decreasing, ecosystem (including genetic stock) and human system (cultural) diversity.

Comment

Environmental impact assessments may provide the scientific data regarding ecosystem diversity; human system diversity requires that such assessments and decision-making fora incorporate and utilise other forms of cultural knowledge. Social impact assessments offer some potential to do so, although such assessments tend to be positivist and to accept *a priori* certain impact categories which reflect certain cultural biases (Rickson and Chu, 1990). How problems are defined and economic activities selected, and the relationship between information and political decision making, may be more important issues than impact assessments *per se.*

Principle 11: nurturing the intangibles

Sustainable development requires that each proposed activity include statements about how it will nurture the intangible quality of life for the citizens affected by it.

Comment

There are many things besides a healthy planet and a healthy body that create the self-actualising experience of human well-being. These things might include aesthetic experiences, feelings of history or continuity in one's family or community, cultural identification, respect for and feelings of oneness with nature, and other spiritual phenomena . . .

As intangibles are identified they become tangible, but never in quite the same way as events that can be represented by data . . . These intangibles, will vary across cultures and communities.

Principle 12: planning across the generations

Sustainable development requires that each proposed activity state how it will ensure equity in future generations, that is, how it will maintain the natural capital and the sustainability of human cultures. It demands that economic activity extend the notion of full-cost accounting across time, as well as across the resource base. . .

Conclusion: the role of health promotion professionals

. . . Health professionals should not wait to be invited into sustainable development discussions. They must invite themselves. As they do so, they should consider that, just as principles are only as good as the actions they generate and the decisions they inform, increased public health participation in sustainable development fora will only be as good as the degree to which health professionals are clear about their unique contributions. These contributions can be summed as:

- The limitations of scientific data, and the ethics of decision-making when epidemiological data are equivocal;
- A broad construction of health, particularly the role of political/ economic equity in creating individual and population health;
- The limitations of 'lifestyle' (individual) based strategies;
- The concept of empowerment, its relationship to personal and community health, and its implication for sustainable development decision-making processes.

Health promotion has emerged in recent years as an attempt to synthesise the relative interplay of biomedical, behavioural and socio-environmental systems in creating health or disease. It represents to the health sector what sustainable development represents to the environment–economy sectors: an effort to articulate value-based strategies that sustain humans. The Ottawa Charter for Health Promotion (WHO, 1986) identifies several strategies that health promotion must address: reorient health services, develop personal skills, build healthy public policy, create supportive environments, and strengthen community action. These can be, and have been, applied to sustainable development; they have also raised political challenges that any sustainable development decision-making process must face.

Reorienting health services speaks to the need to develop more effective and efficient community-based systems of health care. Large health care institutions, predicated on a narrow bio-medical model of disease, often lose the human quality of caring in their relationships with ill people. There is also declining marginal utility in disease treatment, and the amount of public revenue that currently goes into health care services may now be unsustainable . . .

Developing personal skills can be narrowly construed as promoting healthy lifestyles. However, it is being more broadly interpreted by many health promotion practitioners as encouraging skills in community organizing, policy advocacy, political decision-making and other forms of participatory democracy that constitute the larger personal responsibility of citizenship. (Hancock, 1989; Labonté, 1989) It intersects nicely with the rhetoric of broader community participation in sustainable development decision-making . . .

Developing healthy public policies means incorporating human health criteria into all policy sectors. It is a new public health truism that individual and community well-being are determined more by social, environmental and economic systems than by health care provision. Policies in such sectors as transportation, energy, economy, food and agriculture, waste management and urban design can either increase or decrease human health, just as they are either sustainable or not. Health promotion and sustainable development policies intersect in many areas. A low meat, low cholesterol, high fibre diet now recommended as a means of preventing cardio-vascular disease and, perhaps, cancer, requires far less land per capita than do current diets in western industrialised countries. Health concerns are also driving increases in more sustainable, organic forms of agriculture that use fewer toxic petrochemical inputs . . . And so on.

The danger in the concept of healthy public policy is that it might imperialise existing forms of environmental decision-making, and risk further confusion rather than more concerted professional actions . . .

It is likely of greater strategic value for Public Health advocates to expand the parameters of existing environment–economy decision-making fora (such as environmental assessment procedures) to encompass a rigorously broad, social model of health, than to create cumbersome parallel structures.

Creating supportive environments essentially means ensuring that human social organizations enhance well-being . . . Choices are never simply 'personal'. One significant lesson from health promotion has been the importance of public policies in stimulating personal change. Legislated workplace smoking bans are associated with markedly greater smoking cessation and maintenance rates; the carrot without the stick is simply a dangling vegetable.

Creating supportive environments also presumes the existence of a positive experience of community . . . The final strategy, 'strengthening community action', derives from the richer international literature on community development and community organising, and is fundamentally about the re-creation of community . . . These ideas have become driving forces behind the several hundred healthy city/healthy community projects worldwide . . .

Community development successes in health promotion . . . speak to a point salient to sustainable development decision-making. Not only must actions accompany words; local actions are required. . . [Where] citizens can see, speak with and feel less intimidated by their municipal politicians and business leaders. They can also see directly the results of their participation in decision-making political processes.

There is, however, an important caveat to this finding: that of localising global problems, and mystifying macro-level systems of power and decision-making . . . [M]ost economic decision-making is national and transnational in nature.Local decision-making at present can only be within narrow parameters at best, and is unlikely to include substantial control over economic resources. As Lester Brown (1989) of the Worldwatch Institute commented in his 1989 State of the World report, 'Small may be beautiful, but it may also be insignificant'. . .

Unless local actions are integrated with advocacy and political action strategies directed towards higher level government policies, our drive for decentralised decision-making and community development may unwittingly 'privatise', by rendering local, what are much larger issues. We risk mystifying the actual exercise of political power, just as green products mystify the sustainable limits of consumption. Local actions and green products are starting points only, and represent the community organising rule 'to begin where the people are'. But where people are is not necessarily where they should be. The environmental motto to 'Think globally, act locally' may well need amending to 'Start locally, act globally'.

Empowerment, the ability to exercise choice, increasingly informs the individual and community work of health promotion professionals. It does not lack for problems of definition or co-optation, but it speaks to an emergent knowledge that the very act of organising to alter conditions of relative powerlessness enhances individual health. 'Empower' is usually used transitively, as in we (health professionals) need to empower others (poor, marginalised individuals or groups). Empower is also a reflexive verb; the most enduring power (choice) is that which is taken, not that which is given. Health promotion professionals possess a power not yet seized, one that builds upon a discipline specific credibility while capitalising on the relative lack of boundaries defining health promotion . . .

[T]o a considerable extent, health promotion is inherently muti-disciplinary, or a-disciplinary. It incorporates theory and practice from disciplines as diverse as social marketing, education, sociology, psychology, social work, anthropology, ecology, statistics, administration/management, to name only a few. The same might be said for the 'new' public health which, by focusing on the determinants of health, frees itself from the discipline boundaries of medicine and traditional infectious disease control. Few other professionals participating in sustainable development debates share this vague yet liberating generalism.

The most potent role of health promotion professionals in sustainable development decision-making, then, may be that of a cross-discipline interpreter. Using the metaphor of health, which shares its etymology with 'hello' and 'whole', the interpreter does not colonise the other disciplines or sectors with public health imperatives so much as seeks and seeds the commonalities, while raising to the conscious level the conflicts.

References

Brown, L. *et al.* (1989). *State of the World.* New York: Norton.

Daly, H. and Cobb, J. (1989). *For the Common Good.* Boston: Beacon Press.

Hancock, T. (1989). *Sustaining Health: Achieving Health For All in a Secure Environment.* (Conference background paper), Conference on Health–Environment–Economy. York University, Toronto (April 1989).

Labonté, R. (1989). Community empowerment: the need for a political analysis, *Canadian Journal of Public Health, 80,* 87–88.

Levi, L. (1983). Stress. In *Encyclopaedia of Occupational Health and Safety,* vol 2. Geneva: International Labour Organisation, 2106–2111

Rickson, R. and Chu, C. (1990). Social impact assessments and the new public health, *Integrating Health and Environment Workshop Papers.* Nathan, Queensland: Giffith University.

World Commission on Environment and Development (1987). *Our Common Future.* New York: Oxford University Press.

World Health Organisation (1986). *Ottawa Charter for Health Promotion.* Ottawa.

29 Using sponsorship to create healthy environments for sport, racing and arts venues in Western Australia[*]

Billie Corti, C. D'Arcy J. Holman, Robert J. Donovan, Shirley K. Frizzell and Addy M. Carroll

Introduction

Healthway

Healthway is an independent body established under the Tobacco Control Act 1990. Described more fully in Holman *et al.*, (1993a), the main purpose of the Act is the active discouragement of tobacco smoking. Healthway's enabling legislation specifies a number of objectives. These include: funding activities related to the promotion of good health; offering an alternative source of funds for sport, racing and arts activities previously supported by tobacco sponsorship; and sponsoring sport, racing and arts activities that encourage healthy lifestyles and advance health promotion programmes.

As a funding organisation, Healthway does not deliver its own health messages. In Western Australia, there is an active health promotion community with many local agencies involved in programme delivery. Healthway uses these established groups, known as 'support sponsors', to deliver health promotion messages at sponsored events. In 1990–1, some 132 sponsorships were awarded to sport (A$3.4 m), arts (A$ 1.7 m) and racing (A$0.06 m) organisations (Western Australian Health Promotion Foundation, 1992). Each sponsorship organisation is allocated a support sponsor as part of its sponsorship contract. Overall, in 1990–1, support sponsors (including the National Heart Foundation, Cancer Foundation and the Health Department's Smoking and Health Programme) received A$1.3 m to promote health messages at sponsored events including the negotiation of related structural reforms . . .

[*] From *Health Promotion International, 10* (3) (1995), pp. 185–197. Oxford: © Oxford University Press 1995.

Sponsorship

Sponsorship is a relatively new tool to health promotion . . . Sponsorship dollars are exchanged for a range of sponsor 'benefits' designed to promote the sponsor's image and/or products. Examples of negotiated sponsor benefits include naming rights, signage, personal endorsement of a product by a performer or player, programme advertising and editorial, hospitality for sponsor guests and the distribution of promotional materials. For health sponsors, sponsored events provide promotional and educational opportunities for some of the hard-to-impact groups in the community (Egger *et al.*, 1993).

Sponsorship also provides the health sponsor with one additional and potentially powerful sponsor benefit – the introduction of structural reforms that support healthy behaviours at sponsored events. Examples of structural reform include the introduction of smoke-free policies; the provision of healthy food choices; and the introduction of appropriate sun protection for outdoor events (for example, 'legionnaire hats' rather than caps for baseball players). Unlike other sponsor benefits, it is possible that after sponsorship dollars have been depleted, structural reforms introduced during the sponsorship period will remain.

Healthway's approach to sponsorship reflects a broad interpretation of its charter and comprehensive health promotion practice. Taking the lead from the Victorian Health Promotion Foundation, Australia's first health promotion foundation, Healthway requires its sponsored organisations to introduce structural reform at sponsored events, particularly the creation of smoke-free environments.

Health Promotion Development and Evaluation Programme

The Health Promotion Development and Evaluation Program (HPDEP) is an independent academic programme funded by Healthway. The role of the HPDEP is to evaluate Healthway's activities in terms of its legislative mandate . . .

This chapter describes how Healthway has used sponsorship to create healthy environments in sporting and cultural settings. Drawing from results of a HPDEP survey of Healthway-sponsored organisations, it describes the level of structural reform within sport, racing and arts organisations, and the potential reach of these reforms. There are many organisations contributing to structural reform in Australia, particularly in the tobacco control area. Some attempt is made to estimate the extent to which Healthway might have contributed to structural reform in Western Australia. It concludes with a discussion of how a funding body can use healthy public policy to influence intersectoral co-operation and to create healthier environments.

Methods

Sample selection

The sample consisted of sport, racing and arts organisations which had received Healthway sponsorship between May 1991 and June 1992. A questionnaire and an accompanying letter addressed to each organisation's nominated 'contact person' (as specified in the grant application) was posted to 269 organisations. Organisations that failed to respond by a certain date (63 per cent of respondents) were contacted by telephone. Up to three follow-up telephone calls were made.

Survey instrument

The questionnaire, containing 118 separate questions, included eight items about structural reform. Organisations were asked:

(i) which of seven structural reforms they had in place within their groups and, where applicable, in the venues where these groups played, raced or performed: (a) before Healthway started (18 months prior to the survey); and (b) at the time of the survey (referred to hereinafter as 18 months later;
(ii) which structural reforms they had been asked by Healthway to implement; and
(iii) the extent of support for Healthway initiated structural reforms amongst: (a) key people in the organisation; and (b) spectators or audiences of the organisation's activities.

The seven structural reforms investigated were smoke-free areas; safe alcohol practices; sun protection measures; healthy food choices; access for disadvantaged groups; disability access; and safe exercise warm-up practices. The latter two reforms were not priority structural reform areas for Healthway and, although reported . . . in Corti *et al.*, 1993, are not discussed in this chapter.

Organisations also were asked for the number of individual members of the organisation as well as how much Healthway sponsorship they had received, and over what period of time. The latter variables were used to calculate 'average annual sponsorship'.

Methods of analysis

The data were analysed using the Statistical Package for the Social Sciences. The statistical significance of a change in the proportion of organisations exhibiting a particular attribute was assessed by the McNemar Test. Organisations that claimed structural reform was not applicable to their organisation (for example, committees constituted for the sole purpose of mounting a one-off event) and/or that had missing data were excluded from the analysis.

Results

Response rates

Of the 269 questionnaires forwarded to sport, racing and arts organisations, 260 were considered eligible to participate (i.e. excluding those returned-to-sender) and 209 organisations returned completed questionnaires. Response rates achieved were as follows: 81.4 per cent for arts, 80.7 per cent for sport and 70.6 per cent for racing organisations. Of organisations that failed to respond, 90 per cent had received sponsorship of A$15,000 or less from Healthway. The following analysis includes only those organisations that completed the questions relating to structural reform ($n = 171$).

Types of structural reforms in place

Figure 29.1 shows the types of structural reforms in place before Healthway started ($n = 158$, i.e. those for which structural reforms were applicable before Healthway started) and 18 months later ($n = 171$). The results show a substantial increase in the level of reform in all areas.

Eighteen months after Healthway's inception, smoke-free area policies

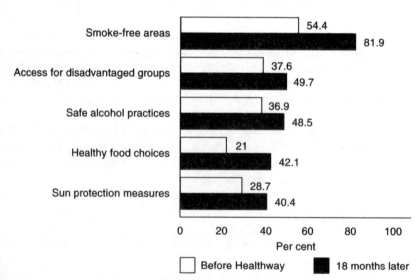

Figure 29.1   *Structural reforms in place before Healthway's inception and 18 months later*

were the most prevalent type of structural reform (81.9 per cent). More than one and one-half (1.65) times as many organisations reported this policy compared with any other (Figure 29.1). Nearly one-half of the organisations surveyed reported having current policies related to access for disadvantaged groups (49.7 per cent) and safe alcohol practices (48.5 per cent).

Changes in the prevalence of structural reform since Healthway's inception

To examine any significant changes in the prevalence of structural reform that may have occurred since Healthway's inception, only organisations that provided data for both time periods (i.e. before Healthway started and 18 months later) were included in the following analysis ($n = 153$).

Since Healthway's inception, there has been a significant increase in the prevalence of structural reforms in all . . . [sponsored organisations]. While the prevalence of smoke-free areas increased the most (27 percentage points), there was also a 21.6 percentage-point increase in the prevalence of healthy food choice reforms.

Structural reform policies were more common among arts organisations. Nearly all arts organisations reported having a current smoke-free area policy (95.6 per cent) 18 months after Healthway's inception. Fewer arts than sports organisations reported having a sun protection policy, however, most arts events are conducted indoors. Arts organisations reported a significant increase in the prevalence of smoke-free policies, safe alcohol practices and access for disadvantage groups.

The majority of sport (69.9 per cent) and racing (60 per cent) organisations claimed to have smoke-free area policies 18 months after Healthway's inception, representing substantial increases since Healthway started. Sport organisations reported a significant increase in the prevalence of smoke-free areas, healthy food choices and sun protection measures.

Structural reforms requested by support sponsors or Healthway

The introduction of structural reform is one of the sponsor benefits negotiated by Healthway or its support sponsors, prior to execution of the contract of grant. Organisations surveyed were asked which, if any, structural reforms they had been requested to implement and which, if any, were not applicable to their organisation (for example, because it was already in place). The results in this section relate to the prevalence of requests amongst organisations that stated a particular policy area was applicable to their organisation.

In accordance with Healthway's legislative mandate, nearly three-quarters of organisations for which a smoke-free policy was applicable claimed that they had been asked to create smoke-free areas (72.8 per cent). Similarly, almost one half of organisations that claimed that healthy food choices were applicable to their organisation, reported they had been asked to make healthy food choices available (46.8 per cent) at their sponsored event(s) . . .

Influence of the level of average annual sponsorship on the likelihood of Healthway requesting reforms

. . . On average, recipients of large sponsorships (i.e. in excess of A$100,000) received 66.5 times more sponsorship than organisations in the smallest sponsorship category (A$154,012 compared with A$2316), they were requested to implement only 13 per cent more structural reforms (1.5 per organisation compared with 1.33). There appeared to be a weak relationship between the amount of sponsorship received and the average number of requests for reform. However, little practical difference existed between groups receiving various levels of funding.

Healthway's contribution to the implementation of structural reform

Figure 29.2 shows the absolute percentage increase in the prevalence of structural reforms since Healthway's inception, comparing organisations

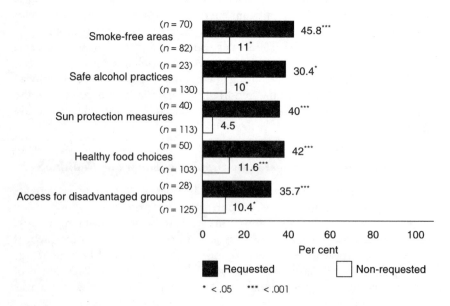

Figure 29.2   *Absolute percentage increase in structural reform (before Healthway started versus 18 months later) for requested organisations and other non-requested organisations*

requested to implement particular policies with other organisations funded by Healthway. Only organisations that provided data for time-points both before and after Healthway's inception were included in the analysis.

Amongst organisations requested to implement reforms, the level of increase was practically and statistically significant. For example, there was an increase of 45.8 percentage points in the prevalence of smoke-free areas and an increase of 30.4 percentage points in the prevalence of safe alcohol practices.

However. Figure 29.2 illustrates that a movement towards the implementation of structural reform existed without Healthway's direct influence. That is, the prevalence of each type of structural reform also increased significantly in organisations not requested to implement changes. The average increases in percentage points were, however, far greater in organisations requested to implement changes compared with organisations not requested to implement reforms: 4.16 times greater for smoke-free areas (45.8 compared with 11 per cent), 3.04 times greater for safe alcohol practices, 8.89 times greater for sun protection measures. 3.62 times greater for healthy food choices, and 3.43 times greater for access for disadvantaged aged groups. These data strongly suggest that Healthway has accelerated the rate of change.

Another way of considering the influence of Healthway on the implementation of structural reform was to examine the prevalence of structural reforms in place 18 months after Healthway's inception in organisations that did not have a reform in place before Healthway started (see Figure 29.3).

The creation of smoke-free areas represented the greatest gain in structural reform. Of organisations that had no such policy before Healthway's inception, 65.9 per cent reported having a policy 18 months later. Substantial gains were made also in the other areas. More than one-quarter of organisations that had no previous policies relating to safe alcohol practice (26.7 per cent), healthy food choices (28.8 per cent), or access for disadvantaged groups (27.2 per cent), claimed to have these reforms in place 18 months later.

The degree of institutionalisation of pre-existing reforms in sporting and cultural venues is also demonstrated in Figure 29.3. As may be seen, the vast majority of organisations that had structural reforms in place before Healthway's inception persisted with the healthy policies 18 months later.

The influence of sponsorship level on the prevalence of structural reform

Regardless of the average amount of annual sponsorship received, significant increases were observed in the prevalence of smoke-free areas and healthy food choice reforms. In organisations receiving A\$50,000 or

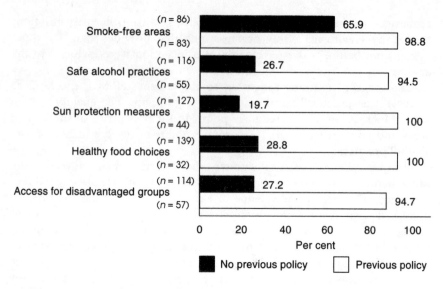

Figure 29.3   *Prevalence of structural reforms 18 months after Healthway's inception: those that had no policy before Healthway versus those that did (excluding those reporting a policy 18 months later that was not applicable)*

more, the percentage point increase in smoke-free area policies was 1.31 times higher than in organisations receiving A\$5000 or less (i.e. 35.7 versus 27.3 per cent), while in the area of healthy food choices the ratio was 2.13 (28.5 versus 13.4 per cent).

In other areas of structural reform, no clear pattern emerged based on the level of sponsorship received. Even organisations receiving A\$5000 or less reported significant increases in the prevalence of four out of the five reform areas.

Potential reach of structural reforms in organisations requested to implement changes

The potential reach of the structural reforms in organisations requested to implement changes (n = 136) was examined by calculating potential member reform-exposures (PMREs). The number of PMREs per organisation was calculated by multiplying the number of reforms by the number of members of the organisation. On average, each organisation had 2.67 structural reforms in place 18 months after Healthway's inception, generating an average of 4584 PMREs.

Regardless of the amount of sponsorship received from Healthway, there was very little difference in the average number of reforms reported. However, as might be expected, there was a considerable difference in the potential reach of these reforms amongst members.

Recipients of small sponsorship (⩽A\$5000), on average, had the potential to generate 2499 PMREs. This was 1.30 times more PMREs than in organisations receiving A$5001–15,000 (1927 PMREs). At the higher levels of sponsorship, the number of PMREs increased to an average of 28,828 for organisations receiving more than A$100,000 per annum. . .

Support for Healthway-initiated structural reform

It was a common view amongst organisations requested to implement reforms ($n = 136$), that all or most key people in the organisation (for example, board members, players, actors) (83.1 per cent) and their spectators or audiences (73.5 per cent) supported Healthway initiated structural reforms . . . Nevertheless, while 45.6 per cent of organisations claimed that *all* of the key people in their organisation supported the changes, only half as many organisations perceived that *all* of their spectators or audience were supportive (22.3 per cent).

Discussion

Structural reform achievement

Although not all of the structural reform observed in this study can be attributed to Healthway, it has, nevertheless, been successful in using sponsorship to create healthier sporting and cultural venues. It has also achieved widespread support for its reform programme. While educational and promotional opportunities are an important component of the negotiated sponsor benefit package, tying the offer of sponsorship to a requirement to implement structural reform has the potential for longer term impact if the reforms become institutionalised.

Considerable structural reform was achieved in all priority areas, but especially the creation of smoke-free areas. While arts organisations appear to be more receptive to reforms, the results also show that it is possible to make considerable progress towards healthier environments in racing and sporting organisations and venues. This is important because promoting health at sport and racing events provides opportunities to contact hard-to-impact audiences, such as blue-collar males (Egger *et al.*, 1993), and to associate health with positive role models and activities (Donovan *et al.*, 1993). A community survey conducted in 1992, found that sporting group members and spectators had above average levels of smoking, low fruit and vegetable consumption, unsafe drinking and physical inactivity spectators only) (Holman *et al.*, 1993b).

Although one might imagine that Healthway has more leverage to encourage recipients of larger sponsorships to implement more reforms, there was very little practical difference in the average number of reforms per organisation amongst groups receiving different levels of funding. This may suggest that Healthway has not capitalised sufficiently on its larger sponsorships, but there are alternative explanations. Larger sponsorships provide greater overall population reach (see below), increased prospects for institutionalisation of reform, and the mix of sponsorship benefits may be designed to take advantage of promotional opportunities associated with large spectator attendances and media coverage.

In addition, Healthway's staff and support sponsors have taken a 'small wins' approach to introducing healthy public policy. Weick (1984, p.43) defines a small win as a 'concrete, complete, implemented outcome of moderate importance'. One small win may seem unimportant, but a series of small wins 'reveals a pattern that may attract allies, deter opponents, and lower resistance to subsequent proposals'. While committed to the creation of supportive environments. Healthway has remained cognisant of real, and potential, opposition to reform amongst its stakeholders. Rather than requiring radical immediate change, or the introduction of multiple reforms at the outset of a sponsorship project, it has moved groups along a continuum. No matter how large or small the sponsorship, or whether it be for a one-off event or a series of events, Healthway's strategy has been to introduce at least one type of reform at the outset and to work towards further reform as a project continues and/or is re-negotiated.

Potential reach of structural reforms

Promoting health through sporting and cultural events and venues has the potential to reach large numbers of people. Some 40 per cent of Western Australians claim to be members of one or more sport, racing or outdoor recreation club, while 1 per cent are members of an arts organisation (Holman *et al.*, 1993b, 1993c).

On average, each Healthway-sponsored organisation had the potential to generate 4584 PMREs, and for every A$10,000 of sponsorship funds expended, 3289 PMRE were generated. Although recipients of larger sponsorships produced many more per organisation, when PMREs were quantified per A$10,000, smaller sponsorship recipients generated 4.44 times as many exposures.

While smaller organisations may represent good value for money in terms of exposure of members, omitted in the estimations of reform-exposures in this chapter is the potential reach among the event's spectators and audiences. Organisations receiving higher levels of sponsorship are more likely to be high-profile organisations and thus more likely to attract larger audiences. In addition, larger sponsored projects are more likely to attract media attention, providing promotional opportunities through television and print media coverage.

Healthway's contribution to reform

Not all of the structured reforms observed in this survey can be directly attributed to Healthway. Many Western Australian health agencies are active advocates of structural reforms related to tobacco control, nutrition and sun protection measures. However, with the exception of limited use by the Health Department of Western Australia prior to Healthway's establishment, no other health organisation used sponsorship as a means of achieving health promotive reforms in recreational and cultural venues. Nor had any other organisation promoted healthy public policy by tying the provision of funding directly to a reformist agenda.

While a sizeable proportion of the organisations surveyed had introduced structural reform prior to their association with Healthway, a substantial contribution was made by Healthway to the rate of policy development amongst 'structural reform laggards'. This is likely to have occurred through direct requests for reform, but also through indirect influence. As Healthway's objectives have become clear to potential recipients of sponsorship, it is possible that they have implemented structural reforms prior to submission of their sponsorship application in an attempt to strengthen their proposal's chance of success. . .

Policy and practice implications

There have been lessons gained from implementing the funding policy described in this chapter, and achieving community support for the introduction of structural reform. Key success factors have included a 'small wins' philosophy of change, developing co-operative working relationships with diverse organisations whose objectives are not related to health; developing an understanding and appreciation of the goals of sponsored organisations; winning over the trust and support of key individuals in the organisations; developing sound policy formation guidelines; working with individuals involved with the organisation and its events at grass roots level (for example, caterers, coaches, front-of-house staff); learning how to promote health appropriately in different settings; and balancing a myriad of conflicting interests. Healthway has used pressure where appropriate, but has also made compromises, and remained committed to a participative model of social reform.

These results suggest that small sponsorship projects represent good value for money in terms of their potential member reform-exposure reach per A$10,000 expended and thus, an investment of A$100,000 in a series of A$5000 sponsorships may yield more than 4-fold the number of structural outputs than one large sponsorship to a single organisation. While having important implications for sponsorship policy, this observation must be interpreted cautiously due to possible qualitative differences in the reforms that are purchased, quantitative differences in reach to spectators and audiences, and the extent to which reforms are enforced . . .

Although these results have been achieved by a system of health grants and sponsorships operating within the context of a relatively affluent developed country, we believe there is no reason to constrain the application of the basic principles outlined in this chapter within certain international borders or systems of health administration. Overseas aid organisations and many community based granting schemes operate in developing countries, and opportunities exist to use these resource flows as a catalyst to facilitate healthy public policy development at the local provincial and state level.

Conclusion

The results indicate that it is possible to work intersectorally to achieve structural reform in sport, racing and arts organisations. Actively encouraging intersectoral co-operation by tying the provision of sponsorship with a requirement to introduce reform is an example of healthy public policy that will create healthier environments. Maximising the institutionalisation of reforms once sponsorship is removed, however, is likely to be achieved only if sponsored groups and the general public support the changes that are taking place. Working in genuine partnership with sponsored organisations, promoting positive community views of the intentions behind the creation of healthy environments, and communicating the results of supportive consumer research is therefore essential.

References

Corti, B., Holman, C. D. J. and Donovan, R. J. (1993). *Survey of the Impact of Healthway on Organisations it Funds 1992*. Health Promotion Development and Evaluation Program. Perth: University of Western Australia.

Donovan, R. J., Corti, B., Holman, C. J. D., West, D. and Petter, D. (1993). Evaluating sponsorship effectiveness, *Health Promotion Journal of Australia*, 3, 63-67.

Egger, G., Donovan, R. J. and Spark, R. (1993). *Health and the Media: Principles and practices for health promotion*. Sydney: McGraw-Hill.

Holman, C. J. D., Donovan, R. J. and Corti, B. (1993a). Evaluating projects funded by the Western Australian Health Promotion Foundation: a systematic approach, *Health Promotion Journal*, 8, 199–208.

Holman, C. D. J., Donovan, R. J. and Corti, B. (1993b). *Survey on Recreation and Health 1992. Volume 1: Participation in Sports and Racing*. Health Promotion Development and Evaluation Program. Department of Public Health and Department of Management. Perth: The University of Western Australia.

Holman. C. D. J., Donovan, R. J. and Corti, B. (1993c). *Survey on Recreation and Health 1992, Volume 2: Participation in the Arts*. Health Promotion Development and Evaluation Program. Department of Public Health and Department of Management. Perth: University of Western Australia.

Weick, K. L. (1984). Small wins: revising the scale of social problems, *American Psychologist*, 39, 40–49.
Western Australian Health Promotion Foundation (1992). *Annual Report 1991–1992*.

30 *An 'insider' looking out: the politics of physical activity in England**

Adrian Davis

Introduction

This chapter examines the debate about 'physical activity' and 'sport' and assesses the progress made in developing a realistic and robust physical activity strategy for England since 1992. The benefits of physical activity in terms of reduced risk of cardiovascular disease and strokes have been documented through studies since the hypothesis was first developed (Morris *et al.*, 1953) and they were identified in the *Health of the Nation* strategy for England (1992).[1] Physical activity was also seen as contributing to reduced accidents and mental health, two of the other four national 'key areas'. The strategy acknowledged the value of targets at a population level in stimulating progress and providing a measure by which it could be assessed.

It also identified that intersectoral working or 'healthy alliances' at all levels were an important element in the reorientation of health policy towards prevention and health promotion.

The role of research in the debate

Shortly before the launch of the *Health of the Nation* the first comprehensive picture of adult fitness levels was published. This reported low levels of physical activity among the majority of men and women aged 16–74. A key finding was that seven out of ten men and eight out of ten women fell below their age-appropriate activity level necessary to achieve a health benefit. Published by the Sports Council and the Health Education Authority (HEA), the Allied Dunbar National Fitness Survey (ADNFS) gave substance to the view that the British adult population is increasingly sedentary, although 80 per cent of those surveyed believed that they were fit and took sufficient exercise (Allied Dunbar National

* Commissioned for this volume.

Fitness Survey (ADNFS), 1992). Reasons given for low levels of activity focused particularly on people not seeing themselves as 'sporty', as well as feeling overweight and embarrassed. The report stimulated further research into barriers to physical activity but also importantly provided a focus for action to address declining levels of activity given the *Health of the Nation* coronary heart disease targets and fears about future burdens to the National Health Service. In this respect the ADNFS provided a benchmark by which efforts to improve physical activity levels among adults could be gauged.

In March 1992 the British Medical Association's (BMA) launched a report promoting cycling which signalled a complete U-turn in policy from a view of seeing cycling as 'dangerous'. Drawing on earlier research the report concluded that:

> even in the current hostile traffic environment, the benefits gained from regular cycling are likely to outweigh the loss of life through cycle accidents for the current population of regular cyclists. (BMA, 1992)

An organised national cycling lobby ensured that the report received maximum publicity. Within six months a leaflet, funded by the BMA, the bicycle industry, and the main cycle campaign body, had been sent to all doctors' surgeries setting out the findings and encouraging the uptake of cycling as an environmentally-friendly means of transport and as part of a healthy lifestyle. In doing this the BMA report was calling for healthy public policies in order that the healthy choice, in this case, cycling, could be an easy choice. As Whitehead noted:

> . . . as well as motivating people to take up cycling there have to be parallel public policies in place making it safer and more pleasant to do so... people cannot be expected to maintain an initial interest in activities such as cycling if conditions on the road do not improve (Whitehead, 1992).

'Physical activity' or 'sport'?

Approaches to fitness and physical activity have been dominated by a sports and leisure led approach. Historically close links between the sports and physical activity lobbies through Universities and research bodies had resulted in a heavy bias and strong lobby which, to a large extent, dominated physical activity research, debate, and policy formulation. This is reflected by a considerable volume of research on physical activity being published within journals associated with sport. This association of sport as physical activity had been particularly promoted through schools. The ADNFS had reported the association of physical activity with 'sporty' images in public perceptions. Further work by the HEA using in-depth discussion groups which sought to compliment the ADNFS identified that 'physical activity' operated as a generic term for sport, exercise and leisure pursuits (HEA, 1993). Images of sport and exercise were associated with youthful men and women with 'rippling muscles', with sport being perceived as particularly male oriented.

An outcome has been that public perceptions are biased towards an understanding that physical activity is largely something that time has to be made available for, something many people claim they cannot find. Together with special clothing, and activity centres that need accessing, this has meant that 'physical activity' has been seen as largely the domain of young, slim and athletic men and women, not attainable by the majority of the adult population as part of their lifestyles. Moreover, research has identified that a significant section of the adult population feel themselves fit enough for the lifestyles they lead, having adapted lifestyles to accommodate low fitness thresholds. This results in a view that: 'I'd say I was fit – well, fit enough to do what I need to do.' This section of the population, 29 per cent of men and 28 per cent of women aged 16–74, lead largely sedentary lifestyles. For them physical activity of all kinds was often viewed as difficult, unpleasant and a little pointless (Killoran *et al.*, 1994).

The perception of physical activity as 'sporty' and an activity beyond the routines of daily life for the majority of the population has resulted in the 'ghettoisation' of physical activity within the sport and physical education sector, with little intersectoral working beyond traditional boundaries. As with all 'sectors' they define boundaries that separate them from the other 'sectors' so framing what is to be excluded, marked out by specialised discourses of knowledge and expertise in seeking their legitimisation and maintenance. Such 'sectoring' is 'oriented towards protecting, if not advancing, the differentiation of one sector from another' (Degeling, 1995). This had resulted in the sports and physical education sectors' reluctance to become involved in wider public policy changes. Operating within a predominantly biomedical disease and lifestyles based approach to health led to a failure to set behavioural change programmes within broader policies for environmental modification (Davis and Jones, 1996). Suggestions for policy changes which would facilitate cycling as part of everyday life, as proposed by the BMA, for example, are infrequent in physical activity research.

This bias linking physical activity with sport and exercise is also evident within health education (Edmunds and Bowler, 1995; Trippe, 1996). Much emphasis, for example, has been placed on GP referrals to exercise schemes managed by staff based in leisure centres. Yet while researchers suggest that physical activity programmes can increase participation sufficiently to achieve long term health gain their research findings 'do not support the increasingly popular *prescription for exercise* schemes . . . we have found no evidence to support the efficacy of facility based inter- ventions'. In contrast, the researchers suggest that physical activity at sufficient frequency and intensity to provide long term health gain 'is best achieved when exercise is home-based, of moderate intensity, can be performed alone or with others, is enjoyable, convenient, and can be completed in three sessions per week. Walking will satisfy all of these criteria.' (Hillsdon, *et al.*, 1995)

Intersectoral collaboration at the national level

The goal of reducing coronary heart disease and promoting physical activity has been progressed by the Department of Health through the establishment of a number of key groupings. A Health of the Nation Cabinet Sub-Committee was established at which all government departments were represented to help enable intersectoral working. In addition a Physical Activity Task Force was established in July 1993. The terms of reference were:

> to develop specific physical activity targets, in the light of available resources: arrange consultation on target and report back to the Chief Medical Officer's Health Priorities Working Group; then develop detailed strategies for the achievement of agreed targets, consider gaps in current knowledge and the means of filling them, reporting back progress to Ministers within one year; and again after developing proposals and recommendations for taking the work forward and for monitoring progress in achieving the specific targets. (Department of Health, 1995)

There were concerns over a sports and exercise bias with the appointment of the Task Force members. The concerns came from those lobby groups who had consistently argued that traditional and narrow sectoral policies were not effective. These were principally the cycling lobby, pedestrian groups, public policy researchers and some public health interest groups. Three of the Task Force members were medically trained (albeit one was a public health director), another three were health education specialists, two were leisure and recreation officers from local government and two were Sports Council executives, one of whom was Chairman. A further grouping of health and sports advisers were available to provide additional assistance as well as officials from Government departments.

The rejection of targets

During the first year of the Task Force's work a considerable amount of time was spent on developing physical activity targets. At a HEA symposium in April 1994, designed to support the Task Force in developing a national strategy, a specific objective was to examine possible targets for physical activity. Three targets at a population level were presented, having been proposed by the Task Force. Based on the latest medical evidence, and the ADNFS, these were focused on reducing the proportion of people who are sedentary, increasing the proportion taking a minimum of 30 minutes of at least moderate physical activity five days a week, and increasing the proportion taking on average three periods of vigorous activity for 20 minutes a week (Fentem and Walker, 1994).

Later that year the Cabinet Sub-Committee rejected a targets oriented approach, perceiving that they might be misconstrued as individual targets, and was concerned to avoid claims of 'nanny-state' inter-ventionism. Targets had previously been set by two other Task Forces, on nutrition, and obesity. More so than these, however, it was recognised by Ministers and officials that physical activity could impact on policies across a wide spectrum of public policies with the potential of raising political and technical impediments. Members of the Task Force were also concerned that targets might be used crudely. The Department of Health's consultation document, which appeared in May 1995, reflected this view, so that 'on balance it has been decided not to set targets for physical activity, but to concentrate instead on promoting the uptake of a more active lifestyle' (Department of Health, 1995).

The consultation paper set out the medical evidence indicating that the greatest health gains would come from shifting the emphasis from regular vigorous to moderate physical activity. This would be a more realistic feat for those currently sedentary and those having low activity levels. Nearly 30 per cent of men and women are sedentary and only 36 per cent of men and 24 per cent of women are sufficiently physically active to achieve health benefits. Essentially, despite omission of 'targets' from the consultation paper the three identified target areas were retained as core goals for the development of a physical activity strategy.

National policy shifts

During the drafting of the consultation paper a range of government departments including Transport, Environment, and Heritage were involved as well as health, sport, leisure, lifestyles, and environmental and transport lobbies reflecting their representation on the Health of the Nation Cabinet Sub-Committee. Pressures to reflect wider public policy changes were important in shaping the paper. The combination of the latest medical evidence with evidence of adult fitness levels gleaned from the ADNFS reinforced the need for a broader policy focus in halting the decline in physical activity and beginning to increase physical activity and fitness. The public health case for focusing on moderate physical activity which could reach a far wider section of the population could only be achieved through a move away from the sport and physical education predominance.

By 1994 policy changes in both the Environment and Transport departments within central government had begun to focus their attention towards the need for more sustainable transport through land use in reducing the need to travel and consequently carbon dioxide emissions (Department of the Environment/Department of Transport, 1994). In the Department of Transport itself, a recognition of the need to shift from seeking to meet 'demand' for road space to 'demand management' led to an increasingly hasty retreat with from a position of opposition to the promotion of cycling. Indeed the BMA report had added extra ammunition for carrying through this change and in June 1995 the Department of Transport announced its intention to develop a national cycling strategy (Department of Transport, 1995).

The influence of lobbying and campaigning

The pressure for a shift in influence away from the sport and physical education sector was strengthened through long term lobbying in the environment policy sphere where environmental campaigners had been arguing the case that environmental as opposed to purely behavioural changes were required in order to reduce environmental impacts. Such concerns were endorsed by the widely publicised Royal Commission on Environmental Pollution's report on *Transport and the Environment* (1994). In this sphere there was a growing recognition of the need for healthy public policies which could enable healthy and environmentally sustainable choices to be made, accelerated by the Bruntland Report *Our Common Future* (1987) and the Earth Summit in Rio de Janeiro (1992) and the Government's response to these *Sustainable Development: The UK Strategy* (1994). The overlapping policy areas of environment and public health increasingly highlighted the need for intersectoral action and public policy responses in tackling both issues (Draper, 1990). The changes in transport policy especially enabled a broader policy focus on physical activity, strengthening the case of those seeking action beyond the traditional sectoral focus for physical activity promotion.

The National Heart Forum, an influential co-ordinating body for an alliance of heart health organisations, played a key role in the physical activity debate. Represented on the Task Force, the Forum took a broad public health view of the need for healthy public policies and to develop a strong intersectoral focus in the development of the physical activity strategy. Its close links with environment and transport groups informed and strengthened their own lobbying of the Task Force. The Forum provided support for the position agreed at the 1994 HEA Symposium and reiterated in the consultation paper that 'successful promotion of physical activity in England amounts to encouraging the reintegration of physical activity into every day life' (p. 3). A copy of the Forum's response was sent to all public health and health departments mid-way through the consultation period to help inform and   influence other responses.

The consultation paper was strikingly similar in emphasis to the statement on the health benefits of exercise developed by a joint committee of WHO and the International Federation of Sports Medicine (FIMS) in 1994 (*Exercise for Health*, 1995). In this daily activity was accepted as being the cornerstone of a healthy lifestyle:

> Physical activity should be reintegrated into the routine of everyday living. An obvious first step would be the use of stairs instead of lifts, and walking and cycling for short journeys. (WHO, 1995)

The statement could be viewed as a logical development of WHO's policy statement given its emphasis in the past decade or so on the need for intersectoral collaboration and healthy public policies. Less expected perhaps was that in its drafting the statement met little resistance from the FIMS members who had come to view physical activity within everyday life as readily compatible with additional exercise for those people seeking additional physical activity. The WHO/FIMS statement highlighted the importance of action across all levels of government, local and central, the need for strong social policies, (re)education of professionals to promote physical activity, and measures to ameliorate the effects of social inequalities on physical activity participation rates. The timing of this statement and the signatories to it which included some of the most prominent public health researchers in this area, added further weight to efforts to promote physical activity through public policies which enable physically active lifestyles.

The publication of the strategy

In March 1996 the Department of Health issued a 'Strategy Statement on Physical Activity' confirming support for the consultation paper's positioning which had found support from the majority of the 200+ submissions from consultees. Much of the Statement focused on the work of other government departments such as Environment, Education and Employment, Heritage, and Transport and external agencies such as the

HEA's 'Active for Life' campaign, launched the same day. The HEA was also given responsibility for taking forward the work of the Task Force, which was concluded, although against the wishes of some members. On the one hand this could be seen as health ministers seeking to extricate themselves from responsibility, while on the other it could be viewed as implementing the Health of the Nation shift of focus towards health promotion.

Although the Statement did not constitute a 'comprehensive physical activity strategy for England' as proposed in the consultation paper the resolution that physical activity should be reintegrated into every day life indicated a recognition of the failure of narrow sectoral policies to promote physical activity and health. Sport, by its very nature tends to involve vigorous activity, recognised to be 'an unrealistic goal for the majority of the population'. Realistically, addressing wider public policy issues was the only way in which declining levels of physical activity could be challenged. In itself this information was not enough, however.

Conclusion

Pressure for policy change came from an alignment of health, environment and physical activity lobby groups who had consistently argued that traditional and narrow sectoral policies were not effective. This was combined with public concerns about the impact of transport on the environment and health. The changing policy direction within both the transport and environment sectors were important leverages. The Department of the Environment's publication of a Sustainable Development Strategy, a parallel to *The Health of the Nation*, combined with specific targets to reduce carbon dioxide emissions through landuse and measures to tackle air pollution, combined with those from the Department of Transport to send a clear signal that policy focus was shifting upstream towards environmental modifications. The recognition by both of these sectors at government level indicated that behavioural change programmes, although ideologically preferable, was not sufficient to contain health damaging lifestyles.

Such factors were endorsed by moves within public health, including the important policy shift made by the BMA in 1992 and evidence of the growth of sedentary lifestyles. The physical activity debate was, therefore, dominated by factors suggesting an unambiguous need for a broader focus on physical activity. This was sufficient to overshadow the in-built bias of the Task Force membership and any reluctance on the part of the sports and physical education sector to relinquish control of the physical activity agenda.

Note

1. While the Health of the Nation only focuses on England similar strategies are being developed elsewhere in the UK in which physical activity is recognised as an important area of health promotion.

References

Allied Dunbar National Fitness Survey (ADNFS): A report on activity patterns and fitness levels. Main findings and summary report (1992). London: Sports Council/Health Education Authority.

British Medical Association (1992). *Cycling: Towards health and safety*. Oxford: Oxford University Press.

Brundtland Report (1987). *Our Common Future: The World Commission on Environment and Development*. Oxford: Oxford University Press.

Davis, A. and Jones, L. (1996). Children in the urban environment: an issue for the new public health agenda, *Health and Place*, 2 (2), 107–113.

Degeling, P., (1995). The significance of 'sectors' in calls for urban public health intersectoralism: an Australian perspective, *Policy and Politics*, 23 (4), 289–301.

Department of Health (1992). *The Health of the Nation: A strategy for health in England*, London: HMSO.

Department of Health (1995). *More People More Active More Often: Physical Activity in England – a Consultation Paper*, London: Department of Health.

Department of Health, (1996). *Strategy Statement on Physical Activity*. London: Department of Health.

Department of Environment/Department of Transport, (1994). *Planning Policy Guidance Note 13: Transport*, London: Department of Environment/Department of Transport.

Department of Transport, (1995). *Norris Says 'Saddle-Up' for New Cycling Century*, Press Release 172 (7 June).

Draper, P. (ed), (1990). *Health Through Public Policy: the greening of public health*. London: Greenprint.

Earth Summit (1992): *The United Nations Conference on Environment and Development, 1992*. London: The Regency Press.

Edmunds, L. and Bowler, I., (1995). *Partners in action*, Health Service Journal (9 February), 27.

Fentem, P. and Walker, A. (1994). Setting targets for England: challenging, measurable and achievable. In *Moving On: International perspectives on promoting physical activity*. London: Health Education Authority.

Health Education Authority, (1993). *Physical activity strategy research* (unpublished).

Hillsdon, M., Thorogood, M., Anstiss, T. and Morris, J., (1995). Randomised controlled trials of physical activity promotion in free living populations: a review, *Journal of Epidemiology and Community Health*, 49, 448–453.

Killoran, A., Cavill, N., and Walker, A. (1994). Who needs to know what? An investigation of the key target groups for the effective promotion of physical activity in England. In *Moving On: International perspectives on promoting physical activity*, London: Health Education Authority.

Morris, J. N., Heady, J. A., Raffle, P. A. B., Roberts, C. G. and Parks, J. W., (1953). *Coronary Heart Disease and physical activity at work*, Lancet, 265, 1111–20.

Royal Commission on Environmental Pollution, (1994). *Eighteenth Report: Transport and the Environment*, London: HMSO.

Sports Council/HEA (1992). *Sustainable Development: The UK strategy* (1994). London: HMSO.

Trippe, H. (1996). Children and sport: Encouraging a healthy attitude to exercise should start in primary school, *British Medical Journal*, 312 (27 January), 199–200.

Whitehead, M., (1992). Editorial, 'Living Dangerously', *Health Education Journal*, *51* (*4*), 156.

World Health Organisation/International Federation of Sports Medicine (FIMS) Committee on Physical Activity for Health, (1995). Exercise for health, *Bulletin of the World Health Organisation*, *73* (*2*), 135–136.

Looking beyond 2000: dilemmas in health promotion

In this section we look beyond the promise of Health for All by the year 2000 to consider an agenda for the 21st century. What are the issues that will grow in importance and how best can we move forward with some confidence without losing sight of key debates and dilemmas? Section Four begins with three contributions relating to the growing focus on risk in health promotion.

The extent to which government should use legislation to limit 'lifestyle' risks is the dilemma addressed by the first article in this section. Dan Beauchamp in Chapter 32, arguing against the anti-paternalism that tends to characterise western democracies, makes out a case for a limited public health paternalism consisting mainly of controls on the market. Striking a balance between individual liberty and the good of the community is a delicate issue and in declaring 'two cheers for paternalism' Beauchamp carefully sketches out one way forward using alcohol as the main example.

Thinking through the implications of advances in diagnostic testing is the task Regina Kenen sets herself in the Chapter 33, 'The At-risk Health Status and Technology'. Challenging the assumption that knowledge is always a good thing, Kenen calls for a greater awareness of the negative as well as positive effects of the 'at-risk' health status. The creation of guidelines and standards to regulate genetic testing is, she argues, an urgent need. Developing the theme of surveillance and risk at a more abstract level, Sarah Nettleton in Chapter 34 explores the intimate relations between surveillance techniques and risk-talk. In the process she presents a challenging critique of the ideological role of health promotion.

Turning to a different area of technological development John Catford in Chapter 35 discerns new possibilities in the ever-expanding world of the mass media. He urges health promoters to position themselves in the middle of the media revolution in order to empower and support consumers.

The persistence of major inequalities forms the theme of Chapters 36 and 37 by Lesley Doyal and Peter Townsend. Pointing to the 'gender blindness' of decision makers and medical researchers Doyal teases out various levels at which men continue to be regarded as the norm and women as the 'other' (for instance, many epidemiological studies relating to coronary heart disease are based on all-male samples). The solution, she concludes, is radical but in one sense quite simple: if women are to optimise their well-being, men will have to share resources and labours more equally. Whether enough are willing to do so remains an open question.

Tackling an even larger canvas, Peter Townsend illustrates and analyses growing inequalities between rich and poor at both global and national levels. Acknowledging that the agenda for the achievement of social justice is dauntingly large, he proposes a set of structural remedies. These include democratisation of international agencies, a minimum wage, modernised social insurance and basic income for child and disability support. To both Townsend and Doyal the way forward is clear: continuing debates and dilemmas reflect a basic lack of commitment to justice.

But where does all this leave visions of Healthy Cities and the project of health promotion in the 21st century? Perhaps the imagination has to be re-awakened if the uncomfortable call for greater social justice is to stand a chance of being heard. The final two chapters briefly look back over the achievements of the health promotion movement as provider of new paradigms for a healthier future before launching into ways of carrying the vision of Health for All beyond 2000.

Arguing that the concept of Healthy Cities and its underlying philosophical principle of Health for All are simply incomprehensible with conventional discipline-led models of scientific research and rational administration, Kelly, Davies and Charlton in Chapter 38 advocate a mood of post-modern celebration. Perhaps the future lies in a confident 'yes' to the open-ended, chaotic and non-rational character of the post-modern world? Those existing at the very bottom of the pile may feel less inclined to celebrate but for believers in the transforming possibilities of the Healthy Cities movement Kelly *et al.* deliver a longed-for word of hope.

The closing chapter by Lowell Levin and Erio Ziglio (Chapter 39) has a more sober but equally optimistic flavour. Combining in some measure the perspectives of the previous two chapters, Levin and Ziglio present 21st century health promotion as an investment strategy that will bring about social, economic, ecological and health returns. Turning upside down the notion that expenditure on health means less money for economic development, the argument here is that economic and social development is dependent upon investment in health. The WHO commitment to a vision of equity, empowerment, sustainability and accountability remains buoyant and new images have surfaced to keep the ship afloat.

31 Lifestyle, public health and paternalism*

Dan Beauchamp

. . . In recent decades it has become a truism that a significant portion (perhaps as much as half) of the disease and early death in industrialised societies stems from personal risk-taking. Dealing with these risks – commonly called lifestyle risks – creates substantial political difficulties in democratic societies.

Questions of what to do about cigarette smoking, alcohol use, or driving without seat-belts arouse great political debate. Policy restrictions for lifestyle choices have in Western democracies been influenced by a strong antipaternalism.

Antipaternalism flourishes in many conditions, but its native soil is political individualism. Political individualism assumes that the political community is an association of self-determining individuals who view the 'purpose of government as confined to enabling individuals' wants to be satisfied, individuals' interests to be pursued and individuals' rights to be protected, with a clear bias toward *laissez-faire* and against the idea that [the government] might legitimately influence or alter their wants, interpret their interests for them or invade or abrogate their rights' . . . (Lukes, 1973)

Moving away from antipaternalism to a democracy that includes some forms of paternalism, especially for public health, does not imply political collectivism or the view that government seeks only to improve the welfare of the community and that the citizenry have only loyalties to the larger interests of society. Democracy that includes some legitimate forms of paternalism is based on the view that government must reconcile two main ends: the rights and interests of the individual taken separately and the good of individuals together – the community – even for lifestyle risks . . .

The case of alcohol problems

What has been the experience of the Western democracies with alcohol problems in the post-war period? With the exception of France, the

* From S. Doxiadis (ed) (1987). *Ethical Dilemmas in Health Promotion*. London: John Wiley, pp. 69–8
© John Wiley & Sons Ltd.

general experience has been that alcohol consumption in the aggregate has increased greatly, reflecting the fundamental increase in economic productivity and personal consumption that occurred in the decades from 1950s to the 1970s (Markela *et al.*, 1981). Alcohol became, during this period, a commodity much like others. Community sanctions over alcohol commerce were gradually but dramatically weakened in many places. Alcohol products like beer became available in general retail outlet chains, which themselves greatly expanded. Regional and local restrictions were relaxed or totally eliminated. The hours of sale expanded. Age limits were often reduced. Drinking patterns became increasingly homogeneous across national and regional boundaries. Advertising and other forms of promotion dramatically increased.

Given these developments, it should come as no surprise that drinking increased – as did alcohol problems. What is surprising is that while alcohol consumption and consequent problems increased, until very recently governments did not strengthen their alcohol control efforts . . .

Just as alcohol problems and drinking were on the rise in Western societies, many governments were abandoning their commitments to alcohol control. The major exception to this pattern has been drunk driving (Markela *et al.*, 1981).

One of forces countering this trend has been the growing influence of public health agencies and public health interests in society. The new public health, and the 'second epidemiological revolution' (Terris, 1985) that undergirds it, call attention not only to the risks of the motor car, the motor cycle, the dangers of the Western diet high in saturated fats, to cigarette smoking, or to alcohol, but also to how commercial practices exacerbate these risks.

The growth of a new alcohol epidemiology stressed the relation of alcohol availability, in price, advertising, and age limits in the genesis of alcohol problems. Several broad principles underlie this new alcohol epidemiology. Increases in total alcohol consumption are likely to mean increases in the number of heavy consumers; heavy consumption and damage to health are highly correlated; therefore, preventive programmes must seek to limit increase in general consumption (Schmidt and Popham, 1980).

The importance of these findings is that they bring into view damages to the community as a whole that arise from changes in the organisation of alcohol commerce – production, availability, price, advertising or promotion of alcoholic beverages. Tax policy is a good example. Cook has reviewed the evidence that tax policy is crucial to preventing alcohol related problems like cirrhosis and even drunk driving, and has statistically verified these relationships for the period 1960–75 in the United States (Cook, 1981) . . .

Tax policy is important not only because of the connection between the price of alcohol, drinking, heavy consumption, and other problems but because tax, along with the number of outlets, the hours of sale, who may sell alcoholic beverages, age restrictions, advertising, and the like are part of the structure of alcohol commerce, and commerce is social in nature, a matter of the common life. But tax policy only partly explains shifts in alcohol consumption. Actually, beer sales increased sharply during the 1970s, while sales of distilled beverages levelled off. The reason for this is that beer is taxed very lightly compared to distilled beverages, and beer is also nationally advertised on American television.

There is little doubt that tax policy and other relaxations on alcohol commerce influence the level of aggregate consumption of alcoholic beverages, including many alcohol-related problems (Cook, 1981). Even J. S. Mill admitted that the market was social:

> [T]rade is a social act. Whoever undertakes to sell any description of goods to the public, does what affects the interests of other persons, and of society in general.

Mill admitted that those who sell alcoholic beverages have an interest in intemperance and therefore restrictions on availability may be justified:

> The interest, however, of these dealers in promoting intemperance is a real evil, and justifies the State in imposing restrictions and requiring guarantees which but for that justification would be infringements of real liberty.

Yet he goes on to rule out taxes for discouraging intemperance as restrictions aimed at the drinker and not at the seller.

But price is little different from restricting the numbers of public houses or supermarkets in a district; both affect availability, the one economic, the other social. And it is this organisation of alcohol commerce that is central to any scheme of balancing the community's interest in temperance with the individual's interest in spending his money how he chooses.

Mill argued that only the individual can know his own particular good:

> He is the person most interested in his own wellbeing: the interest which any other person, except in cases of strong personal attachment, can have in it, is trifling.

But this is precisely the wrong point. Public health paternalism in regulating alcohol commerce seeks to protect the common good, not the good of any particular person. As Richard Flathman (1966) notes, modern governments rarely can be paternalistic in the strict sense of promoting the good of particular persons. The liberalisation of availability of alcoholic beverages affects the broad drinking public. Historically, government has sought to regulate trade when it affects an important community interest.

Two cheers for paternalism

Public health paternalism provides some surprising dividends beyond regulating alcohol commerce and improving the public's health. Strengthening the public health is not only a matter of improving aggregate welfare, it is also encouraging the citizen to share in a group scheme to promote a wider welfare, of which his own welfare is only a part. Seat-belt legislation or signs on the beach restricting swimming when a lifeguard is not present, restrict my liberty for my own good, but only as I am a member of the public and for the general or the common good. From the private viewpoint, the motto for such paternalistic legislation employing the group principle might be, 'The lives we save together might include my own'.

Thus, public health paternalism encourages concern for the wider good, for co-operation, and group solidarity in solving problems. These are community virtues which are needed alongside of the individual virtues of self-reliance and autonomy. National pension schemes may be narrowly paternalistic, but more importantly they encourage group co-operation for the good of everyone alike, stimulating group solidarity. While policies to raise the price of alcohol may seem considerably less concerned with group solidarity than government pension schemes, we should not ignore the possibility that paternalism in lifestyle areas also advances group values and group approaches to solving problems.

This is speculation, but public health paternalism may also help stimulate individual responsibility, at least up to a point. There is often the view that coercion and individual responsibility operate in a zero-sum manner – seat-belt legislation may cause individuals to take less heed for their own safety on the highway. But it may work the other way around. Fluoridation programmes may help stimulate personal dental hygiene, and government pension schemes may establish a secure minimum around which individuals take voluntary actions to purchase annuities. Similarly, and within limits, community restrictions on drinking and smoking may provide a climate that encourages more individual responsibility regarding drinking or smoking, independently of the direct coercive effect on individuals. Indeed, this might be a main way in which many lifestyle limitations work.

Another way in which public health paternalism may help strengthen a sense of group as well as individual welfare is through enlarging the sense that the standards behind regulating commerce and lifestyle choices are based on group norms rather than individual ones. For example, alcohol consumption in most societies for most individuals is far lower than the amount which might be safe for them as private citizens. As a rough yardstick, 'safe drinking' from the individual standpoint is one and a half ounces of absolute alcohol daily, or the equivalent of three glasses of beer. But in the United States, which stands roughly at the mid-point among Western nations in total alcohol consumption, probably less than 15 to 20 per cent of the population drinks that much (Beauchamp, 1980). Community standards are therefore based on solidarity of interest, meant to reduce the number who suffer alcohol problems. Similarly, seat-belt legislation seeks a group level of safety that individuals acting alone find hard to choose.

How do we keep public health paternalism from going too far and threatening individual autonomy? Do we go from regulating alcohol and the promotion of cigarettes to forbidding rock-climbing? The short answer is no. Public health paternalism focusses on the market place and on those areas where private interests can exploit the public interest. This would include limiting commercial corporations who have a stake in low levels of safety and in risk-taking, to also limiting medical practice to protect the common interest in rationing medical care and in controlling medical expenditure. Public health paternalism mixes controls on providers or producers and consumers and does not seem too intrusive. However, requiring each citizen to jog three miles a day, or to maintain an optimum body weight would bring the state far too close to the individual and would threaten personal autonomy. Commercial regulations and regulating public space operate generally and at a distance, not singling out one particular individual or another for moral improvement. Perhaps the key limit to the balance principle is the presumption it usually carries for individual liberty. Liberty is to be preferred unless regulation guarantees a significant gain to the community. The restrictions sought should also be least restrictive measures available consistent with the ends to be achieved. And the burden of proof is on those who desire the restriction of liberty to demonstrate community benefits.

Threatening individual interests

Antipaternalism may actually increase rather than reduce threats to individual interests. It does this in three separate areas: by focussing on blame, by putting undue stress on children and young people otherwise not of legal age, and by raising the risk of prohibition. Policies which balance community and individual interest actually do a better job of protecting individual interests overall by spreading responsibility for prevention more equitably among the affected interests.

Drunk driving has been the main exception to governments' lack of interest in alcohol policy. In the United States, this issue has led the way for increased national and local attention to alcohol policy. The group responsible is Mothers Against Drunk Drivers (. . . [later] renamed Mothers Against Drunk Driving), or MADD which was founded by the charismatic mother of a young girl who was killed by a drunk driver.

Solving social problems by punishing wrongs or crimes is a principal method of those forms of antipaternalism rooted in a strong political individualism. As Mill put it, 'The preventive function of government . . . is far more liable to be abused, to the prejudice of liberty, than the punitory function'. The primary motive behind drunk-driving campaigns is to punish drunk driving as a way of symbolising the community's repugnance for the practice, and secondly, to deter drunk driving by inflicting stiffer penalties and instituting more effective detection methods. These are legitimate and even important governmental interests.

But increasing the legal penalties and certainty of punishment for drunk driving, taken by itself, is not likely to have permanent and long-term results in reducing this problem. The main reason is the difficulty for police forces in detecting drinking and driving. In the United States the risks of detection in most areas is one in 2000 (Reed, 1981). In England the estimate, even during intense enforcement, is only one in 1000 (Reed, 1981). As Lawrence Ross (1973) has noted, campaigns against drinking and driving probably have their effect because they alter the subjective assessment by citizens of the risks of detection. Once the initial wave of publicity passes, the public learns that risk of detection has not increased appreciably, and the previous levels of drunk driving are re-established.

The main problem is that many Western societies have made alcohol so widely available and convenient to the car as to actually constitute a licence to drink and drive. In most Western countries, beer is widely available in most retail establishments, with few government personnel to detect sales to intoxicated or under age people. In many states in the United States it is permissible to drink and drive – only *drunk* driving is forbidden. Western societies have put heavy reliance on detection of drunk driving by the police, with the result that the practice of police stopping drivers randomly to administer sobriety tests is on the increase. What starts out as antipaternalism and legal sanctions winds up as a very serious increase in the level of law enforcement in democratic societies.

Another paradoxical outcome of political individualism is the unusual emphasis given to control and protection of young persons. As Mill argued, the restrictions on limiting society's and the government's power over the adult's private conduct do not apply to young people:

> Society has . . . absolute power over [children and youth] during all the early portion of their existence: it has . . . the whole period of childhood and nonage in which to try whether it could make them capable of rational conduct in life. (1961)

Political individualism puts so much stress on leaving the adult free to choose his own ends that, almost of necessity, the young bear the brunt of social control. Defining the community's interest in alcohol policy as principally that of regulating the behaviour of the young can make them the scapegoat for society's policies. Nils Christie (1981) in Markela *et al.* has warned that increased governmental interest in alcohol policy is likely to take the form of extending 'childhood' for longer and longer periods to legitimise the supervision by the state. Certainly, the . . . experience in the United States, with the federal government's endorsement of a uniform national legal drinking age of 21 years, is partial evidence that this is occurring.

The point is not to ignore the young or punishment for drunk drivers but to balance restrictions and legislation aimed at these groups with broader controls on alcohol commerce that affect the entire population. As Michael Grossman *et al.* (1984) argue, a slight increase in the tax on beer might save as many lives as a one year increase in the age limit for drinking. The other advantage of this policy is that it would also help prevent problems among those who are older as well, and would also make the young feel less singled out. Policies against drunk driving – whether aimed at the young or not – might also include limitation on the availability of alcohol in the retail distribution system, an increase in the level of surveillance of that system by state liquor licence personnel, or an increase in the price of alcoholic beverages, especially beer. Better yet, we could do all three things at once. The growing application of civil liability for retail operators who serve under age or drunk patrons or both is also likely to help reduce the problem, and to shift attention away from the criminal justice system.

There is yet another danger to individual interests from the undue focus on blame in many kinds of antipaternalism. This is the danger of what has come to be called 'victim blaming' (Ryan, 1976) . . . Victim blaming begins by noting that smoking and alcohol abuse add significant social costs to society, especially by lost productivity and increased medical and insurance costs. The next step is to argue that these groups should be held accountable for these costs to the others in society. As one American critic has argued, ' [O]ne man's freedom in health is another man's shackle in taxes and insurance premiums' (Knowles, 1977). But where does this principle of individual responsibility to the larger society end? Are the obese, those with large families, those who fail to exercise also to be similarly burdened? Thus, it is a short step from a position of individual autonomy to a position of social responsibility to the larger society, from a position of individual autonomy to social stigmatisation.

This position of making the risk-taker pay his own way ignores the extent to which drinking and smoking as actions are a complex bundle of voluntary and involuntary features, structural as well as individual causal relationships. While we should not ignore the role of choice, alcohol and cigarettes are also powerfully addictive and heavily promoted by commercial interests. The community position would spread the responsibility more broadly, seeing these problems as *both* community and individual problems, using prevention rather than blame and measures aimed at all who smoke or drink, as well as the industries.

Finally, there is the paradox of prohibition itself. It is striking that the country that experienced the longest period of national prohibition, the United States, is the democracy that comes nearer to a public philosophy of political individualism. Prohibition came to the United States for many complex reasons. One of the reasons is surely that, when problems such as alcohol abuse become so severe that society has to take action, the militant antipaternalist is forced either to revise his antipaternalism or to escalate seriously the threat that alcohol itself poses to the individual. This is what seems to have happened with the shift from the early temperance drives which were voluntary in character, and which met with limited success. Prohibition came next, and it came in significant part because the philosophy of political individualism offered no middle ground for balancing regulation of alcohol use with its continued commercial availability. Antipaternalist philosophies nearly always contain room for substances or conditions which are so inherently dangerous that extreme government regulation and even prohibition is justified. When a balancing approach is not popularly embraced or understood, there is a strong temptation to take a newly problematic set of conditions (the rise of the saloon in the nineteenth century) and a substance (alcohol) and reclassify it in the same group that today is reserved for drugs like heroin. Room for compromise and balance is thus lost, because why should a dangerous drug be allowed in the stream of commerce? This experience might serve as a cautionary tale for commercial interests who defend their interests in the name of political individualism.

So, two cheers for paternalism – public health paternalism. Public health paternalism permits a sharing of responsibility for controlling the impulses of one's life, and for strengthening those motives of cooperation and trust that are the cornerstone of the community (Slater, 1970). As with everything else, this principle has its dangers, but societies which ignore the needs of community and mutual dependency are deeply unwise, encouraging the very threats to private interests that they so noisily and blindly seek to protect.

References

Beauchamp, D. (1980). *Beyond Alcoholism: Alcohol and Public Health Policy*. Philadelphia: Temple University Press.

Cook, P J. (1981). The effect of liquor taxes on drinking, cirrhosis, and auto accidents. In Moore, M. and Gerstein, D. (eds), *Alcohol and Public policy: Beyond the Shadow of Prohibition*. Washington, DC: National Academy Press.

Flathman, R. (1966). *The Public Interest: An essay concerning the normative discourse of politics.* New York: Wiley.

Grossman, M., Coate, D. and Arluck, G. (1984). Price sensitivity of alcoholic beverages in the US, paper presented at the Conference on Control Issues in Alcohol Abuse Prevention: Impacting Communities. South Carolina Commission on Alcohol and Drug Abuse, Charleston, SC 7–10 October.

Knowles, J. H. (1977). The responsibility of the individual. In Knowles, J. H. (ed)., *Doing Better and Feeling Worse.* New York: Norton.

Lukes, S. (1973). *Individualism.* New York: Harper & Row, 79–87.

Markela, K., Room, R., Single, E., Sulkunen, P. and Walsh, B. (1981). *Alcohol, Society and the State: A comparative Study of alcohol control.* Toronto: Addiction Research Foundation, xiv.

Reed, D. S. (1981). Reducing the costs of drinking and driving. In Moore, M. and Gerstein D. (eds), *Alcohol and Public Policy: Beyond the Prohibition.* Washington, DC: National Academy Press, 336–387.

Ross, H. L. (1973). Law, science, and accidents: the British road safety act of 1967, *Journal of Legal Studies, 2,* 1–78.

Ryan, W. (1976). Blaming the Victim. New York: Vintage.

Schmidt, W. and Popham, R. (1980). Discussion of paper by Parker and Harman. In Harford, T. C., Parker, D. A. and Light, L. *Normative Approaches to the Prevention of Alcohol Abuse and Alcoholism,* Research Monograph, *3.,* National Institute on Alcohol Abuse and Alcoholism. Department of Health and Human Services. Washington, DC: United States Government Printing Office.

Slater, P. (1970). *The Pursuit of Loneliness.* Boston: Beacon.

Terris, M. (1985). The changing relationships of epidemiology and society: The Robert Cruikshank lecture, *Journal of Public Health, 6,* 15–36.

32 The at-risk health status and technology: a diagnostic invitation and the 'gift' of knowing*

Regina H. Kenen

Introduction

The at-risk health status differs from just being at risk from a specific health hazard. While every-one is at risk from some health peril, everyone is not expected to adhere to socially approved at-risk health behavior patterns and actions. It is only after at-risk health statuses have been negotiated and accepted that they can be considered as social positions accompanied by expected role performances and norms.

The at-risk health status has professional and societal as well as individual implications. Professional involvement revolves around health education and health promotion. The former operates on the individual level and is concerned with conformity to sociomedical norms regarding a health threat. The latter deals primarily with societal factors and emphasises development of general social awareness and acceptance of the at-risk health status and its role obligations. On the societal level, the media, health care economics and political ideology also influence negotiations regarding the at-risk health status within a primarily market economy, health care system.

The media, a potent socialising agent has also been utilised by the public health community in the United States as a major health promotion tool presenting anti-smoking, anti-drunk driving and safe sex campaigns through advertisements, documentaries and even rock education programmes on MTV. Furthermore, private health care institutions now broadcast on the radio their at-risk messages extolling the latest diagnostic equipment offered by their health care establishments. . .

The at-risk health status is frequently accompanied by what I shall call a diagnostic invitation and the 'gift' of knowing. This technologically oriented invitation presented by some health care professionals to their clients is predicated on the belief that knowledge is intrinsically good,

* From *Social Science and Medicine.* 42,(11) (1996) pp 1545–1553. Oxford: Pergamon Press. © Elsevier Science Ltd 1996.

enabling clients to make more informed decisions. Therefore, the possession of knowledge is equated with empowerment. The down side of this 'gift' is that knowledge is only empowering if it is beneficial. But this may not be so when diagnosis merely reaffirms risk, but offers no cure in the near future. Thus, clients may either embrace the gift of knowing or greet it with ambivalence or even outright rejection depending on both circumstances and individual values. As Nancy Wexler reflected with regard to genetic screening, 'our experience with Huntington's has shown that some things may be better left unknown' (Murray, 1994, p. 30).

The enormous advances in diagnostic technology have dramatically opened the door for a myriad of new possibilities that fit into an at-risk perspective. Physicians have always told patients that they were at-risk for certain medical conditions. But this communication was conducted in the privacy of the doctor's office. What is new is that health care professionals imbued with a preventive perspective are publicly touting the at-risk health status with an agenda for change. The hope is that the public internalises health promotion messages leading to changes in risky behaviour and acceptance of appropriate diagnostic testing. Once the general concept of an at-risk health status becomes institutionalised, an at-risk health role analogous to Parsons' (1951) sick role is likely to develop and newly emerging at-risk categories will be easier to legitimise . . .

Despite some basic differences, there is, however, a relationship between the sick role and the at-risk health role. In the sick role, the patient is supposed to seek physician advice and to try and get better. In the at-risk health role, the doctor's role is not as dominant. The individual is supposed to try to *avoid* becoming ill (instead of trying to get better after they become ill). Depending upon the situation this can be accomplished with the aid of a physician or by self-help in the form of lifestyle changes.

When individuals occupy the sick role (which is temporary), the doctor's task is to heal them so that they can resume their normal obligations. In the case of the at-risk health role, individuals are not entitled to relinquish obligations because they are not sick. But implicit is the assumption that only by fulfilling the at-risk health role (going for diagnostic tests and/or changing behavior, e.g. healthier eating patterns, exercising more frequently, quitting smoking) will individuals be entitled to the rights accompanying the sick role if they were to become ill in the future.

The family and the at-risk role

Accepting the at-risk health role involves complex psycho-social relationships with family members, particularly with those who will become caretakers, if that becomes necessary, and interpersonal relationships, in general, can be particularly problematic when a genetic disease runs in the family. For example, one sibling may want to be open about the at-risk health status which could be stigmatising, while another sibling may not want to reveal any information. In Goffman's (1963) terms, the sibling who wants to be open about the family's genetic history is willing to overtly deal with the possible 'discredited stigma', while the other sibling prefers the stigma to remain 'discreditable' and is willing to manage information so that knowledge about the at-risk health status is not revealed. This individual might then try to relinquish the at-risk health role for fear of discovery, or fulfil the role as surreptitiously as possible. Once a genetic disease has developed, subterfuge no longer works and the person may have little choice but to adopt a chronic illness or acute illness role. Even when genetic testing implicates that the person is *not* at risk, some members of at-risk families find it difficult to renegotiate with themselves a future that no longer includes the expectation of being chronically or acutely ill (Huggins *et al.*, 1992).

Some manifest and possible latent consequences

The existence of applied genetic technology, as well as other diagnostic advances, create both new at-risk health statuses and their antidotes. For example a pregnant woman of advanced maternal age (aged 35+) is labelled as being at high risk for carrying a fetus with a chromosomal defect. At present, the antidotes would be amniocentesis and chorionic villus sampling. If the test results are normal, then this particular high risk status is removed. Partially as a result of this high-risk label, the use of prenatal genetic services – clinical counselling, procedural services and laboratory studies – have soared. Just between 1989 and 1990, the number of women receiving prenatal genetic services in the United States increased by a little more than one third (CORN MDS Report, 1989, 1990).

When prenatal diagnosis was first developed, it was used for serious, untreatable conditions. Now it is also being used to diagnose conditions with little or uncertain impact on health, for which there is treatment, and for conditions that might appear later in life (Lippman, 1992). Prenatal diagnosis is being requested by younger women when the risk for chromosomal abnormalities is very low. Thus, many women may undergo the procedure without gaining any objective benefit. Furthermore, Leuzinger and Rambert (1988) hypothesise that by emphasising the unconscious fears of women and their partners, the medical and genetics professionals may in fact cause women to be seduced into using prenatal technologies. Leuzinger and Rambert further report that when women decide not to inform themselves about the chromosomal and genetic status of their foetus through the use of prenatal tests and reject a diagnostic invitation and the 'gift' of knowing, they must put more energy into actively warding off fear.

While the manifest goal of the at-risk health status is to promote healthier behaviour one latent effect is that the status can also be abused in overt and subtle ways. This can be seen clearly in a few scenarios regarding the reproductive history of women, especially when the health care provider exerts far more power in the negotiation process than does the client.

For example, a pregnant woman who engages in risky behaviours, or does not adhere to medical advice, may be accused of putting her foetus at-risk and sanctioned by a combination of the health care and social control system, particularly if she is poor and a member of a minority group. Attempts have been made to legally punish a woman on the basis of prenatal child abuse (Gallagher, 1989). In a California case, a judge sentenced a woman who had abused drugs during her pregnancy to a jail term unless she agreed to be implanted with Norplant, a long acting contraceptive (Southwick, 1992). In other cases where negotiation of the at-risk health status failed, courts have been asked to order mandatory caesarian sections (Kolder *et al.*, 1987) These actions are reminiscent of eugenic and forced sterilisation policies of the past (Nelkin and Lindee, 1995; Charo and Rothenberg, 1994).

Middle class women, at times, are also left out of the negotiation process in deciding whether to accept the diagnostic invitation and 'gift' of knowing. Many hospitals now give pregnant women a triple marker blood screening test measuring alpha foetoprotein, hCG, and unconjugated estriol in order to detect the possibility of a neural tube defect or Downs Syndrome (Phillips *et al.*, 1992). Many of these women are not told that they are being given this screening test. Instead, it is subsumed under the rubric of routine prenatal care. Only when the test results indicate the possibility of a problem, does the woman realise that an at-risk health status has been thrust upon her. She is offered ultrasound or prenatal diagnosis to determine whether there is a true defect or whether the screening result was a false positive. The expectation is that she accepts the diagnostic invitation and 'gift' of knowing. Some members of the women's health movement and disabilities groups are rejecting routinisation of prenatal screening and testing, emphasising instead the naturalness of pregnancy and childbirth and the diversity of human beings (Kaplan, 1994) – an alternative paradigm to the technologically oriented 'a chance is a chance' perspective (Tymstra, 1989).

The human genome project

While diagnostic technology is expanding in many areas of health care and the acceptance of the at-risk health status is becoming more normative, it is in the area of genetic testing that the most serious discussions of the psychological, ethical, social and legal implications are taking place and will likely be disseminated into other areas. The need to develop accompanying social norms and medical guidelines in tandem with the ability to define the inherent risk in an ever increasing number of genetic conditions was an initial premise of the Human Genome Project (HGP). Although the HGP is aware that the knowledge it generates can be problematical, it emphasises the use of genetic information to ensure that through diagnosis, treatment, and prevention, every human being has the right to health. This sounds benign and even altruistic, but the meaning of health used by the HGP is being questioned. Fox-Keller (1992) calls the premise behind the HGP an 'eugenics of normalcy'. She claims that health is never clearly defined, but only used in relation to the standard of the human genome composite. In contrast, 'unhealth' is indicated by an ever growing list of conditions labelled as genetic diseases. By this definition, there will be a concomitant increase in at-risk health statuses.

Each genetic condition, labelled as a disease, will be accompanied by an at-risk health status. So far most genetic tests have been for single gene diseases. On the horizon are tests for predispositions for diseases such as cancer and cardiovascular disease that are thought to be multifactorial in origin (Sorenson, 1992). Those diagnosed as having a late onset disorder or increased probability of developing a specific genetic disease may spend a lifetime as PPDs (Possibly Potentially Diseased) or DIWs (Diseased in Waiting) (Kenen, 1994) with the accompanying distress and discrimination that might entail. Richards (1993) points out that some genetic conditions may influence intergenerational mobility for non-affected family members as well as those diagnosed as being at risk. If entire families are labelled with an at-risk health status, then all family members might find their marriage and career options limited.

As more and more genetic conditions become diagnosed before any cure is in sight, more and more individuals will be added to the at-risk pool. This trend is accelerating as the time between the introduction of a new technology and its widespread diffusion into standard practice has shortened dramatically (Smith and Benkendorf, 1991). Yet it will be many years until cures are found for more than a relatively few genetic diseases. Meanwhile, the primary medical focus will be on carrier testing, prenatal diagnosis and selective termination of pregnancy and health insurance companies and health maintenance organisation (HMOs) can either require genetic testing, or refuse to pay for it, depending on their estimates of costs and the medical condition involved.

The Ethical, Social and Legal Implications Division of the Human Genome (ELSI) Project has funded several interdisciplinary studies and conferences and has held many working group sessions trying to hammer out consensus in controversial areas of applied human genetics. Several areas of concern are: predictive genetic testing for children (Human Genome News, 1995), the value of prognostic knowledge when treatment is not available (Asch *et al.*, 1992), and job and insurance discrimination against individuals eligible for existing genetic testing and their families (Billings *et al.*, 1992). Some genetics clinics now include discussion of privacy issues and possible insurance and job discrimination as part of the pretesting counselling session, particularly in regard to adult onset genetic conditions.

As a result of efforts to protect genetic testing results from being misused, the Equal Opportunities Commission has interpreted The 1990 Americans With Disabilities Act (ADA) as covering individuals who are carriers of a genetic condition but who are presently healthy. Theoretically, at least, this protection should allow more people to accept the diagnostic invitation and the 'gift' of knowing as they have an avenue of redress against possible workplace and insurance company reprisals. . .

Conclusion

The at-risk health status places the incumbent in a vulnerable position. Therefore, critical questions need to be asked about a diagnostic invitation and the 'gift' of knowing before important financial, ethical and social decisions are made. What kind of reassurance does the person receive from the testing as contrasted with the anxiety provoked by the procedure? At what point between discovery and evaluation of a condition by a new technology should a test be disseminated? How does the advocacy of one type of early diagnostic screening influence the demand for additional early diagnostic tests? How does developing a genetic disease (or bearing a child with a diagnosable genetic condition) affect the person who refused a diagnostic invitation and the 'gift' of knowing? When does the diagnostic invitation and the 'gift' of knowing improve health, when does it place individuals in unwarranted at-risk health statuses, and when may it cause iatrogenic harm?

The increasing expansion of the definition of what constitutes health and the desire to use high technology medicine to achieve this goal supports mainstream America's gluttonous appetite for health care services. Individuals seem to be willing to try anything to improve the quality of their lives and ward off death (Gaylin, 1993). At the same time, insurance companies and HMOs are becoming more reluctant to pay for what they consider to be unnecessary or unproven therapies.

The emphasis on individual responsibility, perceived cost effectiveness of preventive measures combined with the desire to use high technology medicine to achieve these newly expanded definitions of health, make it likely that the concept of the at-risk health status will be integrated into the managed care type of health care system which seems to be evolving in the United States. Acceptance of this status will exert a far-reaching impact on life styles, health practices, ethics, social values and the law. In light of the possible negative, as well as positive, effects of at-risk health labelling American society needs to evaluate the diagnostic invitation and the 'gift' of knowing and establish guidelines and standards for these offerings, especially when the line between prevention and over use is not always clear.

Acknowledgements

1 am grateful to Robin Gregg, Eric Jeungst, Aliza Kolker, Phyllis Langton and Linda Levine for their insightful comments on earlier versions of this paper and to anonymous reviewers for *Social Science and Medicine* whose critiques helped develop my arguments more fully.

References

Asch, D., Patton, J. and Hershey, J. (1992). Knowing for the sake of knowing: the value of prognostic information. *Medical Decision-Making 10*, 47.

Billings, P., Kohn, A., de Cueves, M. *et al.* (1992). Discrimination as a consequence of genetic testing. *American Journal of Human Genetics, 50*, 476.

Charo, R. A. and Rothenberg, K. H. (1994).'The good mother': the limits of reproductive accountability and genetic choice. In Rothenberg, K. H. and Thomson, E. J., *Women and Prenatal Testing: Facing the challenges of genetic technology*. Ohio State University Press, Columbus, Ohio, 105–130.

CORN MDS Report (1989, 1990).

Fox-Keller, E. (1992). Nature, nurture, and the Human Genome Project. In *The Code of Codes: scientific and Social Issues in the Human Genome Project* (Edited by Kevles D. and Hood L.), pp. 281–299. Harvard, Cambridge, MA.

Gallagher, J. (1989). Fetus as patient. In Taub, N. and Cohen, S. (eds), *Reproductive Laws of the 1990s*. New Brunswick: Rutgers University Press, 185–236.

Gaylin, W. (1993). The health plan misses the point, *New York Times*, (15 September), A27.

Goffman, E. (1963). *Stigma: Notes on the management of spoiled identity*. Englewood Cliffs, NJ: Prentice-Hall.

Huggins, M., Bloch, M., Wiggins, S. *et al.* (1992). Predictive testing for Huntington disease in Canada: adverse effects and unexpected results in those receiving a decreased risk, *American Journal of Genetic Medicine, 42*, p. 508.

Human Genome News (1995). Role of media and genome project addressed. March–April, p. 6.

Kaplan, D. (1994). Prenatal screening and diagnosis: the impact on persons with disabilities. In *Women and Prenatal Testing: Facing the Challenges of Genetic Technology* (Edited by Rothenberg K. H. and Thomson E. J.), pp. 49–61. Ohio State University Press, Columbus, Ohio.

Kenen, R. (1994). The human genome project: creator of the potentially sick, potentially vulnerable and potentially stigmatized? In *Social Consequences of Life and Death under High Technology Medicine* (Edited by Robinson, I.), pp. 49–64. Manchester: University of Manchester Press.

Kolder, V., Gallagher, J. and Parsons, M. (1987). Court-ordered obstetrical interventions, *New England Journal of Medicine, 316* (7 May), 1192.

Lenzinger, M. and Rambert, B. (1988). I can feel it – my baby is healthy: women's experiences with prenatal diagnosis in Switzerland. *Reproductive Genetics England* 1.239.

Lippman, A. (1992). Mother matters: a fresh look at prenatal genetic testing, *Issues in Reproductive Genetics in England, 5*, 141.

Murray, M. (1994). Nancy Wexler's test, *The New York Times Magazine* (February 13), pp. 28–31.

Nelkin, D. and Lindee, M. S. (1995). *The DNA Mystique: The gene as a cultural icon.* New York: W. H. Freeman.

Parsons, T. (1951). *The Social System.* Glencoe, IL: Free Press.

Phillips, O., Elias S., Shulman L. *et al.* (1992). Maternal serum screening for fetal Down syndrome in women less than 35 years of age using alpha-fetoprotein, hCG and unconjugated estriol: a prospective 2-year study. *Obstetric Gynecology, 80,* 353.

Richards, M. P. M. (1993). The new genetics some issues for social scientists. *Sociology of Health and Illness,* 569.

Smith, A. C. M. and Benkendorf, J. (1991). Genetic information: impact on counseling, professionals and consumers. *Biotechnology and the Diagnosis of Genetic Disease: Forum on the Technical, Regulatory and Societal Issues.* Georgetown University Medical Center.

Sorenson, J. (1992). What we still don't know about genetic screening and counseling. In *Gene Mapping: Using Law and Ethics as Guides* (Edited by Annas G. and Elias S.), pp. 203–204. Oxford: Oxford University Press.

Southwick, K. (1992). Use Norplan, don't go to jail, *San Francisco Chronicle* (August 2).

Tymstra, T. (1989). The imperative character of medical technology and the meaning of 'anticipated decision regret'. *International Journal of Technological Assessment of Health Care, 5,* 207.

33 Surveillance, health promotion and the formation of a risk identity*

Sarah Nettleton

Contemporary forms of surveillance within the context of health promotion and the new public health are characterised by their emphasis on risk. This chapter explores the relationship between surveillance and risk and suggests that the current emphasis on the construction and monitoring of risk factors has contributed to the formation of a new conceptualisation of 'self' one which is perpetually both cognisant of, and resistant to, risk.[1]

Administering health

To aspire to be healthy is not just a personal goal, it is also a political one. Governments in liberal democratic societies take action to improve the health of their populations. A feature of governments since the 18th century is the way in which they have intensified, developed and refined administrative procedures and technologies to gather data and information on individuals and populations. Data has long been gathered on variables such as levels of morbidity, procreation, life expectancy and mortality (Foucault, 1980). In fact it was this activity that contributed to the development of the discipline that we now call statistics. Foucault (1980) describes how the body became the prime site of political regulation and surveillance: 'the body of individuals and the body of populations – appears as the bearer of new variables' (p.172). This is what he famously describes as 'disciplinary power': the mechanisms of discipline which fashion and train bodies. Alongside the development of procedures for monitoring populations emerged another political preoccupation as Foucault explains:

> This is the emergence of the health and the physical well-being of the
> population in general as one of the essential objectives of political
> power. Here it is not a matter of offering support to a particularly
> fragile, troubled and troublesome margin of the population, but of

---

* Commissioned for this volume.

how to raise the level of health of the social body as a whole. Different power apparatuses are called upon to take charge of 'bodies', . . . *The imperative of health: at once the duty of each and the objective of all.* (Foucault, 1980, pp. 169–70, emphasis mine)

For Foucault, however, such activities constitute only one side of the practical administrative systems by which individuals are governed. Individuals also act upon and govern themselves. Indeed, a liberal democratic society requires the individuals who constitute it to be able to act autonomously as 'good citizens' (Burchell, 1993; Rose, 1993). Thus 'technologies of surveillance' or 'disciplinary power' rely on, and interact with, what Foucault calls *'the technologies of the self'*. Here Foucault is referring to the means by which individuals can act upon their own bodies, minds, souls and their conduct. If health was to be achieved by government it had to be the goal of *both* administrative programmes and of individuals. The desire to be healthy from this perspective, is not an innate aspiration but one that is intimately bound up in the processes of governance. Such a desire forms part of a political aspiration. Following this line of argument, the historian Barbara Duden (1991) argues that health as a 'goal of individual well-being' was derived from the 'administrating and objectivising of the "body politic"' (p.18).

The Enlightenment wrote health onto its banner as a physical-moral category. The concept was politically so effective and so double-edged because the interest of the authorities and the national economy in a self-administered objectification of the self appeared in it as a subjective need of the individual or an act of philanthropy . . . Political medicine cast this desire for a healthy body into a scientifically solid mold of norms and pathologies, thus creating a new image of humankind . . . the human right to the 'pursuit of happiness' (as laid down in the Constitution of the United States) took on concrete form as a right to health. (Duden, 1991, p. 19).

Thus the actions we take to improve our health are bound up with wider political motives and ambitions. The activities, policies and procedures of those authorities who are concerned to promote health reverberate on the activities and desires of individuals. The consequences of public health and health promotion practices should not therefore be underestimated.

The nature of the 'technologies' or administrative mechanisms, which Foucault and others write about invariably change over time. For example, within the context of health and medical care new methods of collecting data are developed, new technologies for observing people's bodies and behaviours are devised and different aspects of peoples social lives are deemed to be relevant. The last few decades have seen a significant change in the mechanisms used to monitor populations and this has occurred alongside a transformation of the philosophical or ideological base of medicine. Furthermore, as we will see, it was this revolution in medicine that generated the political and administrative space for the emergence of health promotion.

From 'dangerousness' to 'risk'

The French philosopher Robert Castel (1991) in a paper titled 'From Dangerousness to Risk' provides a useful way of conceptualising this transformation when he argues that we are entering a new paradigm of health care. He suggests that we are moving from a health care system premised upon 'dangerousness' to one based upon 'risk'. Hitherto, he argues, health professionals have tended to err on the side of caution to prevent the development of disease and, consequently, the illnesses possessed by patients have been treated as being potentially dangerous. However, today the target of health and medical care is shifting from the symptoms of an individual *patient* to the social and behavioural characteristics of the *person*. The 'clinic of the subject' Castel (1991, p. 282) suggests is being replaced by the *'epidemiological clinic'*. Thus we are witnessing the advent of a new mode of surveillance, aided by technological advances which make the calculus and possibilities of 'systematic pre-detection' more and more sophisticated.

Castel suggests that there are two very real consequences of this profound change. First, practitioners' key function will be to assess the social and behavioural characteristics of their clients and on the basis of these assessments provide guidance and advice. In the United Kingdom an example of this would be the requirement of General Practitioners to keep more and more data on their patients 'risk factors' such as their levels of smoking and drinking. A second consequence is that practitioners become subordinate to health care administrators or managers who are charged with tasks such as the profiling of populations and developing health strategies. Whilst Castel labels this new form of health care the 'epidemiological clinic' the medical sociologist David Armstrong (1995) calls it *'surveillance medicine'*. 'A cardinal feature of Surveillance Medicine' he writes ' is its targeting of everyone'. Increasingly health and medical care are not just concerned with those who are ill but with those who are well, it is not just orientated towards treating the symptoms of disease but identifying and monitoring *risk factors* which 'point to' the possibility of a future illness.

A 'risk epidemic'

In recent decades there has been a proliferation of so called 'risk factors' associated with health. One is sometimes left with the impression that whatever one does carries some form of 'risk' or danger. Eating certain foods, drinking alcohol, coca cola or coffee, not doing enough exercise, doing too much of the wrong type of exercise, being overweight, being underweight, watching too much television, not having enough leisure time, smoking cigarettes, in fact doing almost anything now seems to have potential connotations for one's health.

A number of sociologists (Giddens, 1992; Beck 1992; Douglas, 1986) have pointed to the fact that we are living in a society that is characterised by a 'politics of anxiety', indeed that we are living in a *risk society* (Beck, 1992). A point on which all these authors appear to agree is that the risks associated with modern-day living are person made, they are a product of *social* organisation and human actions. Armstrong (1993) contrasts the health risks of today with the health risks present in the 19th century. Whilst in the 19th century health risks were associated with the 'natural' environment and dangers lurked within water, soil, air, food and climate, today the environmental factors that impinge on health, such as acid rain and radiation are the consequence of human actions. Of course not all contemporary health risks are human products, Aids for example is the consequence of a virus. Nevertheless the disease has come to be *conceptualised* within a social matrix; it exists within a wider context of social activities and is envisaged in terms of complex social interactions between gay men, intravenous drug users and those requiring and administering blood transfusions (Armstrong, 1993). In this respect it has increasingly become articulated in the same terms as humanly created risks.

The proliferation of risks is not confined to popular discourse or sociological debates, it has also occurred within the medical literature. A comprehensive analysis of medical journals in Britain, the United States and Scandinavia found that the increase in the use of the term risk has reached 'epidemic proportions' (Skolbekken, 1995). The study looked at journals published between 1967 and 1991, for the first five years the number of 'risk articles' published was around 1000 and for the last five years there were over 80,000. Skolbekken refers to this as a 'risk epidemic' in order to highlight the high prevalence of the term; the fact that there is a degree of contagiousness which 'is indicated by increase in the number of illnesses/disease that are subject to some kind of risk approach' (p.296) and finally, to draw attention to the 'side effects' of the current pre-occupation with the term.

Skolbekken argues further that health promotion provides 'the ideological frame needed to explain the present emphasis on factors regarded as risks to our health. . . Through the ideological frame of health promotion we get a glimpse of some of the functions served by the risk epidemic' (1995, p.296). He cites these functions as: first, to predict disease and death, in other words to gain control over disease which in turn confirms our faith in medical science. Second, it is sometimes assumed that the findings of this type of research may help to save money as people are less likely to require acute and therefore, expensive services. Third, it contributes to medicalisation. Risk factors which are hypothesised to be linked to disease come to be treated as 'diseases to be cured' (Skolbekken, 1995, p.299). Certainly in the public health and health promotion documentation health related behaviours such as smoking or drinking alcohol come to be treated as variables which need to be explained. Whether or not the first function is legitimate or the second function is likely, may be undermined by the third point which draws attention to the 'unscientific' nature of much of this research. Even spurious correlations between risk factors and disease may easily come to be treated as causal (Davey Smith *et al.*, 1992). Certainly, there is considerable controversy within the medical journals about the links between, say, diet and coronary heart disease and the merits and demerits of various interventions, for example the lowering of cholesterol levels (Atrens, 1994; Oliver, 1992; Ravnskov, 1992).

The techniques deployed in the scrutinisation of these 'risk factors' within the context of public health and health promotion are primarily: screening for a range of diseases and symptoms; the collection of information on patients by health professionals; epidemiological studies; social surveys; and qualitative studies. Once a 'factor' such as eating 'fatty foods' is found to be statistically associated with another indicator of ill health (or risk factor) such as cholesterol levels, it is deemed to be a risk. The social aspects of eating this type of food may then be explored by sociologists and anthropologists who aim to answer questions such as: Why do people eat fat? What eating fatty foods means to them? What is the social and symbolic significance of eating fatty foods? This information is considered to be crucial to the development of effective health promotion. The findings of the epidemiologists and the social scientists are drawn upon by health promoters to encourage people to eat less fatty foods. The government will keep an eye on the populations fat consumption and set nutritional targets. For example, *The Health of the Nation* aims:

> To reduce the average percentage of food energy derived by the population from total fat by at least 12% by 2005 (from about 40% in 1990 to no more than 35%. (Department of Health, 1993, p.52)

Thus surveillance techniques and risk go hand in hand. The techniques deployed to survey and monitor populations simultaneously contribute to the construction of more and more risk factors and monitor the extent to which individuals, groups and populations possess them.

The social construction of risk factors

As with any area of medical or scientific research (Wright and Treacher, 1982) the selection of 'factors' to be studied cannot be immune from prevailing social values and ideologies. This is perhaps most overt in relation to Aids where the sexist, racist and homophobic assumptions which underpin epidemiological research have been identified (Bloor *et al.*, 1991; Patton, 1990). It is also evident that so called lifestyle or behavioural factors (such as the holy trinity of risks – diet, smoking and exercise) receive a disproportionate amount of attention. As we have seen the identification and confirmation of risk factors is often subject to controversy and the evidence about causal links is not unequivocal. However, health promotion interventions are developed on the basis of such evidence, and may often gloss over contradictory research findings (Frankel *et al.*, 1991). The recourse to epidemiology by those involved in public health and health promotion results in a veneer of scientific legitimacy and as such the findings of epidemiological research are often taken to be politically neutral (Lupton, 1995, p. 67). However the nature of the dialogue between health promoters and epidemiologists may also be one of 'double standards', as we will see below.

The individualisation of risk

A risk factor which is associated with health is a characteristic of a given population it concerns. Within the context of epidemiological research risks are *calculated* on the basis of *collective* data. Risk factors are not therefore properties possessed by individuals but refer to probabilities which, by definition, can only be derived from the study of a group of people. Confidence in predictions is enhanced by the size of the sample population studied. This conceptualisation of risk is rooted in probability statistics. In fact as Ewald (1991), writing on the subject of insurance, sociology and risk, has pointed out, there is no such thing as an individual risk:

> Whereas an accident, as damage, misfortune and suffering, is always individual, striking at one and not another, a risk of accident affects a population. Strictly speaking there is no such thing as an individual risk; otherwise insurance would be no more than a wager. Risk only becomes something calculable when it is spread over a population. (p.203)

In fact, as Lindsay Prior (1995) points out in his paper 'Accidents as a Public Health Problem' it is entirely feasible to predict the number of accidents for any given population. The *rate* of accidents will vary for subpopulations; for example, working class boys may have more accidents than middle class girls. However, it is not possible to predict with any certainty for an individual working class boy that he, in particular, will have an accident. In many respects this may seem obvious, however, as epidemiological findings become transformed into health promotion discourse this simple fact appears to be lost. Prior points out that we are encouraged to believe two things. First, that we can prevent ill health, or in this case accidents: 'In theory as least, all accidents are preventable' ((Department of Health, 1992, cited by Prior, 1995, p.139). Second, that the maintenance of health, or the prevention of accidents is something which is largely the responsibility of individuals. Prior (1995, p.140) draws attention to the document *The Health of the Nation . . . And You* (1992) which encourages its readers to take due consideration of their own households to: 'fit a smoke detector', 'beware of the chip pan', 'beware of damaged carpets', 'make sure that there is good lighting in hall ways and stairs'. The key point that Prior is making is that there is something of a double standard here. Epidemiological research confirms the fact that accidents are a *collective* phenomena and the accident rate remains fairly constant for given populations, however *individual* and technical solutions are proposed to alleviate the problem.

The interpretation and communication of the results of research is clearly affected by the prevailing political and ideological context. Currently this is a political environment which privileges the individual, and especially an individual who is able to manage and negotiate her or his own risks. Mechanisms of surveillance which focus on individual risk factors may contribute to the formation of a new individual identity, as Armstrong has put it the:

> real significance [of surveillance medicine] lies in the way in which a surveillance machinery deployed throughout a population to monitor a precarious normality delineates a new temporalised risk identity. (1995, p.404)

The formation of the 'risky self'

In recent decades there have been transformations in the 'technologies of self' the means by which we fashion our own thoughts and conduct. Contemporary forms of governance encourage individuals: to be enterprising; to make choices; to seek out and make use of information; to be discerning consumers; and to be accountable. Individuals are encouraged to take care of their own welfare needs and manage their own risks be it in relation to housing, education, pensions, or health. Welfare is no longer provided by government for citizens 'as of right' it is increasingly targeted at those who are deemed to be in 'real need' and everyone else has to insure against, or invest, in their own futures. Contemporary forms of government involves a greater emphasis on self-governance and, associated with this, there has been a proliferation of diverse activities and resources in both the public and the commercial sectors to support individual consumers. Hence the notion of self-governance implies an ongoing project whereby individuals are constantly assessing information and expertise in relation to their selves.

The sociologist Anthony Giddens has labelled this 'project', which he considers to be a key feature of late modern society, as *reflexivity*: 'It is a project carried on amid a profusion of reflexive resources: therapy and self help manuals of all kind, television programmes and magazine articles' (Giddens, 1992, p.30). Few people could be unaware of the explosion of information and advice about health. Barbara Duden was struck by this in the United States some years ago:

> in a bookstore in Dallas I found about 130 manuals that would teach me 'how to be an active partner in my own health.' For many years now the self-care-budget in the United States has been growing at three times the rate of all medical expenses combined. (Duden, 1991, p.20)

Exhortations about healthy living do not only originate in the activities of state sponsored health professionals – public health consultants, health promoters, GPs, nurses, etc. but also in a myriad of other sources such as school teachers, community group leaders, supermarkets, TV, radio, magazines and so on. There has also been an explosion of health 'resources' be it goods, such as healthy foods, exercise bikes, or services such as fitness clubs and therapies, of every kind within the commercial sector. They can all be used by consumers in the construction of their identities. As Lupton succinctly puts it:

> All are directed at constructing and normalising a certain kind of subject; a subject who is autonomous, directed at self improvement, self-regulated, desirous of self-knowledge, a subject who is seeking happiness and healthiness. (Lupton, 1995, p.11)

Indeed, as we have seen those health risks which are identified in the epidemiological literature, and perhaps more importantly those taken up by those involved in 'promoting health' are those which are taken to be within the control of the individual. This, in concert with transformations which have occurred in the psychological and therapeutic sciences, has contributed to the construction of what Jane Ogden (1995) has called the 'risky self'.

In the last decades of the twentieth century, the surveillance machinery, which finds reflection in the individualistic and self reliance ethic of the New Right, has successfully penetrated the spaces of the body to reconstruct an intra-active identity which is increasingly compartmentalised into the controlling self and the risky self. (1995, p.413–14)

Within the context of the 'epidemiological clinic' disease or illness is something that the individual can work to prevent be it through a positive mental attitude or 'healthy lifestyles'. Certain moral and ethical considerations emerge from this. Monica Greco (1993) points out that health which can be 'chosen' represents a very different value and moral dimension to a health which one simply enjoys or has. She writes:

> It testifies to more than just a physical capacity; it is the visible sign of initiative, adaptability, balance and strength of will. In this sense, physical health has come to represent, for the neo-liberal individual who has 'chosen' it an 'objective' witness to his of her suitability to function as a free and rational agent. (Greco, 1993, pp.369–70)

Help is at hand for those individuals who are not able to pursue healthy lifestyles. Health promoters may draw on a range of activities which are orientated towards 'empowering' people to lead healthier lives. For example, those people who do not appear to have a capacity for health can be equipped with all sorts of psycho-social and practical skills to overcome their difficulties.

We have seen that contemporary surveillance techniques and the current proliferation of discourses on risk are mutually constitutive. We have also seen that these processes have helped to forge a new risk identity or risky self. We must however be careful here. This is not the same as saying that humans are simply dupes, shaped by the dominant discourses or ideologies of the day. On the contrary, as we have seen within the context of liberal democratic societies governance requires that individuals are autonomous and free to question the policies and practices of government. This is of course obvious. Lots of people (including those involved in the dissemination of information about health) resist the advice of the health experts - actively, openly, and willingly indulging in 'risky health behaviours'. But such resistance is a necessary prerequisite for the effective functioning of forms of governance which rely on techniques of surveillance or 'disciplinary power'.

Note

[1] This chapter draws upon material published by the author elsewhere see Nettleton (1996, 1997).

References

Armstrong, D. (1993). 'Public health spaces and the fabrication of identity', *Sociology*, 27 (*3*), 393–410.

Armstrong, D. (1995). 'The rise of surveillance medicine', *Sociology of Health and Illness*, 17 (*3*), 343–404.

Aterns, D. (1994). 'The questionable wisdom of a low-fat diet and cholesterol reduction', *Social Science and Medicine*, 39 (*3*), 433–47.

Beck, U. (1992). *Risk Society: Towards a New Modernity*. London: Sage.

Bloor, M., Golberg, D. and Emslie, J. (1991). 'Ethnostatistics and the AIDS epidemic', *British Journal of Sociology*, 42 (*1*), 131–139.

Burchell, G. (1993). 'Liberal governments and techniques of the self', *Economy and Society*, 22 (*3*), 267–281.

Castel, R. (1991). 'From dangerousness to risk'. In Burchell, G., Gordon C. and Miller P. (eds), *The Foucault Effect: Studies in Governmentality*. Brighton, Harvester Wheatsheaf.

Davey Smith, G., Phillips, A and Neaton, J. (1992). 'Smoking as an "independent" risk factor for suicide: illustration of an artifact from observational epidemiology?', *The Lancet*, *340*, 709–712.

Department of Health (1992). *The Health of the Nation . . . And You*. London: HMSO.

Department of Health (1993). *The Health of the Nation*. London: HMSO

Douglas, M. (1986). *Risk Acceptability according to the Social Sciences*. London: Routledge.

Duden, B. (1991). *The Woman Beneath the Skin: A doctor's patients in eighteenth century Germany*. London: Harvard University Press.

Ewald, F. (1991). 'Insurance and risk'. In Burchell, G., Gordon, C. and Miller, P. (eds), *The Foucault Effect: Studies in Governmentality*. London: Harvester Wheatsheaf.

Foucault, M. (1980). 'The politics of health in the eighteenth century'. In Gordon, C. (ed), *Michel Foucault, Power/Knowledge: Selected Interviews and Other Writings 1972–1977 by Michel Foucault*. Brighton: Harvester Press

Frankel, S., Davison, C. and Davey Smith, G. (1991). 'Lay epidemiology and the rationality of responses to health education', *British Journal of GPs*, 41 (*351*), 28–30.

Giddens, A. (1992). *The Transformation of Intimacy*. Cambridge: Polity Press.

Greco, M. (1993). 'Psychosomatic subjects and the "duty to be well": personal agency within medical rationality', *Economy and Society*, 22 (*3*), 357–372.

Lupton, D. (1995). *The Imperative of Health: Public Health and the Regulated Body*. London: Sage.

Nettleton, S. (1996). 'Women and the new paradigm of health and medicine', *Critical Social Policy*, 16 (*3*), 33–53.

Nettleton, S. (1997). 'Governing the risky self: how to be healthy wealthy and wise'. In Bunton, R. and Petersen, A. (eds), *Foucault, Health and Medicine*. London: Routledge.

Ogden, J. (1995). 'Psychosocial theory and the creation of the risky self', *Social Science and Medicine*, 40 (*3*), 409–415

Oliver, M. (1992). 'Doubts about preventing coronary heart disease', *British Medical Journal*, *304*, 393–394.

Patton, C. (1990). *Inventing AIDS*. London: Routledge.

Plummer, K (1988). 'Organising AIDS'. In Aggleton P. and Homans H. (eds), *Social Aspects of AIDS*. London: Falmer Press.

Prior, L. (1995). 'Chance and Modernity: Accidents as a public health problem', In Bunton, R., Nettleton, S. and Burrows, R. (eds), *The Sociology of Health Promotion: Critical analysis of consumption lifestyle and risk*. London: Routledge.

Ravnskov, U. (1992). 'Cholesterol lowering trials in coronary heart disease: frequency of citation and outcome', *British Medical Journal*, *305*, 15–19.

Rose, N. (1993). 'Government, authority and expertise in advanced liberalism', *Economy and Society*, 22, (*3*), 283–299.

Skolbekken, J. (1995). 'The risk epidemic in medical journals', *Social Science and Medicine*, *40* (*3*), 291–305.

Turner, B. S. (1992). *Regulating Bodies: Essays in Medical Sociology*. London: Routledge.

Wright, P. and Treacher A. (eds) (1982). *The Problem of Medical Knowledge: Examining the Social Construction of Medicine*. Edinburgh: Edinburgh University Press.

34 *The mass media is dead: long live multimedia**

John Catford

Considerable experience has emerged over the last 10 years on the value of the various forms of media in health promotion . . . [T]he progress made in theory and practice [has been documented] (for example in recent years Hastings *et al.*, 1991; Booth *et al.*, 1992; Wyllie *et al.*, 1992; Lefebvre, 1993; Stewart *et al.*, 1993; Buchanan et *al.*, 1994; Thomson *et al.*, 1994; Byles *et al.*, 1995). It is clear that the use of mass media approaches has assisted both social advocacy (such as promoting organisational and environmental change) as well as personal education (such as facilitating individual and group behaviour change).

Several distinct roles for the media in health promotion can be identified (Table 34.1). At the moment these are normally utilised through large-scale campaigns to populations of several millions through paid advertising, commissioned programmes and unpaid news items.

Media outlets for health promotion commonly comprise television, radio and newspapers together with posters, leaflets and books. Compared to activity at national or provincial levels, the use of media at local level is not particularly well developed. Co-ordination with community-based interventions (e.g. through schools, workplace, primary health care and

Table 34.1   *Roles of the media in health promotion*

1. Raising public and political awareness
2. Creating a climate of opinion for action at individual and environmental levels
3 Presenting a corporate image/programme identity to win support
4. Providing healthy living information and advice
5 Changing attitudes by presenting examples and role models
6. Introducing skills, encouraging self-confidence
7. Promoting specific 'products' (events, opportunities)
8. Offering triggers and incentives for action and participation
9. Encouraging maintenance of behaviour change
10. Broadcasting achievements, rewarding action

* From *Health Promotion International*, 10, (4) (1995), pp. 247–251. Oxford: © Oxford University Press 1995.

voluntary groups) is increasingly attempted. This, however, often proves difficult because of the logistical and communication difficulties present.

Is this the approach that will continue into the next century, albeit on a more reasoned and results-oriented basis? We think not. Both the media and society as we know it are going through a paradigm shift in the way that information is used. This will have considerable implications for how health may be promoted through the media. What, then, are some of the most important changes that are imminent and how might we respond as health promoters?

First satellite then cable

In Europe there are already over 80 new channels being transmitted on four main satellite systems with consumers in almost 45 million households receiving programmes. One in six households in Britain now have a satellite dish. Satellite coverage varies from prime sports, constant news and current affairs, premium movies to porn and trash. This growth is quite remarkable since it was only 10 years ago that plans for the Sky channel were announced in Europe.

The Pan European Television Audience Research Survey (PETAR) covers Germany, The Netherlands, Sweden, Denmark, Norway and the Flemish region of Belgium. In 1993 the share of satellite television increased from 50 per cent to a staggering 62 per cent in one year. Traditional state-owned, public-service-sector broadcasting – terrestrial television is losing out to commercial television. The market share of terrestrial television varies from 32 per cent in Germany to 56 per cent in Denmark from a time when it would have been 100 per cent.

Commercial channels are now rated higher on enjoyment, entertainment and relaxation but lower on information and education value. Younger adults are more pluralistic and more ready to watch foreign productions. Interestingly, satellite viewing is strongest among manual socio-economic groups. This is true also for ownership of colour television, video tape recorders, camcorders and compact discs. Computer games were in the high street long before Word Perfect.

The most important new technology in television is digitalisation which will replace analogue as the international standard. Digitalisation will not only provide much better picture quality, but will also allow terrestrial transmitters and satellite transponders to split the signal, making it easier to transmit a far greater number of signals. Multimedia is coming fast and the fragmentation of the media will occur at an increasing rate. For example, in the United States, Hughes Communication is introducing a 150-channel system using digitalisation.

Within 10 years, however, satellite television could well be a thing of the past, particularly in towns and cities in Europe. Cable will become the predominent medium, spawning a great number of local stations. This is halted currently because of the high cost of access, but developments are occurring in some countries. For example, in Japan every household will be connected to a fibre-optic grid by 2015 running throughout the country at a cost of $25 billion.

Interactive television is around the corner

Coupled with these changes is also the potential for interactive communication. Mono-media will be overtaken by multimedia, personal-computer-based systems. These will utilise colour pictures (both still and moving), animation and sound. When connected to standard phone lines the interactive opportunities will be immense. These could range from running a business, accessing film libraries, home shopping, learning to fly a plane, explaining symptoms to your doctor and receiving health promotion counselling. The two-way interactive experience between viewer and television set will change product marketing from essentially one-way communication. Television 'soap' programmes will increasingly be used to market products. For example, if you like a particular piece of clothing on a popular programme you could move the television cursor to ask for details, and then order from your armchair.

Advertising will become cheaper through competition between the expanded media outlets. Less information will be provided initially because the consumer will be able to interrogate on demand. Most importantly, there will be less reach as the audience will have been fragmented. On the other hand, targeting will be much easier as niche markets will develop. But, instantaneous, real-time, mass marketing will be much harder. National campaigns will become very much more difficult to manage. They will probably be very costly if large mass audiences are required.

Local media is growing fast

The pattern of standardised nationwide newspapers will also change enormously. The considerable falls in circulation experienced by many developed countries recently is likely to continue due to declining numbers of young readers. This can be attributed to the economic recession but the trend may well be more sinister. For example, in Australia, where the impact of the world recession has not been so evident, there has been a relentless reduction in mass circulation of newspapers over the last decade. The result is that there is now only one national title remaining. In contrast, specialist national magazines have held their readership in most countries. This is another sign of fragmentation, and the development of a more selective audience.

Changes in local press are also interesting; it is now a sizeable market and growing. In the United Kingdom there are now 100 paid daily newspapers and 800 paid weekly newspapers. The number of free papers has also grown dramatically, from 185 in 1975 to over 1000 20 years later. Local newspapers tend to be strongly news-based. They are open, accessible and pluralistic in political view. Improvements in technology are reducing costs and improving quality. Another important feature is the horizontal integration with local radio and in the future with television also. All the evidence suggests that the local media are becoming a very important outlet.

Paper on the back burner

Newspapers as we know them are also under threat from the electronic book. Technology is developing which will dramatically improve the quality of liquid crystal displays to the point where screens become flat and pliant. It will then be possible to make a lightweight but bendable viewing screen making printing unnecessary and paper redundant.

A range of books is already available on compact disc. For example, schools can purchase Grolier's Electronic Encyclopedia on a single disc. Apple Macintosh already has a 'power book computer' similar in size to a traditional book. It can hold several books at one time and is back lit so that you can read it in bed. In the years to come we each will have our own personal palm-top computer. It will be a notepad, an organiser and will be able to accept Email. In the heart of all the other functions will be an electronic book.

Power to the potato

Such developments bring not only advantages but also disadvantages. An important consideration is accountability – how will the international media be regulated? What is to stop, for example, news enhancement? This is already happening in fashion and feature articles. Examples include retroactive repositioning (moving figures closer and further apart) and reverse cropping (extending the image beyond its original frame). The new media could be a powerful method of deceit, since visual images are much more persuasive. Effective regulatory measures will be needed.

This is particularly important when considering the impact of the media on the young. Numerous studies from many countries have shown that television dominates over all other media forms as well as teachers and parents in its ability to communicate with adolescents. Children are considerably influenced by visual images concerning hunger and starvation, environmental issues and 'killing things'. We should be particularly concerned about the possibility of programmes being influenced by vested interests distributing misinformation on health matters, e.g. the tobacco industry.

The consumer has been somewhat disparagingly described as a 'couch potato' – sitting on a sofa and letting the media wash over. The move we are witnessing is the 'couch potato' becoming a 'power potato'. Consumers will increasingly be in control of the media they wish to receive. They will become highly selective from an ever-increasing array of information outlets. They will move from passive to active use of media. For example, soon you will be able to programme your TV computer to scan the news items you are interested in – rather than watching everything. It will be possible to block specific issues such as violent news events. The computer could select the 20 most relevant stories to your needs and play them back to you at your convenience.

Information tidal wave

As Alvin Toffler predicted in his book *The Third Wave* (Toffler, 1980) we are becoming a networked society. We will soon be able to communicate anything, anywhere, anytime. Information energy will be as common place as electrical energy. These new technologies will de-massify the audience, carving it into multiple mini-publics. Their effects will be to create a new human diversity and to breakdown old social institutions.

These major trends in the media revolution (Table 34.2) will provide opportunities as well as challenges. For example, the concerns expressed about a few barons 'owning' the media – the Rupert Murdochs and Lord Beaverbrooks – will dissipate as the consumer takes control. Domination by one group or individual will be difficult as fragmentation will have occurred. As health promoters we too will not be able to be baronial in our mass media work. What then are the implications for health promotion delivery?

Table 34.2   *Trends in the media revolution*

Mass	→	→	Individual
Mono	→	→	Multi
Broad casting	→	→	Narrow casting
Public	→	→	Commercial
Paper	→	→	Electronic
National	→	→	Local

Challenges for health promotion

The media revolution will mean that national campaigns for large populations – as we know them today – will disappear. It will be much harder to reach mass audiences at the same time. However, local action will be more viable. Local radio, television and the press will provide considerable potential to integrate health promotion with local services, e.g. schools, primary care, community groups. This is also much more likely to be effective. The changes will also bring opportunities to reach niche markets at local and national levels. It will be possible to target key groups defined in terms of geography, occupation, economic status, gender, age and interests.

If health promoters wish to reach larger audiences they will need to concentrate on accessing general-interest programmes. In particular this will mean creating news stories – which provide information and have an advocacy emphasis. There is already a growing interest in health news coverage and Ted Turner of CNN has already instructed his staff to prioritise health in terms of 'content'. In some cases it will not be the health promoters convincing the media that they should be doing more about health but the media 'barging' into health – sometimes responsibly, other times not. Entertainment media should also be used more – since these are likely to be accessed by larger groups. The challenge will be to provide a health wash throughout all programming.

We should also be aware of the growing sophistication and diversity of health programmes in the media. Many of these are highly popular, using research, skills, ideas and resources that are often only a pipe-dream in public health education work. In the United States a number of agencies are looking to establish a 24-hour health channel and it is only a question of time before this happens. While specialised health media may only attract smaller audiences, they could be very helpful in empowering opinion leaders and potential role models who will, in time, speed up the diffusion process.

New skills and alliances

Health promoters must be in the middle of these developments. To do this we will need to develop much closer alliances with journalists and producers. Access to them will be harder because of the multiple outlets. It will be important, therefore, to find ways of encouraging them to come and work with us. We will need to be more approachable, supportive and understanding. They will be hungry for stories, ideas, information, funding and even training. We should not refuse them. Win–Win strategies will be important.

A key challenge will be to improve skills and understanding of media work amongst local health promoters. This applies to both professional and lay workers. Alliances also need to be developed with the new technology – cable, interactive media and satellite. Satellite is particularly important for those working in the developing world, where there is likely to be a leapfrogging in media technology. Creative thinking is required to develop new products and packages that support health, for example interactive health games and distance learning programmes.

Increasingly, there needs to be stronger research, planning and pilot work before large investments are made. We should avoid merely copying others' ideas, as experience often shows that this brings poor results. Rather we should continually draw on theoretical principles, scientific studies and practical experience. Evaluation should seek to provide better information on value for money and the returns on different types of investment.

Audiences will not be defined in terms of national boundaries but, increasingly, in terms of content at a global level, e.g. pop music through MTV. Collaboration internationally will therefore be important, for example, if continental-wide coverage through satellite television is to be influenced. WHO, the International Union for Health Promotion and Education and national health promotion agencies could play an important part here. Joint inter-country planning will soon become a necessity.

Above all we need to be aware of the discerning consumer – 'the power potato'. Health promoters should continue to help the consumer acquire skills and understanding – to empower and support rather than to dictate and coerce.

References

Booth. M., Bauman, A., Oldenberg. B., Owen, N. and Magnus, P. (1992). 'Effect of a national mass-media campaign on physical activity participation', *Health Promotion International*, 7, 241–247.

Buchanan, D. R., Reddy, S. and Hossain. Z. (1994). 'Social marketing: a critical appraisal', *Health Promotion International*, 9, 19–57.

Byles, J. E., Redman, S., Sanson-Fisher, R. W. and Bovie, C. A. (1995). Effectiveness of two direct-mail strategies to encourage women to have cervical (Pap) smears', *Health Promotion International*, 10, 5–16.

Hastings, G. and Haywood, A. (1991). 'Social marketing and communication in health promotion', *Health Promotion International*, 6, 135–145.

Lefebvre, C. (1993). 'Public health communication', *Health Promotion International*, 8, 241–242.

Stewart, L. and Casswell, S. (1993). 'Media advocacy for alcohol policy support: results from the New Zealand Community Action Project', *Health Promotion International*, 8, 167–173.

Thomson, A., Casswell, S. and Stewart, L. (1994). 'Communication experts' opinion on alcohol advertising through the electronic media in New Zealand', *Health Promotion International*, 9, 145–152.

Toffler, A. (1980). *The Third Wave*. New York: Morrow.

Wyllie, A. and Casswell, S. (1992). 'Formative evaluation of a policy oriented print media campaign', *Health Promotion International*, 7, 155–161.

35 Gendering health: men, women and wellbeing[*]

Lesley Doyal

Introduction

Differences between men and women are now beginning to receive greater attention in the planning of health services. The appearance of these issues on the health care agenda owes a great deal to the tenacity of the many women who have drawn attention both to the specificity of their reproductive health needs and also to the discrimination they still experience in many of their medical encounters. (Dan 1994; Fee and Krieger 1994; Smyke,1991; White, 1990). More recently, some men have begun to express similar concerns, highlighting their difficulties in obtaining effective and appropriate care for specifically male problems (Carroll, 1994; Sabo and Gordon, 1995). Both women and (latterly) men have also looked at the wider gender dimensions of health and illness, highlighting the different social pressures constructing their lives in unhealthy ways (Doyal, 1995; Harrison *et al.*, 1992).

However, much work remains to be done if these issues are to be taken seriously. First, there are still conceptual confusions about the impact of maleness and femaleness on health and these continue to hamper attempts to develop gender-specific and gender-sensitive policies. On a more practical level, meeting the need for such policies remains low on the agenda of purchasers and providers and attempts to raise it are often frustrated by the continuing 'gender blindness' of decision makers. This article will attempt to clarify some of these underlying theoretical problems. It will also highlight the more practical dilemmas facing those who seek to make health policies in general and health promotion policies in particular, more appropriate for both men and women.

The term 'gender' is now widely used in public sector planning, reflecting the widespread belief that it is simply a more modern or politically correct term for sex. In fact the terms 'sex' and 'gender' have quite specific meanings and it is important that health planners are able to distinguish between them (Birke, 1986; Oakley, 1972). Though they are sometimes difficult to separate in practice, a clear distinction should be

---

[*] Commissioned for this volume.

333

made in principle between biological (or sex) differences and social (or gender) differences. Both are important in understanding human health and illness but their policy implications may be very different.

Understanding sex differences in health and illness

Looking first at the biological dimension, the physical differences between the sexes are of course the most immediately obvious ones and not surprisingly they have dominated both common sense and also biomedical thinking on femaleness and maleness. The differences between their reproductive systems clearly generate particular health promotion needs for both sexes though these issues are more important for women than for men. Unless she is able to control her fertility and give birth safely a woman can determine little else about her life and this is reflected in the greater female use of reproductive health services. In the United Kingdom, for example, contraceptive management is by far the most common reason for women consulting their GPs, with an annual rate of 1406 visits per 10,000 women, compared with the next highest rate of 873 for acute respiratory infections (UK Central Statistical Office, 1995).

These reproductive health needs are important but they do not exhaust the biological differences between the sexes. There is now a growing volume of evidence to suggest that a much wider range of variations may be clinically relevant but as yet these are little understood (LaRosa and Pinn, 1993). It seems likely, for example, that differences between male and female hormonal systems affect both the onset and the progression of coronary heart disease but there has been little research designed to investigate these possibilities (Sharp, 1994). Thus the confinement of 'female problems' to the reproductive speciality of obstetrics and gynaecology leaves important sex differences in biological functioning unexplored. Many of these will be relevant to a broad range of both preventive and curative services and our understanding of them needs to be extended.

Social construction of gender differences in wellbeing

But even if we learn more about these biological variations, this will still give us only a partial picture of the impact of maleness and femaleness on human health and illness. Gender or social differences are also important. The daily lives of men and women often vary dramatically and this can affect their health in very basic ways. Yet these socially constructed variations often receive little attention from those trained within the biomedical tradition, leading to significant limitations on the appropriateness and effectiveness of the services they offer.

To put things simply, all societies are divided along the 'fault line' of gender (Papanek, 1990). This means that men and women are characterised as different types of beings with different responsibilities. The most obvious example of this is the split between the public and the private – the symbolic relationship between women and domesticity that allocates to those who are female the major responsibility for domestic labour (Moore, 1988). It is also significant that in most societies these are not just differences but inequalities, with men and women having unequal access to a wide variety of social resources.

Those things that are 'male' are usually more highly valued than those that are 'female' and men and women are rewarded accordingly. The work women do at home, for instance, is unpaid and usually of low social status compared with waged work. Not surprisingly these gender differences have a major impact on the health of both men and women but so far only their impact on women has been investigated with any degree of precision. We will therefore explore this first and then go on to consider whether a similar analysis can be developed in relation to men.

Economic inequalities mean that many women will have difficulty in acquiring the basic necessities for a healthy life. The degree of deprivation they experience will obviously vary depending on their position in other arenas of stratification; their race, their class, and their geo-political status – whether they live in a rich country or a poor country – will all influence their health status (Doyal, 1995). But underlying these differences is the common thread of gender inequalities in income and wealth – the 'feminisation' of poverty (Jacobson, 1992).

Cultural devaluation is also important though more difficult to map. Because they belong to a group that is seen to be less valuable, women may find it difficult to develop the sense of their own self-worth that is essential for positive mental health (Martin 1987; Usher, 1989). This process begins in childhood with what are often highly gendered educational experiences and continues in later life when activities such as caring are given low status and little reward. Finally lack of power and influence can make it especially difficult for women to effect the changes required either to promote their own health or that of their families.

We have seen that the gender divisions that characterise most societies also constitute a significant constraint on many women's capacity to optimise their wellbeing. Can we say the same about men? Do gender divisions enhance or inhibit men's ability to realise their potential for health? Because it is women and their advocates who have been leading the debate on gender and wellbeing this question has rarely been asked. Instead the focus has been on the ways in which the social structuring of patriarchy leads so many men to behave in ways that damage women's health (Doyal, 1995).

This is not entirely surprising since on the face of it, 'maleness' can only be an advantage, conferring greater power, wealth and status than 'femaleness'. However new questions are now being raised about the possible health hazards of being a man. As we shall see some of these involve a (more or less) radical critique of contemporary constructions of masculinity, arguing that they damage the health of both men and women (Sabo and Gordon, 1995; Harrison *et al.*, 1992). Others take a very different approach, focusing on what they see as destructive and unwarranted attacks on men and their lifestyles (Lyndon, 1992). While these arguments may sometimes appear to overlap, it is important that we recognise them as separate strands running through contemporary debates on masculinities in general and men's health in particular (Hearn, 1993).

What makes men sick?

One of the most obvious links between gender divisions and men's health is to be found in the area of waged work (Waldron, 1995). The emergence of nuclear families and the 'male breadwinner' during the industrial revolution gave many men little option but to continue working in what were often extremely dangerous conditions (Hart, 1988). As a result male rates of industrial accidents and diseases have historically been higher than female rates, with deaths from occupational causes more common among men than among women. Of course many women are now beginning to encounter these traditionally male hazards while men are losing their jobs in some of the most dangerous industries. However waged work continues to pose significantly greater health risks for men than for women (Waldron, 1995).

During the same period men began to adopt unhealthy lifestyles in increasing numbers – smoking and drinking in particular as well as dangerous driving. All of these have contributed to their higher rates of premature mortality, keeping their life expectancy below that of women in the same social group as themselves (Hart, 1988; Waldron, 1995). As yet there have been few attempts to make a clear link between these activities and the ideologies and practices constituting contemporary 'masculinity' but some commentators have begun to stress the pressures young men feel to conform – to 'show they are a man' (Canaan, 1996; Pleck and Sonenstein, 1991).

Similar arguments have been deployed as part of the explanation for the high rates of male on male violence especially in those parts of the world where it is at its most severe. In the inner cities of the United States, for example, young black males have been referred to as an endangered species because they are the only social group with a life expectancy rate that is actually declining (Gibbs, 1988). The interaction of contemporary masculinities with aspects of class and race has been used to explain this phenomenon (Staples, 1995).

In the area of mental health, too, some men are now beginning to make a link between their individual problems and wider gender divisions in society. Women have long complained about what they see as the incapacity of many men to participate fully in intimate and mutually supportive relationships. Some men are now beginning to acknowledge this disability and the constraining effects it has on their capacity to reach their potential as partners and parents. Again the cause of this is said to be the gender stereotyping that narrows the acceptable range of emotional expressivity among those claiming the male identity. Their incapacity to admit weakness, for example, is said to hamper their capacity to seek appropriate health care (Harrison, *et al.*, 1992; Kristiansen, 1989).

The underlying presumption behind many of these arguments is that unreconstructed masculinity can be dangerous to the health of both women and men. This analysis is based in part on ideas from the new field of 'men's studies' which shares much of its theoretical framework with critical feminism (Kimmel and Messner, 1993; Sabo and Gordon, 1995). It needs to be distinguished from the very different argument that men's problems derive not from traditional ideas about masculinity but rather from their disintegration.

One version of this argument stresses the secular changes in society – the rise of male unemployment combined with the entry of more women into the labour market and the increase in single parent families (Sianne and Wilkinson, 1995; Willott and Griffin, 1996). These are said to have challenged men's sense of identity, causing significant mental health problems. The rapid rise in the number of suicides in young males for example has been linked to these trends (Aggleton, 1995; Charlton, 1993).

However, more confrontational writers have placed the major stress not on broader social and economic change but on feminism itself – on women's demands for more resources which are seen as a direct cause of male neglect. The failure to deal effectively with prostate cancer, for example, is blamed on women's demands for higher levels of expenditure on breast cancer research. (Kadar, 1994). More generally, men are said to have been displaced in the family and at work by women's vociferous campaigns for advancement, leaving them vulnerable and damaged (Lyndon, 1992). The solution is seen to lie in a return to traditional values which, it is claimed, could potentially benefit both sexes. It is clear that these are important – but potentially explosive – issues requiring rational debate and careful resolution if health promotion policies are to take gender issues seriously.

Sex and gender bias in medical practice

We have seen that both social (or gender) and biological (or sex) differences may affect health in profound ways that necessitate explicit recognition in the planning of services. Some health problems are unique to one sex – cancer of the cervix or the prostate for example. Some will have more impact on one sex or the other for either biological or social reasons or both. Women are more affected by the ageing process for instance, both because of their greater longevity and also because of the gendered nature of society's response to older people. Hence both their inherited constitutions and the reality of their daily lives will affect the health needs of individuals. It is also clear that gender inequalities in health services themselves may differentially affect the ability of men and women to satisfy these needs. We can explore the implications of this in more detail through looking first at the creation of medical knowledge – at some of the basic assumptions built into the research process – and then at related aspects of the organisation of health care

Sex and gender bias in funding priorities and in the methods of medical research have received a great deal of attention in recent years especially in the United States (US National Institutes of Health, 1992). There have been high visibility campaigns for more money to be spent on topics of specific relevance to women, with breast cancer a particular focus for concern (Batt, 1994). At the same time women's health advocates have stressed the need for mainstream medical research to pay more attention to both sex and gender differences (Auerbach and Figert, 1995).

Most epidemiological studies and clinical trials continue to be based on the unstated assumption that men and women are physiologically similar in all important respects apart from their reproductive systems (Bird, 1994; Freedman and Maine, 1993; Mastroianni *et al.*, 1994). Thus men are treated as the norm and women as the 'other'. This means that many major studies are carried out on all-male samples. Where women are included, the variables of sex and gender are often not treated seriously in the analysis.

The justification for these exclusionary practices usually rests on the argument that women's menstrual cycles may confuse the results or that if they become pregnant during a clinical trial the foetus may be damaged. These are important issues needing careful consideration but they should not result in women being invisible in medical research (Moreno, 1994). The risks of such exclusion are evident since the results from these studies are then applied in the treatment both of men and of women who certainly will menstruate and may get pregnant. This faulty logic results in 'false universalism' where study results are assumed to be unproblematically generalisable to both sexes when it was difference that led to the exclusion of women in the first place (DeBruin, 1994).

This bias can limit the effectiveness both of treatment and of preventive services, as recent debate about coronary heart disease has shown. Many of the major epidemiological studies in both Britain and the United States were based on all-male samples reflecting the perception of heart disease itself as a 'male' problem (Sharp, 1994). As a result we know very little about the sex-specificity of many of the most common health promotion strategies in this field. Doubts have been raised for example about the relative effectiveness of cholesterol lowering drugs in women. Similar concerns have been voiced in relation to both diagnosis and treatment for HIV and AIDS where so much of the early research was (understandably) based on the experience of gay men (Bell, 1992; Denenberg, 1990; Kurth, 1993).

Thus health workers continue to carry out research based on the experiences of a minority of the population. Though some are now beginning to make the case for greater expenditure on specifically male problems such as prostate cancer there can be little doubt that overall the current priorities and practices of medical research show a consistent bias towards male interests. If this is to be remedied, hard decisions will have to be made about the allocation of resources and the accountability of those who spend them.

Who cares for the carers?

Similar concerns have been raised about the patterns of medical treatment and again the major part of the analysis has come from women. In many countries the major problem that has been identified is economic and cultural constraints on access to services (Timyan *et al.*, 1993). In the United Kingdom, these problems have been greatly reduced by the existence of a National Health Service though responsibilities such as child care can still limit women's capacity to use services on their own behalf or to engage in health promoting activities such as exercise. Once they are in the health system there is evidence that the quality of care women receive may be limited by gender bias both in clinical treatment and in the more subjective aspects of the medical relationship itself.

In the case of cardiac surgery one US study showed that men are six times more likely to be given diagnostic catheterisation than women with the same symptoms (Tobin *et al.*, 1987). Women also have a higher operative mortality rate than men for coronary artery surgery and this seems to reflect the more advanced stage of the disease when surgery is undertaken (Feibach *et al.*, 1990). Similar problems have been identified in the United Kingdom where men in one region were found to be 60 per cent more likely than women with the same condition to be given an angiogram (Petticrew *et al.*, 1993). This similarity across two very different health care systems provides a striking illustration of the cross-cultural manifestation of gender bias in the treatment of physical illness.

Turning to the more experiential aspects of care, women have been documenting their concerns about sexism in medical encounters over a long period (Doyal, 1985; Fisher, 1986; O'Sullivan, 1987). There is now a considerable body of evidence to show that women experience particular difficulties in getting enough information from doctors and being able to act on it. This is not of course to suggest that men are always able to do this without difficulty. Working class men and black men in particular could probably report similar experiences as could those whose sexual identities do not conform with what has been called 'hegemonic masculinity' (Connell, 1987). However there is little evidence of systematic bias against men as a group.

Women, on the other hand, continue to be seen as less knowledgeable than men, less competent and less capable of complex decision making. Too many doctors appear to be reluctant to let women speak for themselves and many women feel unable to assert their own wishes (Graham and Oakley, 1981). Women's own experience is devalued by comparison with doctors' 'expert' knowledge and too many doctors are unwilling to admit ignorance and uncertainty (Roberts, 1985). As a result, female patients frequently become the passive victims of doctors' ministrations. For some this will be a distressing and demeaning experience and many of the early criticisms of the medical profession included accounts of this kind of treatment. Current strategies for improving this include greater emphasis on gender issues in medical education, as well as a variety of strategies for empowering women in their encounters with health workers.

The way forward: health for all?

We have seen that both biological differences between the sexes and socially constructed gender differences should be of concern to health planners. Most immediately, issues of gender sensitivity need to be built into all services to make sure that they meet the needs of both women and men. This will mean paying careful attention both to the clinical aspects of services and also to the quality of the human relations that form a central element in the process of health care. Women and men do need to be treated differently – where it is appropriate – but any differential must always be justifiable with reference to its appropriateness in better meeting human need.

However, effective health planning will also need to take some of the more fundamental aspects of social organisation into account. It is evident that if women are to optimise their wellbeing, many men will have to change the ways in which they behave – sharing resources and labours more equally, taking greater responsibility for domestic labour and emotional support and protecting women from the major health risk of physical and sexual abuse (Berer, 1996). This in turn will require a significant restructuring of gender divisions – of the social definitions of femininity and masculinity. Some aspects of these changes might also benefit men themselves. Others most certainly would not and are likely to be strongly resisted as experience in a number of countries has already shown (Faludi, 1992). Whether enough men will accept some loss of power and privilege as a reasonable price to pay for better health both for themselves and for the women in their lives remains to be seen.

References

Aggleton, P. (1995). *Young Men Speaking Out.* London: Health Education Authority.

American Medical Association, Council on Ethical and Judicial Affairs (1991). 'Gender disparities in clinical decision making', *Journal of the American Medical Association, 266 (4)* pp. 559–562.

Auerbach, J. and Figert, A. (1995). 'Women's health research: public policy and sociology', *Journal of Health and Social Behaviour* (extra issue), pp. 115–131.

Batt, S. (1994). *Patient No More: the politics of breast cancer.* London: Scarlet Press.

Bell, N. (1992). 'Women and AIDS: too little too late? In Bequaert Holmes H. and Purdy L. (eds), *Feminist Perspectives in Medical Ethics.* Bloomington: Indiana University Press.

Berer, M. (1996). 'Men', *Reproductive Health Matters, 7,* pp. 7–11.

Bird, C. (1994). 'Women's representation as subjects in clinical studies: a pilot study of research published in Journal of the American Medical Association in 1992'. In Mastroianni, A., Faden R. and Federman D., Women and Health Research: *Ethical and legal issues of including women in clinical studies, 2.* Washington, DC: National Academy Press.

Birke, L. (1986). *Feminism and Biology.* Brighton: Wheatsheaf.

Canaan, J. (1996). 'One thing leads to another': drinking, fighting and working class masculinities'. In Mac an Ghaill M. (ed), *Understanding Masculinities.* Buckingham: Open University Press.

Carroll, S. (1994). *The Which? Guide to Men's Health.* London: Consumers Association.

Charlton, J. *et al.* (1993). 'Suicide deaths in England and Wales: trends in factors associated with suicide deaths', *Population Trends, 71* (Spring).

Connell, R. (1987). *Gender and Power: Society, the person and sexual politics.* Stanford CA: Stanford University Press.

Dan, A. (1994). *Re-framing Women's Health: Multi-disciplinary research and practice.* Thousand Oaks, CA: Sage.

DeBruin, D. (1994). 'Justice and the inclusion of women in clinical studies: a conceptual framework'. In Mastroianni, A,. Faden, R. and Federman, D., *Women and Health Research: Ethical and legal issues of including women in clinical studies, 2.* Washington, DC: National Academy Press.

Denenberg, R. (1990). 'Unique aspects of HIV infection in women'. In the ACF UP/NY Women and AIDS Book Group: *Women, AIDS and Activism.* Boston, Mass: South End Press.

Doyal, L. (1985). Women and the National Health Service: the carers and the careless'. In Lewin, E. and Oleson, V. (eds), *Women, Health and Healing: Toward a new perspective.* London: Tavistock.

Doyal, L. (1995). *What Makes Women Sick: Gender and the political economy of health.* London: Macmillan.

Faludi, S. (1992). *Backlash: The undeclared war against women.* London: Chatto & Windus.

Fee, E. and Krieger, N. (1994). *Women's Health, Politics and Power: Essays on sex/gender, medicine and public health.* Amityville NY: Baywood Publishing Co.

Feibach, N., Viscoli, C. and Horwitz, R. (1990). 'Differences between men and women in survival after myocardial infarction: biology or methodology?', *Journal of American Medical Association, 263 (8),* pp 1092–1096.

Fisher, S. (1996). *In the Patient's Best Interest: Women and the politics of medical decision making.* New Brunswick, NJ: Rutgers University Press.

Freedman, L. and Maine, D. (1993). 'Women's mortality: a legacy of neglect'. In Koblinsky, M. Timyan J. and J. Gay (eds), *The Health of Women: A global perspective*. Boulder, Co: Westview Press.

Gibbs, J. (1988). *Young, Black and Male in America: An endangered species*. Dover, MA: Auburn House.

Graham, H. and Oakley, A. (1981). 'Competing ideologies of reproduction: medical and maternal perspectives on pregnancy'. In Roberts, H. (ed), *Women, Health and Reproduction*. London: Routledge & Kegan Paul.

Harrison, J., Chin, J. and Ficarrotto, T. (1992). 'Warning: masculinity may be dangerous to your health'. In Kimmel, M. and Messner, M. (eds.), *Men's Lives*. New York: Macmillan

Hart, N. (1988). 'Sex, gender and survival: inequalities of life chances between European men and women'. In Fox, A. (ed.), *Inequality in Health within Europe*. Aldershot: Gower.

Hearn, J. (1993). The politics of essentialism and the analysis of the 'Men's Movements', *Feminism and Psychology*, 3, pp. 405–410.

Jacobson, J. (1992). Women's health: the price of poverty. In Koblinsky, M., Timyan, J. and Gay, J. (eds.), *The Health of Women: A global perspective*. Boulder Co: Westview Press.

Kadar, A. (1994). 'The sex-bias myth in medicine', *The Atlantic Monthly*, 274, pp. 66–70.

Kimmel, M., and Messner, M. (eds) (1993). *Men's Lives*, New York: Macmillan.

Kristiansen, C. (1989). 'Gender differences in the meaning of health', *Social Behaviour*, 4, (3).

Kurth, A. (ed.) (1993). *Until the Cure: Caring for women with AIDS*. London and New Haven: Yale University Press.

LaRosa, J. and Pinn, V. (1993). Gender bias in biomedical research, *Journal of the American Medical Women's Association*, 48 (5), pp. 145–151.

Lyndon, N. (1992). *No More Sex Wars: The failures of feminism*. London: Sinclair Stevenson.

Martin E. (1987). *The Woman in the Body: A cultural analysis of reproduction*, Milton Keynes: Open University Press.

Mastroianni, A., Faden, R. and Federman, D. (eds) (1994). *Women and Health Research: Ethical and legal issues of including women in clinical studies*, 1 and 2. Washington, DC: National Academy Press.

Moore, H. (1988). *Feminism and Anthropology*. Oxford: Polity Press.

Moreno, J. (1994). Ethical issues related to the inclusion of women of childbearing age in clinical trials. In Mastroianni, A., Faden, R. and Federman D. (eds), *Women and Health Research: Ethical and legal issues relating to the inclusion of women in clinical studies*, 2. Washington, DC: National Academy Press.

Oakley, A. (1972). *Sex, Gender and Society*. London: Temple Smith.

O'Sullivan, S. (1987). *Women's Health: A Spare Rib reader*. London: Pandora Press.

Papenek, H. (1990). To each less than she needs, from each more than she can do: allocations, entitlements and values. In Tinker. I. (ed). *Persistent Inequalities: Women and world development*. Oxford: Oxford University Press.

Petticrew, M., McKee, M. and Jones, J. (1993). Coronary artery surgery: are women discriminated against?, *British Medical Journal*, 306, pp. 1164–1166.

Pleck, J. and Sonenstein, F. (eds) (1991). *Adolescent Problem Behaviours*. Hilldale, NJ: Lawrence Erlbaum.

Roberts, H. (1985). *The Patient Patients: Women and their doctors*. London: Pandora Press.

Sabo, D. and Gordon, D. (1995). *Men's Health and Illness: Gender, power and the body*. London: Sage.

Sharp, I. (1994). *Coronary Heart Disease: Are women special?* London: Coronary Prevention Group.

Sianne, G. and Wilkinson, H. (1995). *Gender, feminism and the Future*. London: Demos.

Smyke, P. (1991). *Women and Health*. London: Zed Books.

Staples, R. (1995). Health among Afro-American males. In Sabo, D. and Gordon, D., *Men's Health and Illness: Gender, power and the body*. London: Sage.

Timyan, J., Griffey Brechin, S., Measham, D. and Ogunleye, B. (1993). Access to care: more than a problem of distance. In Koblinsky, M., Timyan, J. and Gay, J. (eds), *The Health of Women: A global perspective*. Boulder Co: Westview Press.

Tobin, J., Wassertheil-Smoller, S., Wexler J. *et al.*(1987). 'Sex bias in considering coronary bypass surgery', *Annals of Internal Medicine, 107*, pp. 19–25.

Todd, A. (1989). *Intimate Adversaries: Cultural conflict between doctors and women patients*. Philadelphia PA: University of Pennsylvania Press.

Usher, J. (1989). *The Psychology of the Female Body*. London: Routledge.

UK Central Statistical Office (1995). *Social Focus on Women*. London: HMSO.

US National Institutes of Health (1992). *Opportunities for Research on Women's Health* (NIH Publications no 92–3457). Washington, DC: US Department of Health and Human Services.

Waldron, I. (1995). 'Contributions of changing gender differentials in behaviour to changing gender differences in mortality'. In Sabo, D. and Gordon, D. (eds), *Men's Health and Illness: Gender, power and the body*. London: Sage.

White, E. (1990). *Black Women's Health Book: Speaking for ourselves*. Seattle: Seal Press.

Willott, G. and Griffin, C. (1996). 'Men, masculinity and the challenge of long term unemployment'. In Mac an Ghaill, M. (ed), *Understanding Masculinities*. Buckingham: Open University Press.

36 *Think globally, act locally* *

Peter Townsend

. . . [M]uch of the problem of increasing poverty and instability in the United Kingdom derives from failure to collaborate not just in Europe but more generally in the world to (i) regulate the power of multinational corporations and financial institutions; (ii) democratise international agencies like the World Bank and the International Monetary Fund, and (iii) buttress the living standards (and hence productivity and health) of the poor throughout the world by establishing a new 'International Welfare State' which would include universal services like education and health as well as forms of universal social security. This would offset or balance some of the excesses of the new international market . . .

The trend towards greater social polarisation has first to be slowed and then reversed. Policies for the United Kingdom have to take better account of global causes of local problems, devise new forms of international collaboration to reduce poverty in rich and poor countries alike, and establish equitable conditions of employment and growth . . .

Structural trends

In too many countries in the world, both rich and poor, inequalities have been growing fast during the 1980s and early 1990s. The latest reports from UNDP and the International Fund for Agricultural Development show that a majority of the poorest countries in the world are experiencing an increase in poverty, which is not explained by population changes or flagging growth of their economies. Countries such as Bangladesh, the Philippines, Kenya and Mexico have experienced both an absolute and a proportionate increase in the extent of poverty, as measured by international agencies between 1965 and the end of the 1980s. Their problems are an amalgam of debt, inadequate and misconceived aid policies advocated by the IMF and the World Bank, and stunted opportunities within the international market . . .

In the United Kingdom the richest 20 per cent had disposable income after housing costs in 1979 amounting to 35 per cent of the national total [CSO, 1994]. By 1989 this had grown to 41 per cent and in the next two years, 1990–1, reached 43 per cent . . .

---

* From ELF (Summer 1994), pp. 2–8.

By contrast, the poorest 20 per cent had a disposable income in 1979 amounting to 10 per cent of the national total. This diminished to 7 per cent by 1988–9 and to 6 per cent in 1990–1. This fall represents a loss to the poorest 11 million people of £17 billion a year. For the average household in this group of the population this represents a loss of £3000 each year . . .

Europe

Trends in other European countries have not been so marked. In some there is not much evidence of structural changes, but in others, like the Netherlands, Belgium, Spain and even Sweden, similar trends are beginning to make themselves felt. The point which needs to be seized is that the causes are international as well as national. There is, for example, the growing power of the IMF and the World Bank. Their policies have become increasingly monetarist, and their loans increasingly conditional on national implementation of those policies. The two are embodied in 'structural adjustment' policies which are a prime cause of polarisation and of poverty. There is a close connection between these agencies' policies for the Third World and their policies for the First World. The quasi-monetarist policies of deflation, deregulation, privatisation, cuts in public expenditure, cuts in personal income taxation and withdrawal from the welfare state are being applied in rich and poor countries alike. Governments everywhere have been, and are being, forced to acquiesce. Clear examples in the 1990s are afforded by many Latin American and African countries, but also by the Commonwealth of Independent States and other Eastern European countries.

The rapidly growing power of multi-national corporations, the largest of which now have an annual financial turnover bigger than middle-sized nation states, such as Saudi Arabia, is a related factor. The effects of both these international forces can be seen at local and regional level. For example, the problems of drug addiction in inner cities is directly attributable to the operations of multinational drug empires which the international community shows little capacity to control. Again, hundreds and thousands of redundancies in specific areas are attributable to the closure of modern industrial plants in some of the rich countries, so that they may be reopened in countries where labour costs are smaller. Government intervention to moderate the damage is inhibited by free market ideology . . .

The loss of pension rights provides another example. The growing number of company mergers and take-overs by multinational companies has revealed gaps in national laws which do not provide full protection of occupational pension rights and have had a devastating effect on the pension expectations of thousands . . .

National government policies have reinforced, and in some instances anticipated, deflationary divisive international policies. They have been causing destructive forms of social polarisation. Evidence of the harmful social effects of this polarisation are reported everyday: increases in thefts, burglaries and crimes of violence: high rates of homelessness: increased numbers of bankruptcies and repossessions: unnecessarily high rates of premature mortality and disability: deteriorating public services and deteriorating standards of council housing.

The key strategy

What can be done to halt the international and national slide? A start might be made with a collaborative programme of *social development* . . . Government must act internationally in the first instance to protect economic and social health. This will mean working with European allies to argue for the introduction of forms of regulations for multinational corporations: closing loopholes in cross-national taxation; protecting home based companies and individual employees by means of more democratic company laws nationally and internationally; promoting international trade union links; facilitating the internationalisation of democratic pressure groups; facilitating cross-national links between city authorities; and, in particular, taking new initiatives to foster First–Third World relationships. To such a strategy must be added measures to monitor the development of multinational companies; and to democratise the IMF and the World Bank in ways which are deliberately intended to raise the representation of Third World populations, but also the social interests of poorer groups in all the rich countries. The international problem is not one just of the exclusion of Third World countries It is now also the problem of the exclusion of the poorest fifth or two fifths of the populations of rich countries. The asylum of refugees and the considerate treatment of temporary workers in Europe are prime examples . . .

International social insurance

What can be done in Europe to buttress development and minimise poverty and unemployment? What is needed is a renewed commitment to underpin the security of the waged and non-waged populations. A number of European countries have a deeper commitment to social insurance schemes than does the United Kingdom . . . Levels of benefits are often much higher than in the United Kingdom and were not cut back to the same extent in the 1980s. The change from the earnings related to the price-related formula of the retirement pension, and abolition of earnings related sickness and unemployment benefit, together with the reduction in scope of both sickness and unemployment, are the major examples. While social insurance systems throughout Europe vary widely, it is inconceivable that European economic development will not be predicated upon some harmonisation of existing schemes.

The likelihood is that for both political and economic reasons contributory insurance will be stabilised, with income support or social assistance being reformulated to cope with much larger number of migratory workers and retirees. For reasons of social stability as well as to provide a basis for high productivity, the United Kingdom's strategy should be to emphasise the former.

Universal benefits in the United Kingdom are at a cross-roads. The problem is not that they should be made more selective but that their role should be greatly improved to suit modern conditions. This means better provision for interruptions in employment, part-time employment, migratory labour and populations, and coverage for the hard work of those involved in the care of children, and disabled and elderly persons. The problem is not to defend an old institution for the sake of tradition and familiarity but to use an efficient, economical and socially integrative mechanism to new advantage . . .

A modernised version of social insurance has to be seen as an integral part of a wider policy of economic and .social development. This is partially, but not fully, recognised in the EU's Social Chapter. The Social Chapter provides for workers to have a right to social security benefits of a sufficient level; and for those excluded from the labour market to have a right to a guaranteed level of resources. Inevitably there will be sharp arguments about the definition of these entitlements, but confirmation of the link between contribution and benefits will help to lift some of the downward pressures of fiscal competition. The strengthening of social insurance is a long term and not a short term element of social policy, which will provide partial defence against temporary pressures to undercut wages and employment. Incidentally, social insurance also provides an example of the better usage of the principle of subsidiarity – by allowing connections to be made between national, regional and local schemes affecting relations between governments and subsidiary organisations of workers and employers.

Secure state pensions for the elderly

Income support does not reach more than a million elderly people who are entitled to that support. The basic state pension has already fallen from 20 per cent to 15 per cent of average male earnings. It is predicted to fall to 8 per cent early in the next century unless government policies are changed. European and UK evidence demonstrates public willingness to incur higher taxes to improve the standard of living of the elderly. Some of the evidence from the 9th Report on *British Social Attitudes* and other sources deserves to be quoted:

> not only do the British reject *cuts* in public spending in health and education: a majority claims to support *tax increases* to finance more spending on welfare services . . . Indeed, 1991 saw the largest year-on-year rise in the survey series' history in the proportion of respondents claiming to be willing to see higher taxes to pay for more social spending (Jowell *et al.*, 1992, pp.42–3). (Since 1983 those supporting the idea of increasing taxes and spending more has increased from 32 per cent to 65 per cent).

> The favourite priority for more spending has always been retirement pensions . . . The most striking change in recent years has been an increase in support for more spending on child benefit (Jowell *et al.*, 1992, p. 42) . . .

A key component of policy must be to raise the basic state pension relative to earnings, and then to restore the annual earnings related formula. The increase should be higher for the over 75s and should be related to an increase in the disability living allowance for those who are moderately or severely disabled. At ages 65–74 a higher rate of tax should be applied to those with a disposable income of more than three times the basic state pension. The privatisation of the state earnings-related pension scheme should also be opposed, but a phased introduction of a regionalised and locally accountable successor for younger age groups should be investigated as a priority.

The additional costs of a modernised and revitalised scheme for social insurance could be met partly by extending the national insurance contribution to the top of the earnings scale, partly by selective cuts in tax expenditure . . .

Basic income for child and disability support

If modernised social insurance can play a new part in providing security and protection for those in the labour market in a form which is both proven and popular, and yet also serves the social and economic objectives of European union, the needs of the larger number who are outside the labour market have to be recognised. There are elderly and disabled people, especially women whose benefit is very small and whose income needs to increased. But there are also many younger people providing many hours of support to families and to disabled relatives and others whose work, and financial needs, are not recognised in the market economy. An organised and industrious society must be based on principles which go much wider than the vagaries of the market. Levels of reward for work performed in the interests of society and of economic growth deserve public scrutiny, discussion and approval. This feature of democracy has hitherto attracted too little attention. The extent of inequalities in the wage system, and trends in those inequalities, of course deserve regular examination. But other inequalities cannot be ignored. The provision of social insurance for those in the wage system has to be balanced by adequate child care and disability care payments to those engaged in equally demanding, if not more demanding work, despite the fact that they do not receive a conventional wage . . .

Minimum wage

The features of social polarisation which have been documented in this chapter show how different are the conditions of the, 1990s compared, say, with the 1950s and 1960s. In the aftermath of action on the Beveridge Report social insurance (together with social assistance in a subsidiary role) was believed to meet the problem of poverty. Today the depression of low wages, together with the casualisation of employment and the much larger numbers holding part-time employment, highlights the importance of minimum wage, or minimum earnings guarantee, legislation. A decent minimum wage is a necessary condition of productive and good quality work, but also of employment incentives and social stability. In the conditions of the so-called secondary labour market it is a particular necessity.

But, like proposals targeted on the poorest outside work, proposals for the poorest inside work are not enough. Schemes for a minimum wage have to be related to the evolution of the national (and international) wages system. Action on one cannot be effective without action on the whole. All wages and salaries are part of a hierarchy of earnings. Action at any level will only be effective if action is taken (by corporations no less than by governments) to modify the entire structure. This applies especially to topmost earnings – which set the pace, or the example, for the evolution of the entire structure. The justification for absurdly high salaries and substantial perks is too rarely debated. The problem of the undeserving rich is treated lightly, when in fact it is far more of a threat to social order and responsibility than the problem of the so-called 'undeserving poor'.

In the 1970s criticisms of narrowly conceived incomes policies were just. In today's conditions, when multinational companies are creating greater wage inequalities among their workforces, and when the bargaining rights of unions have been greatly reduced, the formulation of any statutory (and maybe international) incomes policy has to be very different . . . Proposals for a minimum wage are meaningless unless set within a reconstituted and modern income policy. This has to include guidelines in principle for the structure of wages and their development in a democracy.

In conclusion

National strategy to enhance economic and social development should therefore take full account of the problems being created by international market and financial forces, including the role of the international agencies:

A national and European social contract

This would be a UK version of the European Social Chapter which would extend as well as illustrate, in nationally specific form, the agreements involved in that chapter. It would specify proposals for the integration of international company law, the monitoring of information about multinational companies, revision of the democratic constitutions, and principles of accountability, of international agencies, and the rights and responsibilities of citizens and employee and employer organisations, as well as develop a national model of collaborative action within Europe to promote social development.

Democratisation of international agencies as well as of rich and poor nation states

The representation of the nations who are not members of the G7 nations – which account for only 12 per cent of world population – on the executive and other committees of the agencies should be increased. The G7 nations currently account for more than 50 per cent of the voting powers of the executive boards of the World Bank and the IMF. There is also the well-documented problem of the 'democratic deficit' of the European Parliament, and the weak powers as well as representativeness of many national Parliaments. Renewed efforts to strengthen democratisation at local level are also necessary to social development. In the United Kingdom, local government has been seriously weakened since 1979, and quangos have been created without adequate elected representation on governing bodies. The rights of citizens must be reinforced in both respects. Democratisation is part and parcel of social development

Modernised social insurance

This would build on the basic state pension, the state earnings related pension, the disability living allowance, and child benefit. Costs would be met by raising the national insurance earnings ceiling, targeting of mortgage income tax relief and of the married couples allowance (and the restriction of subsidy for personal pensions), and the restructuring of tax expenditures generally to leave the tax system itself more progressive and more logical. Savings in income support would be made from an expansion of social insurance.

Basic income for child and disability support

In modern conditions of greater equity between men and women the skills of women can only be recognised by ensuring a basic participation income outside as well as inside paid employment, as conventionally defined. In the interests of economic and not only social development a basic income for both child care and disability care has to be paid. That income has to be complemented with a more adequate level of child benefit and disability income.

[The last two] recommendations would of course need to be implemented in conformity with the earlier recommendations. The contributory element of social insurance would be widened to cover more comprehensively those with intermittent, part-time and occasional earnings, those seeking asylum, and visitors and migrant workers. There would be non-contributory rights to benefit on the part of those working in occupations of national importance but not attracting a conventional wage, or only attracting a wholly inadequate wage. Once childcare, disability care and other care payments are introduced or improved, non-contributory rights for those attracting those payments would be reduced.

Minimum and Maximum Earnings

In the interests of maximising revenue as well as conditions and quality of work, guidelines for the evolution of the wage system need to be laid down. This could take the form of a minimum earnings guarantee and conditions for increases in high earnings.

A new charter of collective and individual worker rights

More account would have to be taken of the collective as well as individual interests of workers. These would have to be framed in relation to general worker-rights within the European Union – as they are implemented during the 1990s and the early years of the next century. The individualisation of pay in rich countries through schemes for performance-related and skills-related pay, have tended to depreciate employee rights, as well as lower already low levels of pay. The restoration of definitions of collective worker rights will be a necessity in the middle and late 1990s . . .

The agenda for the achievement of social justice is indeed dauntingly large. An international perspective is inescapable.

37 Healthy cities: a modern problem or a post-modern solution*

Michael P. Kelly, John K. Davies and Bruce G. Charlton

If the Healthy Cities movement retains a commitment to conventional, discipline-bound research methods and paradigms, it will not only remain irrelevant to mainstream delivery of acute and chronic medical services, but also, and more importantly, it will not succeed even in its own intersectoral and participative mission. Research for Healthy Cities, the new public health or community development may become marginalised (Davies and Kelly, 1993). It will be difficult to avoid this, even when research concerned with Healthy Cities is not sidelined (Davies and Kelly, 1993). We suggest that the reasons for this lie not in a conspiracy to disparage this type of research. Rather, we argue that the concept of Healthy Cities and its underlying philosophical principle of Health for All are simply incomprehensible with conventional discipline-led models of scientific research and rational administration. We also suggest that the implications of that incompatibility must be grasped for the vision of Healthy Cities to be realised.

Modernity, post-modernity and health

Social theorists have attempted to analyse social formations by perceiving the traditional world as being stable and fixed, set firmly under the control of religion and magic. In contrast, the modern world is seen as dynamic and constantly developing, based on concepts of rationality legitimised by the pursuit of scientific truth (Kellner, 1988). Modernity uses conventional scientific research and rational administration to solve social or physical problems. In late modernity (Giddens, 1991), or more fundamentally post-modernity, social and cultural processes become increasingly subject to constant change and reorganisation, rather than progress.

'The modern world is a "runaway world": not only is the *pace* of social change much faster than in any prior system, so also is the *scope* and the *profoundness* with which it affects pre-existing social practices and behaviour'. (Giddens, 1991, p. 16).

---

* Commissioned for this volume.

Post-modernity as a sociological, philosophical, cultural and artistic idea has many meanings (Giddens, 1992). However, for the present purposes, it refers to a major social and cultural disjunction that has happened in various fields of human cultural and scientific endeavour, particularly in the twentieth century. It involves the growth of a new social totality with distinct emerging principles (Featherstone, 1988). Post-modernism is basically a critique of modernity's reliance on the assumption that knowledge and science are inextricably linked and science therefore can reveal or produce ultimate truth and/or human happiness (Seidman and Wagner, 1992). Reality is not rational, but chaotic, uncertain and open-ended (Featherstone, 1988). In post-modernity, rationality and irrationality merge together, along with truth and falsehood, lay beliefs with expert knowledge (Kelly and Charlton, 1995). Biomedically-based health and healthcare (i.e. professionally/expert led, biological, institutionally-based, high tech/high resource, passive individual patients) has been seen as modernist. In contrast, the new public health and health promotion, based on Health for All (i.e. preventative, multi-sectoral, multi-disciplinary, socio-ecological, low resource, participative and community empowering) reflects late or post-modernity, 'oriented towards the social body' (Bunton and Burrows, 1995, p. 207). The latter approach acknowledges that positive health is a quality of individuals and social groups that is self-defined, not externally imposed. Idealist definitions of health, such as the original WHO definition, are meaningless when considered in rationalist terms. What is complete social wellbeing? How do we measure it? It is subjective and belongs to, and is the property of, the individual or group and not the property of some scientist or administrator who wants to control or operationalise it. Once this is grasped, the fact that it cannot be measured in the same way that pathology can be measured ceases to be a problem.

Through this process of modernisation, the social structures of modernity are being replaced by a radically new set of arrangements. The traditional forms of social control are being eroded, with the consumer rather than producer being the driving force. Experimentation in cultural, artistic and life forms becomes the dominant force (Lyotard, 1984; Bauman, 1992; Featherstone, 1988). The Healthy Cities movement is one such experiment. The core idea of post-modernity is that the social and moral conditions pertaining in the world at the present time mark a fundamental break with the past. In art, form displaces content; in philosophy, interpretation replaces system; in politics, pragmatism displaces principle; and in science chaos displaces order. To be paradoxical: the core idea of post-modernity is that there are no core ideas! In Healthy Cities, an emphasis on health displaces an emphasis on disease, in research for Healthy Cities the focus becomes the origins of health rather than the origins of disease.

Albeit unwittingly, the depiction of health established in the WHO

1946 definition (WHO 1946) – a state of complete physical, mental and social well-being, and not merely the absence of disease or infirmity – created the original post-modern motif for health. We say 'unwittingly' because WHO in its practice and its personnel has generally been an ultra-modernist organisation, favouring technical expertise as a means of solving clearly defined problems. It is true that advocates of the health promotion movement frequently describe their activities as constituting a decisive break with the medically dominated model of health (De Leeuw, 1989), yet they may have identified the wrong decisive break! Conventionally the social model of health is contrasted with the traditional medical model in this context. We contend, following Antonovsky (1984; 1985; 1987; 1996 [see Chapter 1 in this volume]), that both the social *and* medical models remain locked in a pathogenic (modernist) world-view. Pathogenesis seeks out the underlying causes of *system breakdown*. Both the social and medical models are united by the commitment to the existence of a system that is capable of being destroyed, broken down and analysed. The fact that one model identifies microbiological pathogens, and the other social pathogens, is not a fundamental difference (Antonovsky, 1987; Kelly, 1989, 1990). Both models are based upon a causal epistemology whereby bad outcomes have bad precursors and the job of the scientist – social or medical – is to identify the ways of eliminating, or controlling, the pathogen.

The post-modern approach does not see or seek systems. It views physical and social life as chaotic and their understanding as contingent. Antonovsky (1996) highlights the continued dominance of the disease/risk factor model, and his work challenges us to address not the origins of pathology, but the origins of health. How is health created? This Antonovsky calls salutogenesis, the need to study those who survived rather than succumbed to disease. It's orientation is proposed as a viable paradigm for health promotion research and practice through initiatives such as the Healthy Cities movement (City of Copenhagen, 1994). Cities which are largely the result of human planning with their urban sprawls, their pollution, their social problems and their inequalities in health seem to give the lie to the fact that rationalist planning can produce human happiness. The salutogenic approach is critical for Healthy Cities for two reasons. First, it defines the goal or purpose as understanding the origins of health. It's success is seen in terms of enhanced quality of life. Second, its focus upon survival in spite of inbuilt tendencies to chaos, disorder and fragmentation is capable of uniting disciplines as diverse as Sociology and Anatomy and Anthropology and Epidemiology. Science in the post-modern condition is concerned with discipline integration not discipline imperialism. Antonovsky's 'Sense of Coherence' theory relates to the link between person and environment that enables the individual to make sense of his or her world (Antonovsky, 1987, 1996).

Our premise, then, is that it is not the social model of health which is the basis of the difference between conventional approaches and the new public health and the Healthy Cities movement. The social and medical models are both system-based, and built upon the assumption that an underlying system is open to systematic scientific explanation and investigation. We suggest that the distinction between this and the philosophy of Healthy Cities, Health for All and health promotion more generally, is the emphasis on *positive health*. Positive health is the key and post-modern concept in this regard. But positive health is not amenable to conventional scientific investigation, or to conventional (modern) scientific discussion (Charlton and Kelly, 1992a, 1992b).

The paradigm which stalks much work on Healthy Cities, health promotion and the new public health is that of 'normal' science. Normal science is convergent and has a defined object, methodology and procedure for validation (Kuhn, 1970). It is hardly surprising that normal science is so seductive to Healthy Cities, given that normal science has such a long and distinguished track record. For many purposes, including most medical ones, it is the best available (Charlton, 1993). Normal science is based on the assumption that if enough time, energy and resources are expended on a problem, then, inevitably, a scientific solution will be forthcoming. Normal science is a puzzle-solving exercise which works within a strong and accepted paradigm where we know what the problem is, and that there is an answer to it. The scientist's task is working out that answer.

A variety of attempts, some using normal science and some attempting to break out of normal science practice, have recorded the tensions, the difficulties and the problems of bringing together communities, researchers, policy-makers, and planners (Davies and Kelly, 1993). This is partially because Healthy Cities work is not a puzzle. Once communities are brought into the research process in a meaningful way, and scientists and other stake holders no longer define conventional research problems, the nature of what the question should be and whose version of the truth should be applied to evaluate the answer immediately become a matter of dispute. The normal science paradigm is shattered. It is not clear what the answer might look like, whether we would know it if we found it or even whether the answer exists at all! This is not puzzle solving, it is not even a paradigm shift. It is turning the scientific enterprise upside down.

Dubos (1962) defined health as a pattern of adjustment or adaptation within the environment:

> Health is the expression of the extent to which the individual and social body maintain in readiness the resources required to meet the exigencies of the future.

According to Nutbeam (1986), within the context of health promotion, health has been considered less as an abstract state and more in terms of the ability to achieve potential and to respond positively to the challenges of one's environment. In these terms, health is seen as a resource for everyday life, not merely the object of living. It is a positive concept emphasising social and personal, as well as physical, capabilities. Such a view emphasises the interaction between individuals and their environment and the need to achieve some balance between the two (De Leeuw 1989). The post-modern vision of health is founded, therefore in aesthetics and in moral values. Health like pleasure is personal and individualistic:

> Asceticism has been transformed into practices which promote the body in the interests of commercial sensualism. (Turner, 1996, p. 234).

In the post-modern condition, therefore, such aesthetic considerations are, whether we like it or not, paramount in determining how we choose to lead or shape our own lives and how we assess what is a good life (Shustermann, 1988, p. 335). If we are to develop a post-modern healthy city in which we can practice Health for All and in which the new public health can thrive, the importance of this definition must be recognised, although the whole notion of producing a healthy city by rational planning is precisely, of course, what is at issue!

The definitions of Dubos and Nutbeam amount to a rejection of the notion of health as the opposite of disease. Health and disease are not to be conceptualised as two ends of continuous spectrum. Disease and health belong to quite separate universes of discourse, one modern, the other post-modern. Healthy Cities will, therefore, sit most uneasily within that most modern of scientific discourses, namely scientific medicine. Historically speaking, the definitions of positive health gained popularity precisely when the critique of rationalist medicine reached a crescendo in the 1960s and 1970s. Writers as diverse as Illich (1975), Szaz (1972), McKeown (1976) and others in their different ways questioned the underlying rationalist and normative principles of medical advance. Sociologists in particular highlighted the role of medicine as an instrument of social control (Friedson, 1970). The arguments about medical dominance, medical imperialism, the limitations of high technology medicine and so on, were vigorously debated a generation ago. Much of the debate eventually metamorphosed into doctor bashing. In practice, much of this doctor bashing was probably misguided, not because doctors did not deserve criticism, but because it missed the main point (Kelly, 1990b). What the Healthy Cities vision offers is a way out of the now sterile debates of the 1960s and a genuinely integrated approach to health promotion. The role of research in such an endeavour hinges not on its methodology and whether such methodology is qualitative or quantitative. The role of research depends first, on its ability to embrace its objects of study (i.e. ordinary people) into its own processes; second, its capacity to work across traditional and conventional discipline boundaries; and third, its willingness to recognise the chaotic, contingent and non-systematic nature of social and physical reality.

The point of departure for the unification of research and practice in Healthy Cities is an emphasis on health as a phenomenon which is subjectively defined and must include biological, social, psychological and environmental factors. What the Healthy City must articulate rapidly, is a means of integrating these levels of analysis in a way which the modernist boundaries between sociology, medicine, psychology and the environmental sciences are dissolved. This dissolution is entirely in line with the spirit of the post-modern condition in which the very subject matter is contingent. Here the existence of a systematic universe governed by underlying laws amenable to scientific investigation is rejected in favour of a view of knowledge which must constantly modify itself, must be tentative, probabilistic and reversible (Kellner, 1988). Such knowledge changes and develops but does not have a transcendental goal.

Modernity was the attempt to impose structures on a disorderly world (Bauman, 1992). Post-modernity is the celebration of disorderliness and the recognition of the impossibility of anything other than imperfect and temporary structures of meaning being imposed upon the disordered world. This history of the delivery of health services and the organisation of towns and cities has been precisely the searching after human systems of perfection in the face of individual people with their own minds, and patterns of social and medical problems which defy easy solution of any kind. The Healthy Cities project and the Health for All movement must acknowledge that systems of perfection (including their own) are modern utopian inventions, and that human happiness is not so much a product of human institutions, but more a product of human relationships. In pessimistic mood Bauman argues that post-modern society is one in which the place previously dominated by human work is now dominated by consumer life (Bauman, 1992, p. 51). Pleasure is no longer a diversion from reality, pleasure *is* reality, and freedom is the choice between greater and lesser satisfactions in the market place. Fashion has a pervasive role in post-modern society and the market is based upon meeting the needs of rapidly changing fashion. If society is based on desire including the desire for physical, psychological and social wellbeing then desire must be refreshed and sharpened by novelty. The fads for healthy foods, diets, aerobics are also part of the search for novelty. In these circumstances, health is not so much an economic good, but a private choice (Charlton and Kelly, 1992b). It is not something which is imposed on individuals by some national or local organisation (the traditional public health model), but something which people choose for themselves from a range of goods on offer – 'making healthy choices the easy choices' in the jargon of healthy public policy, or the bottom-up approach.

Healthy Cities and Health for All are political as well as scientific activities. The principles of the Ottawa Charter for Health Promotion (WHO, 1986) are political principles, not conventional scientific ones; demands for the prerequisites of health are political not scientific, and the doctrine of positive health is an aesthetic and moral principle not a scientific one! In such political processes, meta-narratives (Lyotard, 1984) must give way to 'micro-narratives'. More precisely the post-modern science for Health for All and Healthy Cities must attempt to describe the lives of men and women as they live and experience them (Kelly, 1990a, 1990b, 1992). It must grasp the complexities of their thoughts and actions as they move through stressor-rich environments and attempt to come to some kind of accommodation with them. That accommodation with them will be micro-biological and internal. It will also be macro-biological *vis-à-vis* the external world. It will be psychological and interpersonal. It will be a political, economic and geological process more akin to the flexible, goal-directed micro-analysis of advertising and marketing than to the abstract, principled analysis of science. For the purposes of understanding these adaptation processes, it is useless to abstract. Abstraction is a modernist principle. The post-modern solution integrates the holistic involvement in all these spheres of human existence and states that they must be understood in themselves and in the way the individual understands them him or herself. Only then may micro-narrative goals be successfully achieved.

Healthy Cities could be viewed as merely yet another separate rationality which, while distinctive, follows a pattern discernible from the time of the Enlightenment. Its attack on inequalities and its scientific credo strongly suggest that many of its advocates see it in precisely these terms, as a superior rationalist solution to a set of hitherto inseparable problems. If that were, or is, the case, when the history of the delivery of health care comes to be written a hundred years from now, Healthy Cities will merit at best a footnote in the avalanche of late twentieth century attempts to get things right. However, if the truly post-modern conception of Healthy Cities is grasped with its emphasis on the values of locality and community, aestheticism, relativism and private behaviour, then it will mark a turning point in the history of our understanding of health.

These kinds of ideas are not new. The philosophy of Schultz (1967), the ecology of Dubos (1980), the sociology of Antonovsky (1985) and the psychology of Lazarus (1980) all in their ways, contribute to this view. The fundamental break with conventional science that each of these writers make, and the implications of their work for Healthy Cities, has not made great progress yet. But there is hope. In recent attempts to develop ways round the difficulties of applying research to practice, prominence has been given to the work of Antonovsky (1996) with his Sense of Coherence framework being offered as a useful theory for taking a salutogenic approach to health research. We would like to see further development of models and theories of change – for Healthy Cities is a movement about change – which have an integrated approach to the potential contributing disciplines, being developed. Recent attempts have been made to explore theory in health promotion (McQueen, 1996; Levin and Ziglio, 1996; Milburn, 1996 [see Chapter 38 in this volume]) but we have a long way to go. We would like to see many more experiments of involvement and participation, not in narrow partisan ways, but in ways that allow the wit and wisdom of ordinary men and women to sit comfortably with the knowledge accumulated by conventional scientific methods.

Of course, post-modernity is only one part of the picture. Boundaries and limitations will remain in science, in medicine and even in artistic and political discourse (Charlton 1993). But the post-modern mood is powerful and pervasive. If the Healthy Cities movement is to come to terms with the post-modern condition – both in exploring its inner possibilities, and in becoming aware of its inherent contradictions – this can only strengthen its available strategies for future development. A consideration of post-modernity can teach us *not* so much the right answers, but how *not* to ask the wrong questions.

Health promotion and its most visible offspring, the Healthy Cities movement, are at a cross-roads, as we move towards the Millenium. Health for All will not be achieved at our current pace by the year 2000. We are living in a rapidly changing, turbulent era of post-modern industrial change. Traditional approaches are only tinkering with the complex health-related problems that we face. Health promotion and Healthy Cities, from humble beginnings, have achieved a great deal by challenging the dominant biomedical conception of health ideologically and have offered a new paradigm to cope with such problems. Yet they have to prove themselves as practical strategies that are effective, productive and worthy of further investment, both economic and political. But pressures on funding are increasing all the time – 'the window of opportunity for health promotion to prove itself *scientifically* may not even be five years', (O'Neil *et al.*, 1994, p. 385 emphasis, mine). This is the challenge that we face – the pressing need to develop new and adapt existing methods and related indicators to demonstrate that the Healthy Cities approach is of value and is worthy of further investment. In the meantime Healthy Cities will need to remain flexible and creative enough to continue to exist and redevelop, as fitting as new social movement that seeks to transform our modern societies towards Health for All.

References

Antonovsky, A. (1984). The sense of coherence as a determinant of health, *Advances 1*, 37–50.
Antonovsky, A. (1985). *Health, Stress and Coping*. San Francisco: Jossey Bass.

Antonovsky, A. (1987). *Unravelling the Mystery of Health: How People Manage Stress and Stay Well*, San Francisco: Jossey Bass.

Antonovsky, A. (1996). The salutogenic model as a theory to guide health promotion, *Health Promotion International 11*, (*1*), 11–18.

Bauman, Z. (1992). *Intimations of Postmodernity*. London: Routledge.

Bunton, R. and Burrows, R. (1995). Consumption and health in the 'epidemiological' clinic of late modern medicine. In Bunton, R., Nettleton S. and Burrows, R. (eds), *The Sociology of Health Promotion: Critical analyses of consumption, lifestyle and risk*. London: Routledge.

Charlton, B. G. (1993). Medicine and post-modernity, *Journal of the Royal Society of Medicine*, 86, (*9*), 497–499.

Charlton, B. G. and Kelly, M. P. (1992a). Profit and loss on the pulse of a nation, *The Times Higher Education Supplement*, (7 February) 1005–1019.

Charlton, B. G. and Kelly, M. P. (1992b). Paying for an off-the-peg life, *The Times Higher Education Supplement*, , (22 May), 1020.

City of Copenhagen (1994). *Healthy City Plan of the City of Copenhagen, 1994–1997*. Copenhagen: Copenhagen Health Services.

Davies, J. K. and Kelly, M. P. (eds) (1993). *Healthy Cities: Research and practice*. London: Routledge.

De Leeuw, E (1989), *The Sane Revolution: Health promotion: background, scope and prospects*, Assen: Van Gorcum.

Dubos, R. (1962). *Torch of Life*. New York: Simon and Schuster.

Dubos, R. (1980). *Man Adapting*, New Haven: Yale University Press.

Featherstone, M. (1988). In pursuit of the post-modern: an introduction, *Theory, Culture and Society*, 5, 195–221.

Friedson, E. (1970). *Professional Dominance: The Social Structure of Medical Care*, Chicago: Aldine.

Giddens, A. (1991). *Modernity and Self-Identity: Self and Society in the Late Modern Age*. Cambridge, Polity.

Giddens, A. (1992). Uprooted signposts at the century's end, *The Times Higher Education Supplement* (17 January), 21–22.

Illich, I. (1975). *Medical Nemesis*. London: Calder and Boyars.

Kellner, D. (1988). Post-modernism as social theory: some challenges and problems, *Theory, Culture and Society*, 5, 239–269.

Kelly, M. P. (1989). Some problems in health promotion research, *Health Promotion*, 4, 317–330.

Kelly, M. P. (1990a). The role of research in the new public health, *Critical Public Health*, 3, 4–9.

Kelly, M. P. (1990b). A suitable case for technik: behavioural science in the post-graduate medical curriculum, *Medical Education*, 24, 271–279.

Kelly, M. P. (1992). Foreword to A. Kennedy, *Local Voices Local Lives – the story of the Kendoon Community Health*, Glasgow: Drumchapel Community Health Project.

Kelly, M. P. and Charlton, B. G. (1995). The modern and post-modern in health promotion. In Bunton, R., Nettleton S. and Burrows R. (eds). *The Sociology of Health Promotion*. London: Routledge.

Kuhn, T. (1970). *The Structure of Scientific Revolutions*, 2nd edn. Chicago: University of Chicago Press.

Lazarus, R. (1980). The stress and coping paradigm. In Bond L. and Rosen J. (eds). *Competence and Coping during Adulthood*. Boston: University Press of New England.

Levin, L. and Ziglio, E. (1996). Health promotion as an investment strategy: considerations on theory and practice, *Health Promotion International*, 11, (*1*), 33–40.

Lyotard, J. F. (1984). *The Post-modern condition: A report on knowledge* (trans G. Bennington and B. Massumi), Manchester: Manchester University Press.

McKeown, T. (1976). *The Role of Medicine: Dream, Mirage, Nemesis?* London: Nuffield Provincial Hospitals Trust.

McQueen, D. (1996). The search for theory in health behaviour and health promotion, *Health Promotion International, 11*, (*1*), 27–32.

Milburn, K. (1996). The importance of lay theorising for health promotion research and practice, *Health Promotion International, 11*, (*1*), 41–46.

Nutbeam, D. (1986). Health promotion glossary, *Health Promotion, 1*, 113–127.

O'Neil, M., Rootman, I. and Pederson, A. (1994). Beyond Lalonde: two decades of Canadian health promotion. In Pederson, A., O'Neil, M. and Rootman, I. (eds), *Health Promotion in Canada: Provincial, national and international perspectives*. Toronto: W. B. Saunders.

Schulz, A. (1967). *The Phenomenology of the Social World*. Evanston: North Western University Press.

Seidman, S. and Wagner, D. G. (eds) (1992). *Post-Modernism and Social Theory*. Oxford: Blackwell.

Shustermann, R. (1988). Post-modernist aestheticism: a new moral philosophy, *Theory, Culture and Society, 5*, 337–355.

Szaz, T. (1972). *The Myth of Mental Illness: Foundations of a Theory of Personal Conduct*, London: Paladin.

Turner, B. S. (1996). *The Body and Society* 2nd edn. London: Sage.

WHO (1946). *Constitution*. New York: World Health Organisation.

WHO (1986). *The Ottawa Charter for Health Promotion*. Ottawa: WHO, Canadian Public Health Association, Health and Welfare Canada.

38 Health promotion as an investment strategy: a perspective for the 21st century*1

L. S. Levin and Erio Ziglio

Introduction

Health promotion should be positioned at the heart of social and economic development and be increasingly perceived as a health investment strategy. This is the approach chosen by the Health Promotion and Investment programme of the European Office of the World Health Organization (WHO/EURO) to position health promotion for the 21st Century (Ziglio, 1993; WHO, 1995; Ziglio and Krech, 1996).

The Ottawa Charter's action domains

Over the last decade the Ottawa Charter for Health Promotion (WHO, 1986) has had remarkably wide acceptance as a strategic 'checklist' for health promotion, if not as a formal strategy. The Charter incorporates elements of traditional concern (personal health skills) with the more recent attention given to community action and environmental and public policy issues. Further, the Charter focuses on the key functions of en-abling, advocacy, and mediation. The five action domains are: building healthy public policy; creating supportive environments; strengthening community action; developing personal skills; and re-orienting health services.

Beyond the principles set out in WHO documents such as the *Health for All* strategy and in the *Ottawa Charter for Health Promotion* lies the real challenge to apply them in practice in increasingly complex societies (WHO/EURO, 1996). These societies invariably have immediate priorities, such as economic competitiveness and fiscal soundness, and their social institutions are directed towards achieving those priorities. Specifically, the challenge is therefore to find ways of deploying investment for health to reinforce such priorities and, conversely, to

---

* Commissioned for this volume.

enhance people's health – equitably and sustainably – through the medium of social and economic development.

For 21st century health promotion, our energy can therefore be most productively applied to figuring out how health promotion can be integrated effectively into mainstream social development and have its influence visible in relevant programmes, regulations and a wide-ranged public policies. The success of this strategy will quite clearly depend heavily on health promotion expertise which is based on the most valid theoretical constructs of the social and behavioural sciences, organisational behaviour and social development sciences.

There is no useful benefit in seeking a single, united, independent theory of health promotion. What would be useful, indeed critical, for 21st century health promotion, is to organise an international record of intervention efforts, including their contextual circumstances, strategies applied, logistical and technical aspects, and observations of their impact, e.g. cost benefit, cost effectiveness, diffusion, etc. Without such a knowledge base, health promotion will lack the traction necessary to move forward toward a strategic theme that could guide its general advance and at the same time encourage national and regional variations.

Such a knowledge base would be requisite for research which would have known denominators (populations) and numerators (resources) and known independent variables (interventions, programmes or policies) and dependent variables (health and socio-economic change). Since health promotion is conceptually framed in broad terms of social development, well beyond the limits of a bio-clinical model, it is necessary to document its impact on a wide range of decisions in diverse policy areas. Here, it is not only a matter of documentation, but justification for sustainable intersectoral involvement.

The goal is to demonstrate the synergistic contribution of its component parts to an holistic and equitable improvement in the health and wellbeing of the population. The focus should not be on evaluating the impact of isolated interventions as end points, but rather on the relationship of a given intervention to the other components of the health promotion strategy. Such an analysis may indeed provide a fresh assessment of the validity of theories underlying its several components.

Re-framing communication

Health promotion at this moment of rapid change in the world's political and economic order must define its potential in a way strong enough to withstand the vagaries of shifting political boundaries and populations, international and civil conflicts and fearful, sometimes cynical, withdrawal of people from sharing their resources or committing themselves to co-operative social action. In both developed and developing countries, there is an atmosphere of uncertainty and anomie that dampens enthusiasm for long term investments to secure health and wellbeing.

The challenge now is to adapt the Ottawa Charter strategy to 21st century realities. This is the case when the opinions and perspectives of new partners in health promotion must command attention; particularly those of the lay community, legislators and policy-makers (see Levin *et al.*, 1994, pp. 1–4). These new partners may possess little or no sophistication or primary interest in health *per sè*. Nevertheless, it is *their* construction of reality that must frame health promotion action.

The exchange of ideas, experiences, and information among these partners in health promotion is often far from ideal. Indeed, there are often substantial miscommunications between parties of unequal social status or political power or between groups with different demographic characteristics such as age, gender, ethnicity and race.

Differences in conceptual language are often daunting. Consider the conceptual vocabularies of educators, environmentalists, policy analysts, and community organisers. Where is the common denominator of meaning they may assign to such notions as empowerment, equity, participation, or even health? What aspects of communication theory or social marketing theory pertain here?

Clearly, health promotion will have to be inventive, will of necessity have to test a variety of new techniques and fora for dialogue and consensus building. What is presented here is an exceptional opportunity to create what may be called collaborative or adaptive communication; namely communication that leads to a common understanding and harmonious, mutually beneficial interaction between action domains of the Ottawa Charter and their link with public policy sectors.

Many experts in health promotion feel uneasy about working in policy and programme sectors where concepts and technologies are unfamiliar and/or where they perceive a potential ethical conflict of values (e.g. saving money versus saving lives). Misunderstandings on both sides of the equation have limited tests of health promotion's potential in key areas of public policy. Can health promotion respond opportunistically without jeopardising its integrity? What aspect of social change theory pertains here? What strategic advice is available to increase the possibility of success? What are the implications for preparing the health promotion workforce to have an effective influence on public policies outside the health sector?

New thinking for multisectoral action

The current 'Investment for Health' programme and related demonstration projects of WHO/EURO are designed to explore collaborative communication, option appraisals and other issues mentioned earlier. These demonstration projects began in 1994. They have as their primary goal strengthening the capacity of national, regional and local authorities to identify public policy areas relevant to the solution of priority health concerns and modify those policies, singly or in concert, to achieve and sustain health gains (WHO/EURO, 1994, 1995a, 1996).

In brief outline, the health investment strategy involves the following processes. Community groups and health authorities contribute perspectives on health concerns and opportunities, prioritise them, and then break down the agreed list of priorities into their more detailed aspects. Each aspect is then 'located' on a 'health gain map' which relates them to the most relevant policy areas (e.g. education, transportation, housing, communications, income maintenance, medical care, agriculture, tourism, environment). Finally, possible policy intervention choices are assessed against criteria that include matters of equity, empowerment, sustainability, accountability, acceptability, fiscal feasibility, amongst others (WHO/EURO, 1995a, 1996). The aim is to identify mutual concerns and policy options to seek grounds for conflict resolution.

A variant of the above health investment strategy was first developed by WHO/EURO (Health Promotion and Investment Programme) in Slovenia in 1996 (WHO/EURO, 1996). The objective was to undertake a systems-wide assessment of health promotion resources (current and potential) at country level: human resources, management infrastructure, financial resources and political support. The assessment, undertaken as a demonstration, was commissioned by the Slovenian Parliament and was thus free of any bias or obligation to any ministry or special group. The proposals for health investment which resulted, while reflecting the options of a vast array of agencies and voluntary interest groups, were independently arrived at and were assiduously politically neutral.

It is clear that we need more investment-for-health approaches which can respond to a wide range of circumstances: political, cultural and at the level of socio-economic development. The task is to make the investment process empowering of those involved, and a process which will have long-lasting development benefits beyond immediate health investment decisions.

The WHO/EURO Investment for Health projects are helping to clarify, and in some important respects redefine, the role of the health sector in promoting health. It is essentially an oversight role where the prime concern is to ensure that a holistic approach to health promotion takes into account the social determinants of health, be they at the individual, community, or policy level. These determinants are referenced in operational terms by the Ottawa Charter (WHO, 1986; see also WHO/EURO, 1984). Indeed there are few precedents for a managerial role in social, much less health development, where multiple public policy and agency inputs are orchestrated. Even the World Bank's 'structural adjustment' strategy provides only limited oversight confined to economic and fiscal policies and their related programmes (World Bank, 1993, 1995).

The circumstances of promoting health in an open system with multiple players, agendas, and citizen participation, simply make the application of most of the existing management theories inappropriate (see Grossman and Scala, 1993; see also Bennis *et al.*, 1994; Ray and Ritzler, 1993; Senge, 1990). Experience with the Investment for Health demonstration projects offers an unique opportunity to build a theory of management within the open system approach to health promotion (see Ashton, 1992; WHO/EURO-CEC-CE, 1992; Jensen and Schnack, 1994; Ziglio *et al.*, 1995). Some insights into such a managerial role have been organised for the above-mentioned projects, but these remain largely anecdotal.

The task now is to standardise observations relevant to the management role in comprehensive health promotion efforts. Thus we can begin to generate testable hypotheses as a basis for forming a theoretical perspective as a practical tool for advancing this role. We are seeking defining management strategies that empower populations; reduce health inequities; estimate available resources; respond to consumer preferences; set programme and policy priorities; assign intersectoral action; design interventions; organise collaborative efforts; build professional capacity; and assess cost-benefit and cost-effectiveness as well as peripheral impact. This is a formidable paradigm shift from current management in public and private sectors!

Get ready for the 21st century

Now is a propitious time for health promotion to position itself for the 21st century. In doing so, there is a need to play a stronger and more effective role in examining the options for health promoting investments and recommending the appropriate legislative and other relevant initiatives to achieve a truly comprehensive and sustainable health-promoting policy. Is health promotion prepared to accept this challenge in Europe and elsewhere? (In Europe, the World Health Organization is taking no chances with the answer to these questions, (WHO/EURO 1995b.)

The vision is there. Now we need to inventory the analytic and political skills available; upgrade professional education programmes; and undertake the research and demonstrations required to bring the health promotion resource up to an appropriate standard.

In the light of the above, there are a number of tough questions which people committed to 21st century health promotion should address. Some of the most relevant are:

• Where are those health investments in public policies with the greatest promise of benefits?

- Who will identify them?
- What kind of data and policy-relevant information will be required?
- What new analytical skills will be needed to evaluate the cost and benefits implications for health investments?
- How will investment options be presented in order to ensure political acceptability?
- How will public policies be monitored and publicised to achieve public review and critique of their health implications?

Conclusions

Health promotion, since the promulgation of the Ottawa Charter in 1986. has advanced considerably in all the Charter's five action areas. Emerging most strongly is the focus on building healthy public policies. The major determinants of population health lie in diverse public policy areas including, but going well beyond, traditional health care policy.

The task now for health promotion is to identify those aspects of public policy that contribute to a health problem or its resolution, assess the resources needed and/or assets available to support corrective action, identify the politically attractive policy options, and enable or mediate an effective resolution in the best interest of the population health.

There are exciting new prospects for health promotion, particularly as we consider these within the context of economic and social development. Health, we must recognise, is influenced heavily by decisions made in this context. It is the responsibility of health promotion to ensure that these decisions are health friendly while at the same time supportive of the main developmental goals.

As the investment for health perspective becomes a major orientation for health promotion, additional research and training needs will become obvious. Fewer distinctions will be made between the concepts of health and general wellbeing and thus we can expect a more productive and harmonious integration of efforts among all relevant public policies. Health, and particularly the speciality of health promotion, can serve as the nexus for this new convergence of policy resources in health investment. Health promotion has to respond to and influence a rapidly changing world. The catalogue of disciplines upon which it must base its practice must expand to meet new challenges, new opportunities.

Note

1 This chapter is based on an article 'Health promotion as an investment strategy: considerations on theory and practice', published in *Health Promotion International, 11, (1),* (1996), pp. 33–39. Oxford: Oxford University Press.

References

Ashton, J. (1992). *Healthy Cities*. Buckingham: Open University Press.

Bennis, W., Parikh, J. and Lessem, R. (1994). *Beyond Leadership: Balancing economics, ethics and ecology*. Cambridge, MA: Blackwell Publishers.

Grossman, R. and Scala, K. (1993). Health promotion and organizational development. *European Health Promotion Series, 2*. Copenhagen: World Health Organization, Regional Office for Europe.

Jensen, B. B. and Schnack, K. (eds) (1994). Action and action competence. *Studies in Educational Theory and Curriculum, 12*. Copenhagen: Royal Danish School of Educational Studies.

Levin, S. L., McMahon, L. and Ziglio, E. (eds) (1994). *Economic Change, Social Welfare and Health in Europe*. Copenhagen: World Health Organization, Regional Office for Europe.

Ray, M. and Ritzler, A. (eds) (1993). *The New Paradigm in Business – Emerging strategies for leadership and organizational change*. New York: The Putnam Publishing Group.

Senge, P.M. (1990). *The Fifth Discipline – The art and practice of the learning organization*. New York: Dubleday.

World Bank (1993). *Investment in Health. The World Bank in action*. Washington, DC: The World Bank.

World Bank (1995), *Investing in People: The World Bank in Action*. Washington, DC: The World Bank.

World Health Organization (WHO) (1986). *Ottawa Charter for Health Promotion*. World Health Organization, Health and Welfare Canada, Canadian Public Health Association. Ottawa Charter for Health Promotion, Ottawa, Ontario, Canada (November 21) (available through: Copenhagen: World Health Organization, Regional Office for Europe).

World Health Organization (1995). *Health in Social Development*. (WHO Position Paper, World Summit for Social Development, Copenhagen, March). Geneva: WHO.

WHO/EURO (1984). *Health Promotion: A discussion document on the concept and principles*. Copenhagen: World Health Organization, Regional Office for Europe.

WHO/EURO (1994). *Investment in Health in the Valencia Region: Mid-Term Report*. Copenhagen: World Health Organization, Regional Office for Europe (Health Promotion and Investment Unit).

WHO/EURO (1995a). *Securing Investment in Health: Report of a demonstration project in the provinces of Bolzano and Trento*. Copenhagen: World Health Organization, Regional Office for Europe (Health Promotion and Investment Unit).

WHO/EURO (1995b). *First Meeting of the European Committee for Health Promotion Development – Dublin, Ireland, 14–16 March 1995. Summary Report*. Copenhagen: World Health Organization, Regional Office for Europe (Health Promotion and Investment Unit, ICP/IVSP 94 01/MT 04).

WHO/EURO (1996). *Investment for Health in Slovenia*. Copenhagen: World Health Organization (Intersectoral Health Development Unit, Health Promotion and Investment Programme).

WHO/EURO–CEC–CE (1992). *The European Network of Health Promoting Schools*. Copenhagen: World Health Organization, Regional Office for Europe (Health Promotion and Investment Unit).

Ziglio, E. and Krech, R. (1996). Brüchenschlag zwischen Politik und Forschung in der Gesudheitsförderung. In Rütten, A. and Rausch, L. (eds), *Gesunde Regionen in Internationaler Partnerschaft: Konzepte und Perspektiven*. Werbach-Gamburg, Germany: G. Conrad, Verlag für Gesundheitsförderung.

Ziglio, E., Rivett, D. and Rasmussen V. (1995). *The European Network of Health Promoting Schools: Managing innovation and change. Report prepared by the Technical Secretariat of the European Network of Health Promoting Schools*. Copenhagen: World Health Organization, Regional Office for Europe (Health Promotion and Investment Unit).

Index

371